MARRIOTT'S
Practical
Electrocardiography

TENTH EDITION

Galen S. Wagner, M.D.

Associate Professor
Department of Internal Medicine
Duke University Medical Center
Durham, North Carolina

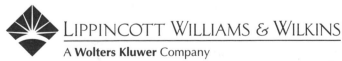

LIPPINCOTT WILLIAMS & WILKINS
A **Wolters Kluwer** Company
Philadelphia • Baltimore • New York • London
Buenos Aires • Hong Kong • Sydney • Tokyo

Acquisitions Editor: Ruth W. Weinberg
Developmental Editor: Raymond E. Reter
Production Editor: Jonathan Geffner
Manufacturing Manager: Benjamin Rivera
Cover Designer: Patty Gast
Compositor: Maryland Composition
Printer: World Color

© 2001 by LIPPINCOTT WILLIAMS & WILKINS
530 Walnut Street
Philadelphia, PA 19106 USA
LWW.com

Printed in the USA

Library of Congress Cataloging-in-Publication Data

Wagner, Galen S.
    Marriott's practical electrocardiography.—10th ed. / Galen S. Wagner.
      p. ; cm.
    Includes bibliographical references and index.
    ISBN 0-683-30746-0
      1. Electrocardiography. I. Title: Practical electrocardiography. II. Marriott,
Henry J.L. (Henry Joseph Llewellyn), 1917-Practical electrocardiography. III. Title.
     [DNLM: 1. Electrocardiography. 2. Heart Diseases—diagnosis. WG 140
W133m 2000]
    RC683.5.E5 M3 2000
    616.1′207547—dc21

00-057609

---

10 9 8 7 6 5 4 3 2 1

To Marilyn Bell Wagner,
who nurtures my happiness and humility
with the double-edged reminder:
"The only thing you do well is reading ECGs."

Contents

I. Basic Concepts

II. Abnormal Wave Morphology

III. Abnormal Rhythms

Preface

Barney Marriott created *Practical Electrocardiography* in 1954 and nurtured it through eight editions. After assisting him with the 8th edition, I enthusiastically accepted the challenge of writing the subsequent editions. The 9th edition had extensive revisions to the text, and the 10th edition has further text revisions and almost completely new illustrations.

One of the strengths of *Marriott's Practical Electrocardiography* has been its lucid foundation for understanding the basis for ECG interpretation. In this revision, I have attempted to retain the best of the Marriott tradition—emphasis on the concepts required for everyday ECG interpretation and the simplicities, rather than complexities, of the ECG recordings.

The chapters are in the same order as in the 9th edition, and each is divided (as indicated in the table of contents) into discrete, compact "learning units." Each learning unit begins on a new page. Space is provided for the reader's notes. The purpose of the learning units is to make this book easier to use by allowing the reader to be selective regarding the material to be considered at a particular time.

The three chapters in Section I ("Basic Concepts") provide an introductory orientation to electrocardiography. I have expanded the first chapter to provide a more basic perspective for those with no previous experience in reading ECGs. The reader is asked to consider "What can this book do for me?" and, further, "What can I expect from myself after I have 'completed' this book?" Also, in Chapter 1 ("Cardiac Electrical Activity"), the magnetic resonance images of the normal heart *in situ* provide orientation to the relationship between the cardiac structures and the body surface ECG recording sites. Color has been added to many of the illustrations throughout this section to enhance their clarity.

In the eight chapters of Section II ("Abnormal Wave Morphology"), the format for presenting the standard 12-lead ECG recordings has been modified. Single cardiac cycles are included for each of the leads to show how the morphology of the ECG waveforms characteristically appear in each of these 12 different views of the cardiac electrical activity. There is particular emphasis on the four chapters on myocardial ischemia and infarction (Chapters 7–10) because of the many recent advances in understanding of these common cardiac conditions. Many and varied health care providers are being challenged to learn the ECG interpretive skills required for rapid prehospital diagnosis and management of patients with "acute coronary syndromes."

The Marriott legacy is particularly strong in Section III ("Abnormal Rhythms"). Barney and I worked extensively in the preparation for the 9th edition to retain his methodical and innovative approach while including the more recent concepts. In the 10th edition, I have included perspective from clinical electrophysiologists into a practical classification of the various tachyarrhythmias. Ten-second rhythm strips from three simultaneously recorded ECG leads are used as often as possible for the illustrations. Chapter 21 ("Artificial Cardiac Pacemakers") has been entirely rewritten because of the current availability of a wide variety of sophisticated systems.

Many friends and colleagues guided me in the revisions I have made in the 10th edition. Rick White, Director of Cardiac Imaging at the Cleveland Clinic, provided the magnetic resonance images of the normal heart in Chapter 1. For Chapters 1–3 in Section I ("Basic Concepts"), and those on chamber enlargement, intraventricular conduction abnormalities and ischemia, and infarction (Chapters 4, 5, and 7–10), Ron Selvester of Long Beach Memorial Hospital and Editor of *Journal of Electrocardiology* provided his unique perspectives on myocardial electrical activation.

Jerry Liebman of Rainbow Babies Hospital of Case Western Reserve Medical Center freely gave his insights and example ECGs to elucidate the normal changes during the pediatric years and congenital abnormalities.

My long-time colleagues in teaching electrocardiography—Barry Ramo of the New Mexico Heart Institute; and Bob Waugh, Bob Warner, and Joe Greenfield of Duke—were continually available to address my questions and to offer their critique.

Marcel Gilbert of Laval University in Quebec provided the ECG illustrations for all of the chapters on tachyarrhythmias. During long evening calls, Marcel explained the interventions he performed on these patients to stimulate the changes in rhythm that revealed the clinical diagnosis.

Ken Haisty and his Cardiology Fellow, Scott Robertson, of Wake Forest University share authorship of Chapter 21 ("Artificial Cardiac Pacemakers") with me. It had become clear that advances in pacing had made the chapter in the 9th edition obsolete. Since I do not implant pacemakers, I asked Ken to completely develop this section for the 10th edition. During long evening phone calls, we talked through the interrelationships among illustrations, text, and legends.

Throughout the two years of manuscript development, I was assisted daily by Paul Leibrandt and Sam Bell. This was Paul's major project during his year between college and medical school. Paul did the primary editing during the manuscript production. Sam then coordinated my communication with Lippincott Williams & Wilkins personnel, which included Ruth Weinberg, Acquistions Editor; Ray Reter, Developmental Editor; and Jonathan Geffner, Senior Production Editor.

My approach to publishing is based on advice from a long ago consultation with Dr. Seuss (Ted Geisel). I tried to attain the "personal attention to all details" approach he developed over his years of publishing with Random House. Thus, I appreciate all of the patience and attention to details that everyone at LW&W provided.

A special thanks goes to Diana Andrews who coordinated the entire art program for the 10th edition. This was complicated by our movement to color ECG production. Diana faithfully reproduced my illustration concepts, often improving greatly on my original plan. No quantity of my revisions discouraged her, and we both are proud of the quality of the finished product.

Finally, and most importantly, I recognize the tremendous input into this volume by my friend and colleague Olle Pahlm of Lund University in Sweden. Olle recruited his colleagues Jonas Petterrson and technologist Kerstin Brauer to locate the needed ECGs from their Clinical Physiology ECG files, and then to prepare the recordings in the required format. Olle also provided the wonderful support of reading and editing the complete manuscript—twice.

My goal for both the 9th and 10th editions has been to preserve the "spirit of Barney Marriott" through the many changes in words and images. He has been my toughest but most helpful critic as I attempt to justify maintenance of the title "Marriott's Practical Electrocardiography."

Galen S. Wagner, M.D.
Durham, North Carolina

MARRIOTT'S
Practical
Electrocardiography

TENTH EDITION

I

BASIC CONCEPTS

CHAPTER 1

Cardiac Electrical Activity

THE BOOK: MARRIOTT'S PRACTICAL ELECTROCARDIOGRAPHY, 10TH EDITION

What Can This Book Do for Me?

This 10th Edition of *Marriott's Practical Electrocardiography* has been specifically designed to provide you with a practical approach to reading electrocardiograms (ECGs). No previous text or experience is required. You should consider how you learn best before deciding how to approach this book. If you are most comfortable acquiring a basic understanding of a subject even before being faced with a need to use the subject information, you will probably want to read the first section (*Basic Concepts*) carefully. However, if you have found that such understanding is not really helpful to you until you encounter a specific problem, you probably will want to quickly scan this first section.

All medical terms are defined in a glossary at the end of each chapter. Each individual "practical concept" is presented in a "Learning Unit." Arrows in the margins of the text indicate the beginning and end of each Learning Unit. The Learning Units are listed in the Table of Contents, and are presented on varying numbers of full pages. This book will be more useful to you if you provide your own annotation, and blank space is provided for this purpose.

The illustrations are fully integrated into the text, eliminating the need for extensive figure legends. A pink background is used for the ECG examples, to provide contrast with the recordings, which appear in black. Since ECG reading is a visual experience, typical examples of the various clinical situations for which ECGs are recorded constitute most of the book's content. Reference to these examples should provide you with capability for accurately reading the ECGs you encounter in your own clinical experience.

What Can I Expect from Myself When I Have "Completed" This Book?

This book is not intended for you to "complete." Rather, it is intended as a reference for the ECG problems you encounter. There will be evidence that this is your book, with dog-eared pages and your own notes in the sections you have already used. Through your experience with this book, you should develop confidence in identifying a "normal" ECG, and be able to accurately diagnose the many common ECG abnormalities. You should also have an understanding of the practical aspects of the pathophysiologic basis for each of these common ECG abnormalities.

THE ELECTROCARDIOGRAM

What Is an Electrocardiogram?

An ECG is the recording ("gram") of the electrical activity ("electro") generated by the cells of the heart ("cardio") that reaches the body surface. This electrical activity initiates the heart's muscular contraction that pumps the blood to the body. Each ECG recording *electrode* provides the view of this electrical activity that it "sees" from its particular position on the body surface. Observation of the 12 views provided by the routine clinical ECG allows you to "move around" this electrical activity just as though you were seeing the heart from various viewpoints. You should probably have your own ECG recorded, and then ask an experienced ECG reader to explain it to you. This experience will remove the mystery surrounding the ECG and prepare you for the "Basic Concepts" section of this book.

What Does an Electrocardiogram Actually Measure?

The ECG recording plots voltage on its vertical axis against time on its horizontal axis. Measurements along the horizontal axis indicate the overall heart rate and regularity, and also the time intervals required for electrical activation to move from one part of the heart to another. Measurements along the vertical axis indicate the voltage measured on the body surface. This voltage represents the "summation" of the electrical activation of all of the cardiac cells. Some abnormalities can be detected by measurements on a single ECG recording, but others become apparent only by observing serial recordings over time.

What Medical Problems Can Be Diagnosed With an Electrocardiogram?

Many cardiac abnormalities can be detected by ECG interpretation, including enlargement of heart muscle, electrical conduction blocks, insufficient blood flow, and death of heart muscle due to a blood clot. The ECG can even identify which of the heart's coronary arteries contains this clot when it is still only threatening to destroy a region of heart muscle. The ECG is also the primary method for identifying problems with heart rate and regularity. In addition to its value for understanding cardiac problems, the ECG can be used to diagnose medical conditions throughout the body. For example, the ECG can reveal abnormal levels of ions in the blood, such as potassium and calcium, and abnormal function of glands such as the thyroid. It can also detect potentially dangerous levels of certain drugs. All of this information can be determined by the careful observations of an experienced electrocardiographer.

Would It Be Helpful to Have My Own Electrocardiogram Recorded?

In the process of learning electrocardiography, it may be useful to have your own ECG recorded. Here is a list of possible reasons why:

- You will be able to understand the orientation of the ECG leads because you have experienced the electrodes being placed on your body.
- You can carry your ECG with you as reference if an abnormality is ever suspected.
- You can compare it to someone else's ECG to see normal variations.
- You can compare it at different times of your life to see how it changes.
- You can exercise while your ECG is being recorded to see the increase in your heart rate.
- You can take deep breaths to see how the resulting slight movement of your heart affects your ECG.
- You can move the electrodes to incorrect positions to see how this distorts the recording.

ANATOMIC ORIENTATION OF THE HEART

 The position of the heart within the body determines the "view" of the cardiac electrical activity that can be observed from any site on the body surface. The atria are located in the top or base of the heart, and the ventricles taper toward the bottom or apex (Fig 1.1A). The long axis of the heart, which extends from base to apex, is tilted to the left at its apical end in the drawing of this frontal-plane view (Fig 1.1B).

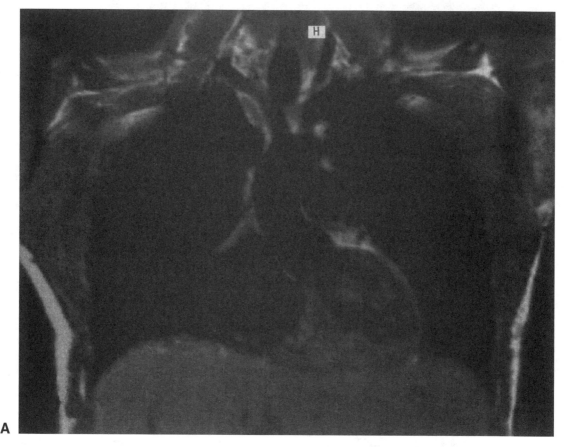

A

Figure 1.1. **A.** Frontal-plane magnetic resonance image (MRI) of the heart within the thorax. **B.** Schematic drawing showing the tilt of the long axis of the heart and the orientation of the heart's chambers: right atrium (*RA*), left atrium (*LA*), right ventricle (*RV*), and left ventricle (*LV*). The large arteries and veins seen prominently on the MRI have been omitted from the schematic to better illustrate the relative positions of the cardiac chambers (see also Fig. 1.2).

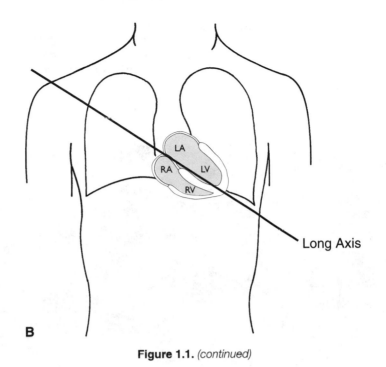

Figure 1.1. *(continued)*

However, the right atrium/right ventricle and left atrium/left ventricle are not directly aligned with the right and left sides of the body (Fig 1.2A). The right-sided chambers of the heart are located anterior to the left-sided chambers, with the result that the inter-atrial and interventricular septa form a diagonal in this transverse-plane view (Fig 1.2B).[1,2]

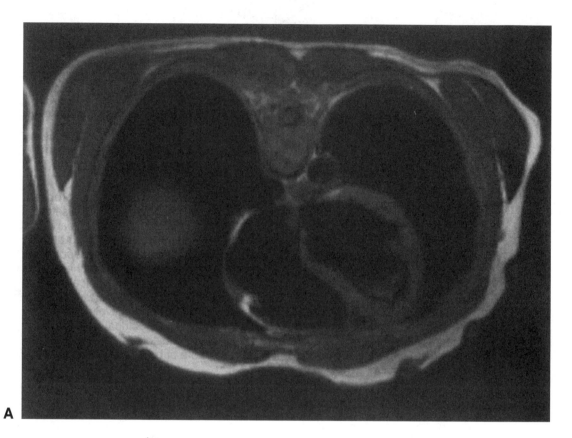

A

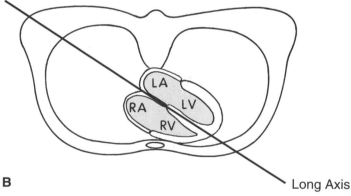

B

Long Axis

Figure 1.2. **A.** Transverse-plane magnetic resonance image of the heart within the thorax, viewed from above. **B.** Schematic drawing showing how the right atrium (*RA*)/right ventricle (*RV*) is oriented more anteriorly than the left atrium (*LA*)/left ventricle (*LV*).

THE CARDIAC CYCLE

The mechanical pumping action of the heart is produced by cardiac muscle ("myocardial") cells that contain contractile proteins. The timing and synchronization of contraction of these myocardial cells are controlled by noncontractile cells of the *pacemaking* and *conduction system*. Impulses generated within these specialized cells create a rhythmic repetition of events called *cardiac cycles*. Each cycle includes electrical and mechanical activation (*systole*) and recovery (*diastole*). The terms commonly applied to these components of the cardiac cycle are listed in Table 1.1. Since the electrical events initiate the mechanical events, there is a brief delay between the onsets of electrical and mechanical systole and of electrical and mechanical diastole.

Table 1.1. Terms Describing Cardiac Cycle

	Systole	Diastole
Electrical	Activation	Recovery
	Excitation	Recovery
	Depolarization	Repolarization
Mechanical	Shortening	Lengthening
	Contraction	Relaxation
	Emptying	Filling

The electrical recording from inside a single myocardial cell as it progresses through a cardiac cycle is illustrated in Figure 1.3. During electrical diastole, the cell has a *baseline* negative electrical potential and is also in mechanical diastole, with separation of the contractile proteins. An electrical impulse arriving at the cell allows positively charged ions to cross the cell membrane, causing its *depolarization*. This movement of ions initiates electrical systole, which is characterized by an *action potential*. This electrical event then initiates mechanical systole, in which the contractile proteins within the myocardial cell slide over each other, thereby shortening the cell. Electrical systole continues until the positively charged ions are pumped out of the cell, causing its *repolarization*. The electrical potential then returns to its negative resting level. This return of electrical diastole causes the contractile proteins within the cell to separate. The cell is then capable of being reactivated if another electrical impulse arrives at its membrane.

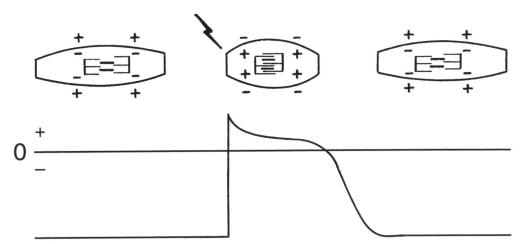

Figure 1.3. At top, a single cardiac cell is shown at three points in time, during which it is relaxed, contracted, and relaxed again. An electrical impulse (the *lightning bolt*) causes transport of positive (+) ions into the cell. Below the cell is a representation of an internal electrical recording. The *horizontal line* indicates the level of zero (*0*) potential, with positive (+) values above and negative (–) values beneath the line. (Modified from Thaler MS. The only EKG book you'll ever need. Philadelphia: JB Lippincott, 1988:11.)

The electrical and mechanical changes in a series of myocardial cells as they progress through a cardiac cycle are illustrated in Figure 1.4. In Figure 1.4A, the four representative cells are in their resting or repolarized state. Electrically, the cells have negative charges, while mechanically their contractile proteins are separated. An electrical stimulus arrives at the second myocardial cell in Figure 1.4B, causing electrical and then mechanical systole. The wave of depolarization in Figure 1.4C has spread throughout all the myocardial cells. In Figure 1.4D, the recovery or repolarization process begins in the second cell, which had been the first to depolarize. In Figure 1.4E, the wave of repolarization has finally spread throughout all of the myocardial cells, and they await the coming of another electrical stimulus.[3–6]

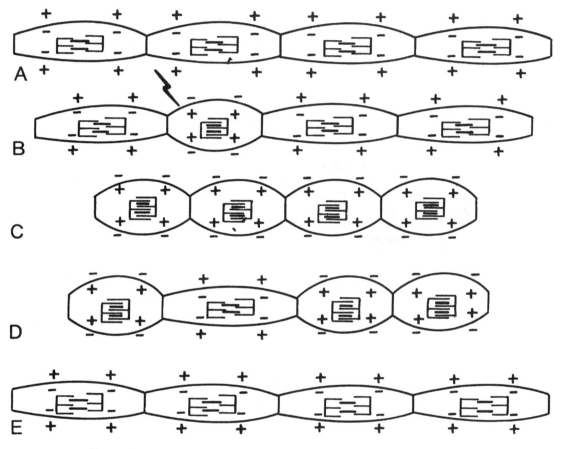

Figure 1.4. The symbols are the same for these four myocardial cells aligned end to end as for the single cell in Figure 1.3. (Modified from Thaler MS. The only EKG book you'll ever need. Philadelphia: JB Lippincott, 1988:9.)

In Figure 1.5, the relationship between the intracellular electrical recording from a single myocardial cell presented in Figure 1.3 is combined with an ECG recording from positive and negative electrodes on the body surface. The ECG recording is the summation of electrical signals from all of the myocardial cells. There is a flat baseline when the cells are in their resting state electrically, and also when the summation of cardiac electrical activity is directed perpendicular to a line between the positive and negative electrodes. The onset of depolarization of the cells produces a relatively high-frequency ECG *waveform*. Then, while depolarization persists, the ECG returns to the baseline. Repolarization of the myocardial cells is represented on the ECG by a lower frequency waveform in the opposite direction from that representing depolarization.

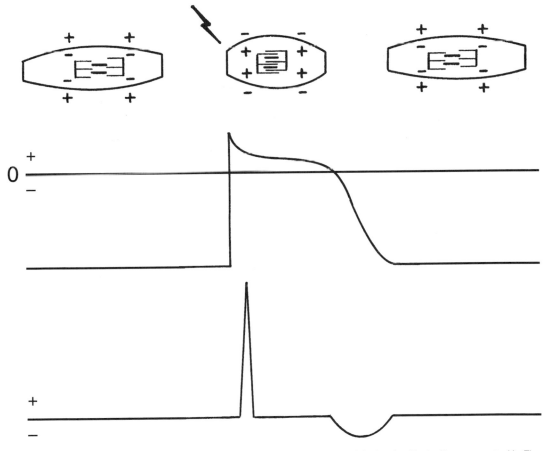

Figure 1.5. The schematic ECG recording beneath is added to the illustration presented in Figure 1.3. (Modified from Thaler MS. The only EKG book you'll ever need. Philadelphia: JB Lippincott, 1988:11.)

In Figure 1.6, positive and negative electrodes have been placed on the body surface and connected to a single-channel ECG recorder. The process of production of the ECG recording by waves of depolarization and repolarization spreading from the negative toward the positive electrode is illustrated in the figure. In Figure 1.6*A*, the first of the four cells shown has been electrically activated, and the activation has then spread into the second cell. This spread of depolarization toward the positive electrode produces a positive (upward) *deflection* on the ECG. In Figure 1.6*B*, all of the cells are in their depolarized state, and the ECG recording has returned to its baseline level. In Figure 1.6*C*, repolarization has begun in the same cell in which depolarization was initiated, and the wave of repolarization has spread into the adjoining cell. This produces the oppositely directed negative (downward) waveform on the ECG recording.

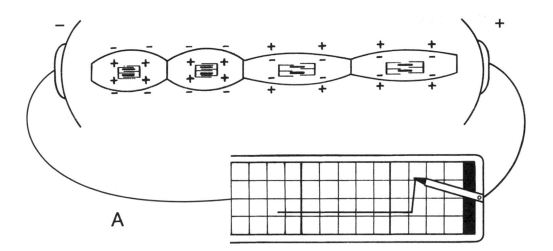

A

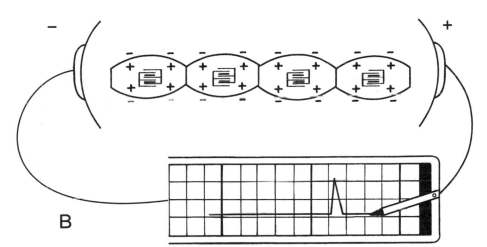

B

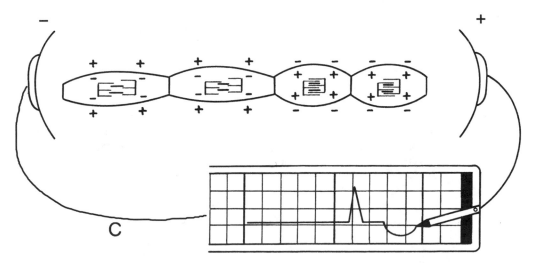

C

Figure 1.6. Negative (−) and positive (+) electrodes on the body surface are connected to an ECG machine that records the depolarization and repolarization waveforms generated by the heart as they spread from left to right toward the positive electrode. (Modified from Thaler MS. The only EKG book you'll ever need. Philadelphia: JB Lippincott, 1988:29,31.)

CARDIAC IMPULSE FORMATION AND CONDUCTION

The electrical activation of a single cardiac cell or even of a small group of cells does not produce enough voltage to be recorded on the body surface. Clinical electrocardiography is made possible by the activation of large groups of atrial and ventricular myocardial cells whose numbers are of sufficient magnitude for their electrical activity to be recorded on the body surface.

Myocardial cells normally lack the ability for either spontaneous formation or rapid conduction of an electrical impulse. They depend for these functions on special cells of the cardiac pacemaking and conduction system that are located strategically through the heart (Fig. 1.7). These cells are arranged in *nodes*, *bundles*, *bundle branches*, and branching networks of *fascicles*. The cells that form these structures lack contractile capability, but can generate spontaneous electrical impulses (act as pacemakers), and can alter the speed of electrical conduction throughout the heart. The intrinsic pacemaking rate is most rapid in the specialized cells in the atria and slowest in those in the ventricles. This intrinsic pacemaking rate is altered by the balance between the sympathetic and parasympathetic components of the autonomic nervous system.[7-10]

Figure 1.7 illustrates the anatomic relationships between the cardiac pumping chambers and the specialized pacemaking and conduction system. The *sinoatrial (SA)* or *sinus node* is located high in the right atrium, near its junction with the *superior vena cava*. The SA node is the predominant cardiac pacemaker, and its highly developed capacity for autonomic regulation controls the heart's pumping rate to meet the changing needs of the body. The *atrioventricular (AV) node* is located low in the right atrium, adjacent to the interatrial *septum*. Its primary function is to slow electrical conduction sufficiently to synchronize the atrial contribution to ventricular pumping. Normally, the AV node is the only structure capable of conducting impulses from the atria to the ventricles, because these chambers are otherwise completely separated by nonconducting fibrous and fatty tissue.[11-13]

In the atria, the electrical impulse generated by the SA node spreads through the myocardium without the need for being carried by any specialized conduction bundles. However, rapidly conducting bundles with branches and fascicles are present in the ventricles, so that activation of the myocardium at the base can be delayed until the apical region has been activated. Since the pulmonary and aortic outflow valves are located at the bases of the ventricles, this sequence of electrical activation is necessary to achieve the most efficient cardiac pumping.

The intraventricular conduction pathways include a common bundle (*Bundle of His*) that leads from the AV node to the summit of the interventricular septum, and the right and left bundle branches of the Bundle of His, which proceed along the septal surfaces of their respective ventricles. The left bundle branch fans out into fascicles that proceed along the left septal surface and toward the two papillary muscles of the mitral valve. The right bundle branch remains compact until it reaches the right distal septal surface, where it branches into the interventricular septum and proceeds toward the free wall of the right ventricle. These intraventricular conduction pathways are composed of fibers of *Purkinje cells* with specialized capabilities for both pacemaking and rapid conduction of electrical impulses. Fascicles composed of Purkinje fibers form networks that extend just beneath the surface of the right and left ventricular endocardium. After reaching the ends of these Purkinje fascicles, the impulses then proceed slowly from endocardium to epicardium throughout the right and left ventricles.[14-16]

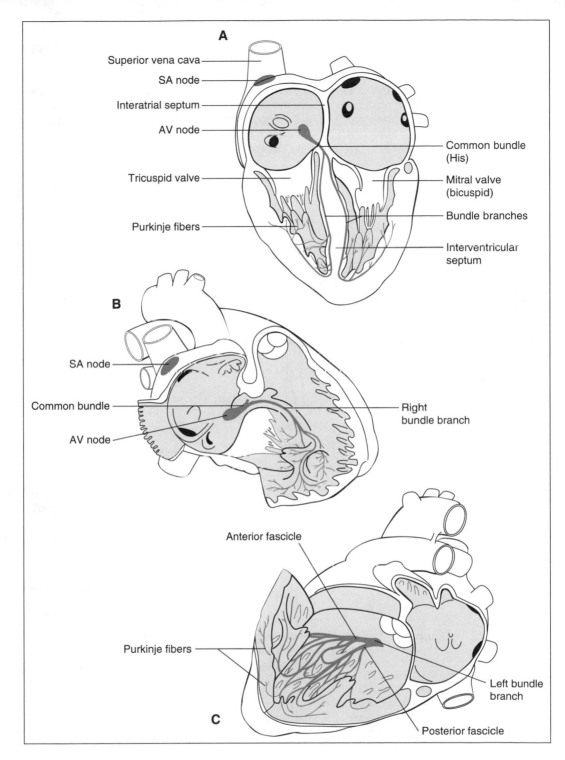

Figure 1.7. Three views of the anatomic relationships between the cardiac pumping chambers and the structures of the pacemaking and conduction system. **A.** From the anterior precordium, as in the frontal-plane MRI and schematic of Figure 1.1, but with less tilt. **B.** From the right anterior precordium looking onto the interatrial and interventricular septa through the right atrium and ventricle. **C.** From the left posterior thorax looking onto the septa through the left atrium and ventricle. (Modified from Netter FH. In: Yonkman FF, ed. The Ciba collection of medical illustrations. vol 5. Heart. Summit: Ciba–Geigy, 1978;13,49.)

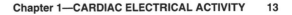

RECORDING LONG-AXIS (BASE–APEX) CARDIAC ELECTRICAL ACTIVITY

   The optimal body-surface sites for recording long-axis (base–apex) cardiac electrical activity are located where the extensions of the long axis of the heart intersect with the body surface (Fig. 1.8). A negative electrode on the right shoulder and a positive electrode on the left lower chest produce predominantly upright *waveforms* on the ECG, as will be discussed in Chapter 2, "Recording the Electrocardiogram."

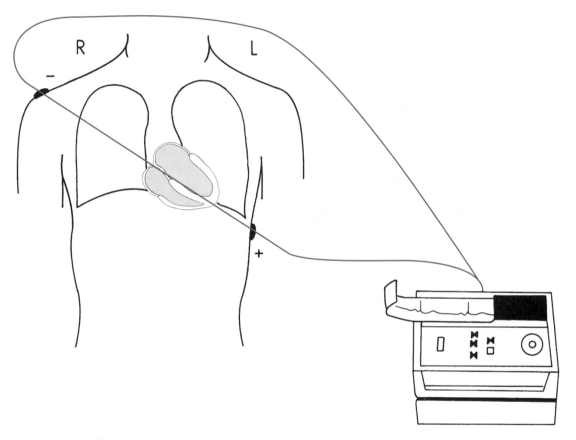

Figure 1.8.   The schematic frontal-plane view of the heart in the thorax from Figure 1.1*B*, with electrodes where the long axis intersects with the body surface. The positive electrode on the left lower thoracic wall and the negative electrode on the right shoulder are aligned from the cardiac base to apex parallel to the interatrial and interventricular septa, and are attached to a single-channel ECG recorder. The ventricular repolarization wave is positively oriented, as explained later in this unit and illustrated in Figure 1.11.

The initial wave of a cardiac cycle represents activation of the atria and is called the *P wave* (Fig. 1.9). Since the SA node is located in the right atrium, the first part of the P wave represents the activation of this chamber. The middle section of the P wave represents completion of right-atrial activation and initiation of left-atrial activation. The final section of the P wave represents completion of left-atrial activation. Activation of the AV node begins by the middle of the P wave and proceeds slowly during the final portion of the P wave. The wave representing electrical recovery of the atria is usually too small to be seen, but it may appear as a distortion of the PR segment. The His bundle and bundle branches are activated during the PR segment but do not produce ECG waveforms.

The next group of waves recorded is the *QRS complex*, representing the simultaneous activation of the right and left ventricles. On this long-axis recording, the P wave is entirely positive and the QRS complex is predominantly positive. Minor portions at the beginning and end of the QRS complex may appear as negative waves.

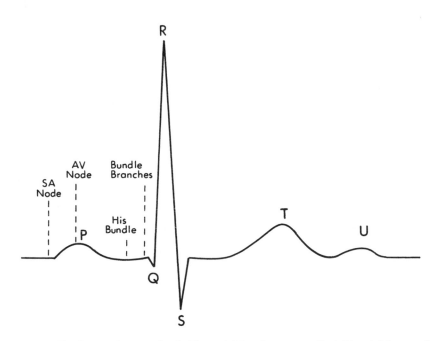

Figure 1.9. The long-axis recording in Figure 1.8 has been magnified. The visible waveforms represent activation of the atria (*P*) and ventricles (*Q*, *R*, and *S*) and recovery of the ventricles (*T* and *U*). The timing of activation of the structures of the pacemaking and conduction system is also indicated.

The QRS complex may normally appear as one (*monophasic*), two (*diphasic*), or three (*triphasic*) individual waveforms (Fig. 1.10). By convention, a negative wave at the onset of the QRS complex is called a *Q wave*. The predominant portion of the QRS complex recorded from this long-axis viewpoint is normally positive and is called the *R wave*, regardless of whether or not it is preceded by a Q wave. A negative deflection following an R wave is called an *S wave*. When a second positive deflection occurs, it is termed R'. A monophasic negative QRS complex should be termed a *QS wave*. Occasionally, more complex patterns of QRS waveforms occur, as will be discussed in Chapter 3, "Interpretation of the Normal Electrocardiogram."

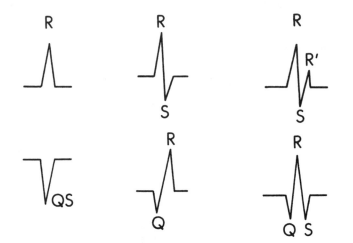

Figure 1.10. Examples of QRS complex waveforms and their alphabetical terms. Monophasic R and QS complexes are on the left, biphasic RS and QR complexes are in the center, and triphasic RSR' and QRS complexes are on the right. (From Selvester RH, Wagner GS, Hindman NB. The development and application of the Selvester QRS scoring system for estimating myocardial infarct size. Arch Intern Med 1985;145:1879, with permission. Copyright 1985, American Medical Association.)

The wave in the cardiac cycle that represents recovery of the ventricles is called the *T wave*. Since recovery of the ventricular cells (repolarization) causes an ion flow opposite to that of depolarization, one might expect the T wave to be inverted in relation to the QRS complex, as shown in Figures 1.5 and 1.6. However, epicardial cells repolarize earlier than endocardial cells, thereby causing the wave of repolarization to spread in the direction opposite that of the wave of depolarization (epicardium to endocardium) (Fig. 1.11*A*). This results in a T wave deflected in a similar direction as the QRS complex (Fig. 1.11*B*). The T wave is sometimes followed by another small upright wave (the source of which is uncertain), called the *U wave*, as seen in Figure 1.9.

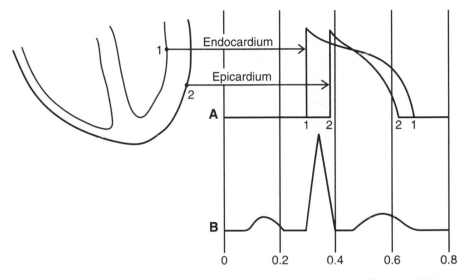

Figure 1.11. The frontal-plane view of the right and left ventricles (as in Figure 1.7*A*) is presented along with schematic recordings from left-ventricular myocardial cells on the endocardial (*1*) and epicardial (*2*) surfaces in (*A*), and the long-axis body surface ECG waveforms (as in Figure 1.9) are shown in (*B*). The numbers below the recordings refer to the time (in seconds) required for these sequential electrical events.

The time from the onset of the P wave to the onset of the QRS complex is called the *PR interval*, whether the first wave in this QRS complex is a Q wave or an R wave (Fig. 1.12). This interval measures the time between the onset of activation of the atrial and ventricular myocardium. The designation *PR segment* refers to the time from the end of the P wave to the onset of the QRS complex. The QRS interval measures the time from the beginning to the end of ventricular activation. Since activation of the thick left-ventricular free wall and interventricular septum requires more time than does activation of the right-ventricular free wall, the terminal portion of the QRS complex represents the balance of forces between the basal portions of these thicker regions.

The *ST segment* is the interval between the end of ventricular activation and the beginning of ventricular recovery. The term "ST segment" is used regardless of whether the final wave of the QRS complex is an R or an S wave. The junction of the QRS complex and the ST segment is called the *J point*. The interval from the onset of ventricular activation to the end of ventricular recovery is called the *QT interval*. This term is used regardless of whether the QRS complex begins with a Q or an R wave.

At low heart rates in a healthy person, the PR, ST, and TP segments are at approximately the same level (*isoelectric*). The PR segment is typically used as the *baseline* for measuring the amplitudes of the various waveforms.[17–19]

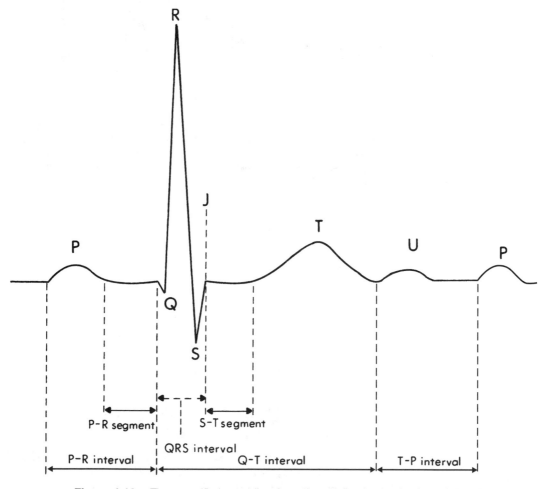

Figure 1.12. The magnified recording from the cardiac long-axis viewpoint in Figure 1.9 is again presented, with the principal ECG segments (*P-R and S-T*) and time intervals (*P-R, QRS, Q-T,* and *T-P*) indicated.

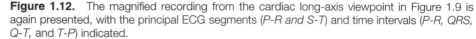

RECORDING SHORT-AXIS (LEFT–RIGHT) CARDIAC ELECTRICAL ACTIVITY

It is often important to determine whether an abnormality originates from the left or the right side of the heart. The optimal sites for recording left- versus right-sided cardiac electrical activity are located where the extensions of the short axis of the heart (perpendicular to the interatrial and interventricular septa) intersect with the body surface (Fig. 1.13). A negative electrode on the left posterior thorax and a positive electrode on the right anterior thorax produce waveforms similar to those indicated on the ECG recording.

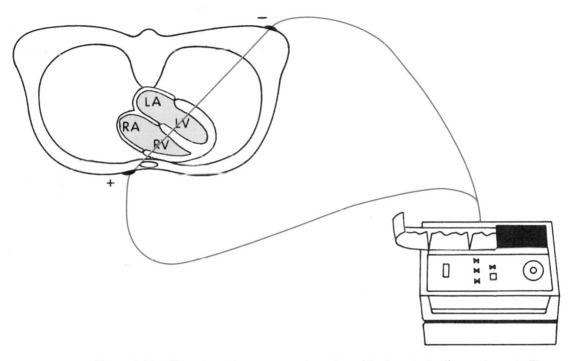

Figure 1.13. The schematic transverse-plane view of the heart in the thorax shown in Figure 1.2B, with electrodes where the short axis intersects with the body surface. The positive electrode to the right of the sternum and the negative electrode on the back are aligned perpendicular to the interatrial and interventricular septa, and are attached to a single-channel ECG recorder. The typically diphasic P and T waves and the predominately negative QRS complex recorded by electrodes at these positions are indicated on the ECG.

These ECG waveforms are magnified in Figure 1.14. The initial part of the P wave, representing right-atrial activation, appears positive at this site because of the progression of electrical activity from the interatrial septum toward the right-atrial free wall. The final part of the P wave, representing left-atrial activation, appears negative because of progression of electrical activity from the interatrial septum toward the left-atrial free wall. This activation sequence produces a diphasic P wave.

The initial part of the QRS complex represents the progression of activation in the interventricular septum. This movement is predominately from the left toward the right side of the septum, producing a positive (R wave) deflection at this left- versus right-sided recording site. The midportion of the QRS complex represents progression of electrical activation through the left and right-ventricular myocardium. Since the posteriorly positioned left-ventricular free wall is much thicker than the anteriorly placed right-ventricular free wall, its activation predominates over that of the latter, resulting in a deeply negative deflection (S wave). The final portion of the QRS complex represents the completion of activation of the left-ventricular free wall and interventricular septum. This posteriorly directed excitation is represented by the completion of the S wave. The T wave is typically biphasic in this short-axis view, and there is no U wave.

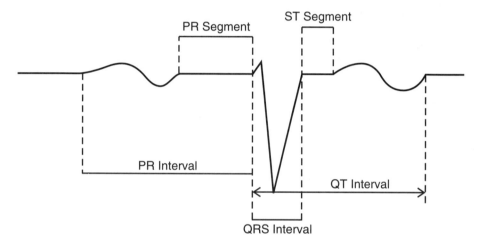

Figure 1.14. Magnified view of the recording from the cardiac short-axis viewpoint in Figure 1.13, with the principal ECG segments and time intervals indicated as in Figure 1.12 for the long-axis view.

This short-axis-oriented recording provides the key ECG view for identifying enlargement of one of the four cardiac chambers and localizing the site of a delay in ventricular activation (Fig. 1.15). Right-atrial enlargement produces an abnormally prominent initial part of the P wave (A), while left-atrial enlargement produces an abnormally prominent terminal part of the P wave (B). Right-ventricular enlargement produces an abnormally prominent R wave (C), whereas left-ventricular enlargement produces an abnormally prominent S wave (D). A delay in conduction through the right bundle branch causes right ventricular activation to occur after left ventricular activation is completed, producing an R' deflection (E). A delay in conduction through the left bundle branch markedly postpones left-ventricular activation, resulting in an abnormally prominent S wave (F).

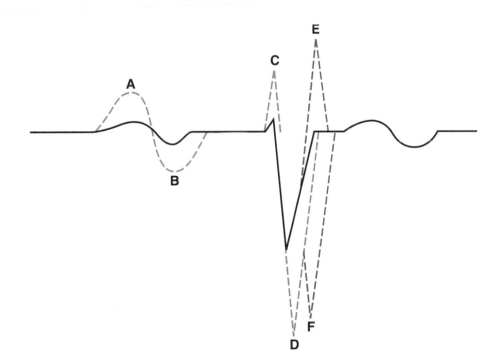

Figure 1.15. The ECG waveforms from Figure 1.14 are reproduced with the alterations, indicated by *dashed lines*, that would typically result from enlargements of the right (A) and left (B) atrial chambers and the right (C) and left (D) ventricular chambers, and from right-sided (E) and left-sided (F) intraventricular conduction delays.

GLOSSARY

Action potential: the electrical potential recorded from within a cell as it is activated by an electrical current or impulse.

Anterior: located toward the front of the body.

Apex: the region of the heart where the narrowest parts of the ventricles are located.

Atrioventricular (AV) node: a small mass of tissue situated in the inferior aspect of the right atrium, adjacent to the septum between the right and left atria. Its function is to slow impulses traveling from the atria to the ventricles, thereby synchronizing atrial and ventricular pumping.

Atrium: a chamber of the heart that receives blood from the veins and passes it along to its corresponding ventricle.

Base: the broad top of the heart where the atria are located.

Baseline: see **Isoelectric line**.

Bundle branches: groups of Purkinje fibers that emerge from the common bundle (of His); the right bundle branch rapidly conducts electrical impulses to the right ventricle, while the left bundle branch conducts impulses to the left ventricle.

Cardiac cycle: a single episode of electrical and mechanical activation and recovery of a myocardial cell or of the entire heart.

Cardiac pacemaking and conduction system: Groups of modified myocardial cells strategically located throughout the heart and capable of forming an electrical impulse and/or of conducting impulses particularly slowly or rapidly.

Common bundle (of His): a compact group of Purkinje fibers that originates at the AV node and rapidly conducts electrical impulses to the right and left bundle branches.

Depolarization: the transition in which there becomes minimal difference between the electrical charge or potential on the inside versus the outside of the cell. In the resting state, the cell is polarized, with the inside of the cell markedly negative in comparison to the outside. Depolarization is then initiated by a current that alters the permeability of the cell membrane, allowing positively charged ions to cross into the cell.

Deflection: a waveform on the ECG; its direction may be either upward (positive) or downward (negative).

Diastole: the period in which the electrical and mechanical aspects of the heart are in their baseline or resting state: electrical diastole is characterized by repolarization and mechanical diastole by relaxation. During mechanical diastole the cardiac chambers are filling with blood.

Diphasic: consisting of two components.

Distal: situated away from the point of attachment or origin; the opposite of proximal.

Electrode: an electrical contact that is placed on the skin and is connected to an ECG recorder.

Electrocardiogram (ECG): the recording made by the electrocardiograph, depicting the electrical activity of the heart.

Endocardium: the inner aspect of a myocardial wall, adjacent to the blood-filled cavity of the adjacent chamber.

Epicardium: the outer aspect of a myocardial wall, adjacent to the pericardial lining that closely envelops the heart.

Fascicle: a small bundle of Purkinje fibers that emerges from a bundle or a bundle branch to rapidly conduct impulses to the endocardial surfaces of the ventricles.

Inferior: situated below and closer to the feet than another body part; the opposite of superior.

Isoelectric line: a horizontal line on an ECG recording that forms a baseline; representing neither a positive nor a negative electrical potential.

J point: junction of the QRS complex and the ST segment.

Lateral: situated toward either the right or left side of the heart or of the body as a whole.

Monophasic: consisting of a single component, being either positive or negative.

P wave: the first wave depicted on the ECG during a cardiac cycle; it represents atrial activation.

PR interval: the time from onset of the P wave to onset of the QRS complex. This interval represents the time between the onsets of activation of the atrial and the ventricular myocardium.

PR segment: the time from the end of the P wave to the onset of the QRS complex.

Purkinje cells or fibers: modified myocardial cells that are found in the distal aspects of the pacemaking and conduction system, consisting of the common bundle, the bundle branches, the fascicles, and individual strands.

Q wave: a negative wave at the onset of the QRS complex.

QRS complex: the second wave or group of waves depicted on the ECG during a cardiac cycle; it represents ventricular activation.

QRS interval: the time from the beginning to the end of the QRS complex, representing the duration required for activation of the ventricular myocardial cells.

QS: a monophasic negative QRS complex.

QT interval: the time from the onset of the QRS complex to the end of the T wave. This interval represents the time from the beginning of ventricular activation to the completion of ventricular recovery.

R wave: the first positive wave appearing in a QRS complex; it may appear at the onset of the QRS complex or following a Q wave.

R′ wave: the second positive wave appearing in a QRS complex.

Repolarization: the transition in which the inside of the cell becomes markedly positive in relation to the outside. This condition is maintained by a pump in the cell membrane, and it is disturbed by the arrival of an electrical current.

Septum: a dividing wall between the atria or between the ventricles.

Sinoatrial (SA) node: a small mass of tissue situated in the superior aspect of the right atrium, adjacent to the entrance of the superior vena cava. It functions as the dominant pacemaker, which forms the electrical impulses that are then conducted throughout the heart.

ST segment: the interval between the end of the QRS complex and the beginning of the T wave.

Superior: situated above and closer to the head than another body part.

Superior vena cava: one of the large veins that empties into the right atrium.

Systole: the period in which the electrical and mechanical aspects of the heart are in their active state: electrical systole is characterized by depolarization and mechanical systole by contraction. During mechanical systole, blood is being pumped out of the heart.

T wave: the final major wave depicted on the ECG during a cardiac cycle; it represents ventricular recovery.

Triphasic: consisting of three components.

U wave: a wave on the ECG that follows the T wave in some individuals; it is typically small and its source is uncertain.

Ventricle: a chamber of the heart that receives blood from its corresponding atrium and pumps the blood it receives out into the arteries.

Waveform: electrocardiographic representation of either the activation or recovery phase of electrical activity of the heart.

REFERENCES

1. De Vries PA, Saunders. Development of the ventricles and spiral outflow tract of the human heart. Contr Embryol Carneg Inst 1962;37:87.
2. Mall FP. On the development of the human heart. Am J Anat 1912;13:249.
3. Hoffman BF, Cranefield PF. Electrophysiology of the heart. New York: McGraw–Hill, 1960.
4. Page E. The electrical potential difference across the cell membrane of heart muscle. Circulation 1962;26:582–595.
5. Fozzard HA, ed. The heart and cardiovascular system: scientific foundations. New York: Raven Press, 1986.
6. Guyton AC. Heart muscle; the heart as a pump. In: Guyton AC, ed. Textbook of medical physiology. Philadelphia: WB Saunders, 1991.
7. Rushmer RF. Functional anatomy and the control of the heart, Part I. In: Rushmer RF, ed. Cardiovascular dynamics. Philadelphia: WB Saunders, 1976:76–104.
8. Langer GA. Heart: excitation–contraction coupling. Ann Rev Physiol 1973;35:55–85.
9. Weidmann S. Resting and action potentials of cardiac muscle. Ann N Y Acad Sci 1957;65:663.
10. Rushmer RF, Guntheroth WG. Electrical activity of the heart, Part I. In: Rushmer RF, ed. Cardiovascular dynamics. Philadelphia: WB Saunders, 1976.
11. Truex RC. The sinoatrial node and its connections with the atrial tissue. In: Wellens HJJ, Lie KI, Janse MJ, eds. The conduction system of the heart. The Hague: Martinus Nijhoff, 1978.
12. Hecht HH, Kossmann CE. Atrioventricular and intraventricular conduction. Am J Cardiol 1973;31:232–244.
13. Becker AE, Anderson RH. Morphology of the human atrioventricular junctional area. In: Wellens HJJ, Lie KI, Janse MJ, eds. The conduction system of the heart. The Hague: Martinus Nijhoff, 1978.
14. Meyerburg RJ, Gelband H, Castellanos A, et al. Electrophysiology of endocardial intraventricular conduction: the role and function of the specialized conducting system. In: Wellens HJJ, Lie KI, Janse MJ, eds. The conduction system of the heart. The Hague: Martinus Nijhoff, 1978.
15. Guyton AC. Rhythmic excitation of the heart. In: Guyton AC, ed. Textbook of medical physiology. Philadelphia: WB Saunders, 1991.
16. Scher AM. The sequence of ventricular excitation. Am J Cardiol 1964;14:287.
17. Graybiel A, White PD, Wheeler L, Williams C, eds. The typical normal electrocardiogram and its variations. In: Electrocardiography in practice. Philadelphia: WB Saunders, 1952.
18. Netter FH. Section II, The electrocardiogram. The CIBA collection of medical illustrations. vol 5. New York: CIBA, 1978.
19. Barr RC. Genesis of the electrocardiogram. In: Macfarlane PW, Lawrie TDV, eds. Comprehensive electrocardiology. vol I. New York: Pergamon Press, 1989:139–147.

CHAPTER 2

Recording the
Electrocardiogram

EVOLUTION OF FRONTAL PLANE LEADS

Examples have been provided in Chapter 1 ("Cardiac Electrical Activity") of two viewpoints for recording cardiac electrical activity: base–apex (long axis) and left–right (short axis). The standard electrocardiogram (ECG) used for clinical diagnosis includes these two plus 10 other viewpoints. Each view is provided by recording the electrical potential difference between a positive and a negative pole, referred to as a *lead*. Six of these leads provide views in the *frontal plane* and six provide views in the *transverse* (*horizontal*) *plane*. A single recording electrode on the body surface serves as the positive pole of each lead; the negative pole of each lead is provided either by a single recording electrode or by a "central terminal" that averages the input from multiple recording electrodes. The device used for recording the electrocardiogram is called the *electrocardiograph*.

One hundred years ago, Einthoven[1] placed recording electrodes on the right and left arms and the left leg and called the recording an "Elektrokardiogramme" (EKG), which is replaced by the anglicized "ECG" throughout this book. Einthoven's work produced three leads (I, II, and III), each consisting of a pair of the limb electrodes, with one electrode of the pair serving as the positive and the other as the negative pole (Fig. 2.1). The positive poles of these leads were positioned to the left and inferiorly, so that the cardiac electrical waveforms would appear primarily upright on the ECG. This waveform direction results because the summations of both the atrial and ventricular electrical forces are generally directed toward the apex of the heart. For lead I, the left-arm electrode provides the positive pole and the right-arm electrode provides the neg-

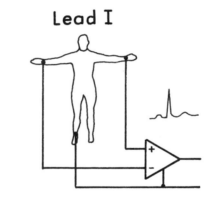

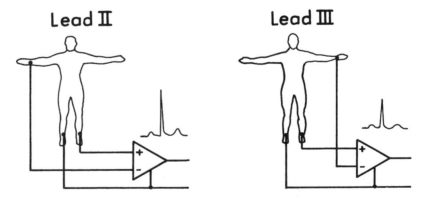

Figure 2.1. The method of ECG recording of Einthoven's three original limb leads is illustrated, with an example of a typical recording from each. An electrode placed on the right leg is used to ground the system. The distal limb sites for positive (+) and negative (–) electrodes are indicated. (Modified from Netter FH. The Ciba collection of medical illustrations. vol 5. Heart. Summit, NJ: Ciba–Geigy, 1978:51.)

ative pole. Lead II, with its positive electrode on the left leg and its negative electrode on the right arm, provides a long-axis view of the cardiac electrical activity similar to that presented in Figures 1.8, 1.9, and 1.12. Lead III has its positive electrode on the left leg and its negative electrode on the left arm.

The three leads used to produce the ECG form the *Einthoven triangle* (Fig. 2.2A), which constitutes a simplified model of the true orientation of the leads in the frontal plane. Consideration of these three leads so that they intersect in the center of the cardiac electrical activity but retain their original orientation provides a triaxial reference system for viewing the cardiac electrical activity (Fig. 2.2B).

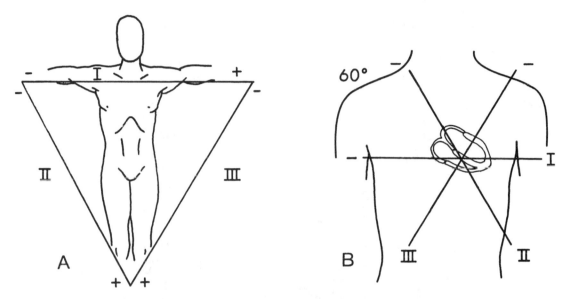

Figure 2.2. **A.** The equiangular (60-degree) Einthoven triangle formed by leads I, II, and III is shown with positive (*I, II, III*) and negative poles (−) of each of the leads indicated. **B.** The Einthoven triangle is shown in relation to the schematic view of the heart presented in Figure 1.1B, and the three leads are shown to intersect at the center of the cardiac electrical activity.

The 60-degree angles between leads I, II, and III create wide gaps among the three views of the cardiac electrical activity. Wilson and coworkers[2] developed a method for filling these gaps without additional body-surface electrodes: they created a central terminal by connecting the three limb electrodes through resistors. An ECG lead using this central terminal as its negative pole and a recording electrode on the body surface as its positive pole is termed a *V lead*.

However, when the central terminal is connected to a recording electrode on an extremity to produce an additional frontal-plane lead, the resulting electrical signals are small. This occurs because the electrical signal from the recording electrode is partially cancelled when both the positive electrode and one of the three elements of the negative electrode are located on the same extremity. The amplitude of these signals may be increased or "augmented" by disconnecting the central terminal from the electrode on the limb that is serving as the positive pole. Such an augmented V lead is termed an *aV lead*. For example, lead aVR fills the gap between leads I and II by recording the potential difference between the right arm and the average of the potentials on the left arm and left leg (Fig. 2.3). Lead aVR, like lead II, provides a long-axis viewpoint of the cardiac electrical activity, but with the opposite orientation from that provided by lead II. Lead –aVR would be more useful for ECG interpretation. The gap between leads II and III is filled by lead aVF, and the gap between leads III and I is filled by lead aVL. The three aV frontal-plane leads were introduced by Goldberger and colleagues.[3]

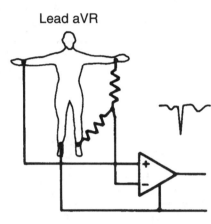
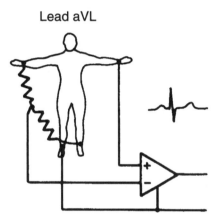

Figure 2.3. The method of ECG recording of the augmented limb leads is illustrated along with an example of a typical recording of each. The alternating lines indicate resistors on the connections between two of the recording electrodes that produce the negative poles for each of the aV leads. (Modified from Netter FH. The Ciba collection of medical illustrations. vol. 5. Heart. Summit: Ciba–Geigy, 1978:51.)

Addition of the three aV leads to the triaxial reference system produces a hexaxial system (Fig. 2.4) for viewing the cardiac electrical activity in the frontal plane, with the six leads of this system separated by angles of only 30 degrees. This provides a perspective of the frontal plane similar to the face of a clock. By convention, the degrees are arranged as shown. With lead I (located at 0 degrees) used as the reference lead, positive designations increase in 30-degree increments in a clockwise direction to +180 degrees, and negative designations increase by the same increments in a counterclockwise direction to −180 degrees. Lead II appears at +60 degrees, lead aVF at +90 degrees, and lead III at +120 degrees, respectively. Leads aVL and aVR have designations of −30 degrees and −150 degrees, respectively. The negative poles of each of these leads complete the "clock face."

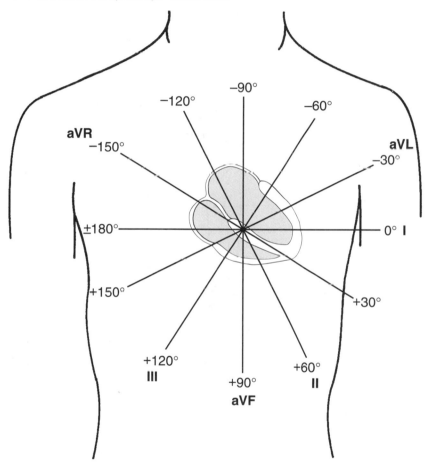

Figure 2.4. Figure 2.2B is reproduced with the lines of the three added leads superimposed on the lines of the three original leads. The locations of the positive and negative poles of each lead around the 360 degrees of the "clock face" are indicated, with the names of the six leads appearing at their positive poles.

Modern electrocardiographs, using digital technology, record leads I and II only, and then calculate the voltages in the remaining limb leads in real time on the basis of Einthoven's law: I + III = II.[1] The algebraic outcome of the formulas for calculating the voltages in aV leads from leads I, II, and III are:

$$aVR = -\tfrac{1}{2}(I + II)$$
$$aVL = I - \tfrac{1}{2}(II)$$
$$aVF = II - \tfrac{1}{2}(I)$$

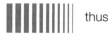 thus

$$aVR + aVL + aVF = 0$$

TRANSVERSE-PLANE LEADS

 The standard 12-lead ECG includes the six frontal-plane leads of the hexaxial system and six additional leads relating to the transverse plane of the body. These additional leads, introduced by Wilson, are produced by connecting the central terminal of the hexaxial system to a recording electrode placed at various positions on the anterior and left lateral chest wall.[4–8] Since the positions of these latter leads are immediately in front of the heart, they are termed *precordial*. The six additional leads used to produce the 12-lead ECG are labeled V1 through V6, because the central terminal connected to the average of all three of the limb electrodes provides their negative poles (Fig. 2.5). The figure shows lead V1, with its positive pole on the right anterior precordium and its negative pole in the center of the cardiac electrical activity, since this lead provides the short-axis view of cardiac electrical activity useful for distinguishing left versus right cardiac activity as described in Chapter 1 (Fig. 1.13).

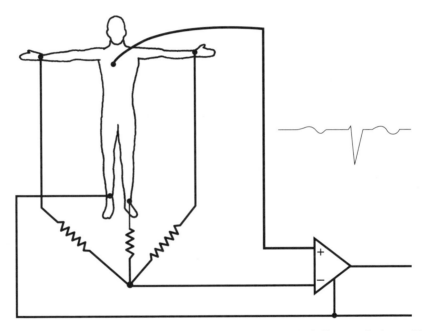

Figure 2.5. The method of ECG recording of the precordial leads is illustrated, along with an example of lead V1. The *wave-like lines* indicate resistors in the connections between the recording electrodes on the three limb leads that produce the negative poles for each of the V leads. (Modified from Netter FH. The Ciba collection of medical illustrations. vol 5. Heart. Summit, NJ: Ciba–Geigy, 1978:51.)

Each of the sites of the recording electrode is determined by bony landmarks on the precordium (Fig. 2.6). The clavicles should be used as a reference for locating the first rib. The space between the first and second ribs is called the first *intercostal space*. Lead V1 is placed in the fourth intercostal space just to the right of the sternum. Lead V2 is placed in the fourth intercostal space just to the left of the sternum (directly anterior to the center of cardiac electrical activity), and lead V4 is placed in the fifth intercostal space on the *midclavicular line*. Placement of lead V3 is then halfway along a straight line between leads V2 and V4. Leads V5 and V6 are positioned directly lateral to lead V4, with lead V5 in the *anterior axillary line* and lead V6 in the *midaxillary line*. In adult females, leads V4 and V5 should be positioned on the chest wall beneath the breast.

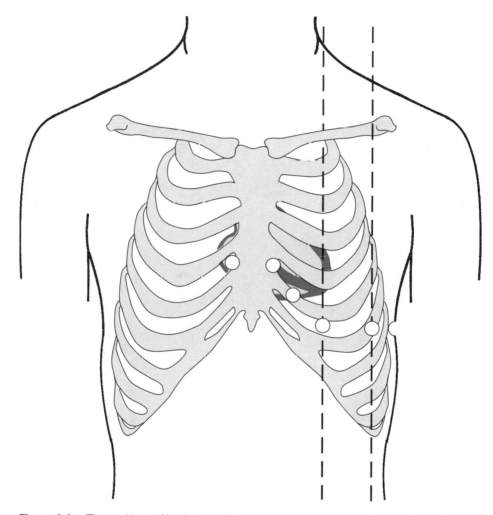

Figure 2.6.   The positions of leads V1 to V5 are indicated by *circles*, and the position of lead V6 is indicated by the *semicircular indentation* to the left of the V5 position. The *dashed vertical lines* signify the midclavicular (through lead V4) and anterior axillary (through lead V5) lines. The schematic drawing of the external cardiac outline from Figure 1.1 B is shown within the thorax. (Modified from Thaler MS. The only EKG book you'll ever need. Philadelphia: JB Lippincott, 1988:41.)

The angles between the six transverse-plane leads are approximately the same 30 degrees as in the frontal plane (Fig. 2.7).

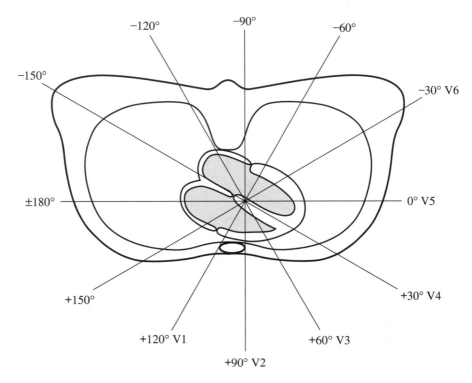

Figure 2.7. Figure 1.2*B* is shown with the orientation of the six precordial leads indicated by *solid lines* from each of their recording sites through the approximate center of cardiac electrical activity indicated in Figure 2.3. Extension of these lines through the chest indicates the opposite positions, which can be considered the locations of the negative poles of the six precordial leads. The same format as in Figure 2.3 indicates the angles on the "clock face."

CORRECT AND INCORRECT LEAD PLACEMENT

A single cardiac cycle from each of the standard 12 ECG leads of a healthy individual, recorded with all nine recording electrodes positioned correctly, is shown in Figure 2.8A. An accurate electrocardiographic interpretation is possible only if the recording electrodes are placed in their proper positions on the body surface. The three frontal-plane electrodes (right arm, left arm, and left leg) used for recording the six limb leads should be placed at distal positions on the designated extremity. It is important to note that when more proximal positions are used, particularly on the left arm,[9] marked distortion of the QRS complex may occur. The distal limb positions provide "clean" recordings when the individual maintains the extremities in "resting" positions.

The other panels of Figure 2.8 present examples of ECG recordings produced by incorrect placement of either a limb (Fig. 2.8B–E) or a precordial (Fig. 2.8F) electrode on the same individual as described above. The most common error in frontal-plane recording results from reversal of two of the electrodes. One example of this is reversal of the right and left arm electrodes, as illustrated in Figure 2.8B. In this instance, lead I is inverted, leads II and III are reversed, leads aVR and aVL are reversed, and lead aVF is correct. Another example that produces a characteristic ECG pattern is reversal of the right leg grounding electrode with one of the arm electrodes. Extremely low amplitudes of all waveforms appear in lead II when the grounding electrode is on the right arm (Fig. 2.8C), and in lead III when the grounding electrode is on the left arm (Fig. 2.8D). These amplitudes are so low because the potential difference between the two legs is almost zero. Left arm and leg electrode reversal is the most difficult to detect: lead III is inverted and leads I and II, and aVL and aVF are reversed (Fig. 2.8E). It is also possible for the positions of the precordial electrodes to be reversed, as illustrated for leads V1 and V2 in Figure 2.8F.

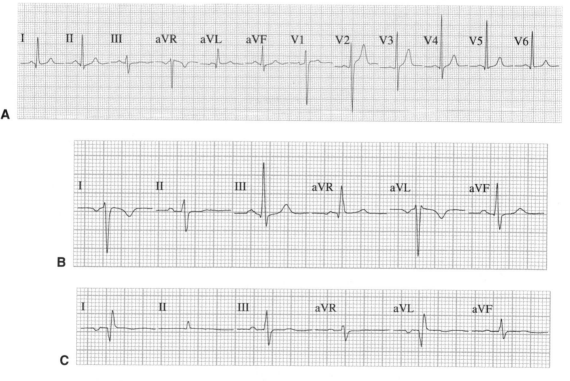

Figure 2.8. All 12 leads are shown for the normal example **(A)**. The six frontal plane leads are contrasted for the limb lead reversals **(B–E)**, and the six transverse plane leads are contrasted for precordial lead reversal **(F)**.

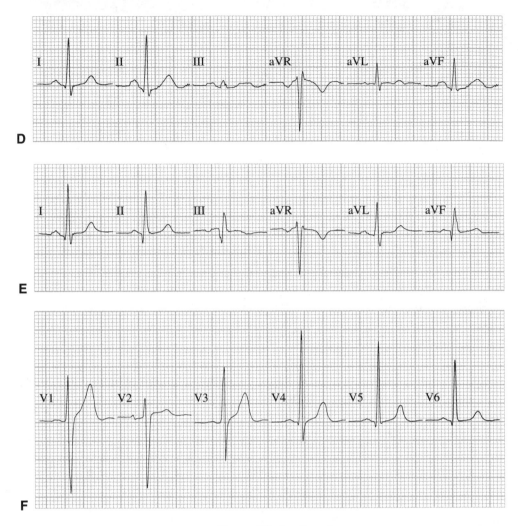

Figure 2.8. *(continued)*

However, a more common error in transverse-plane recording involves failure to place the individual electrodes according to their designated landmarks (Fig. 2.6). Precise identification of the bony landmarks for proper electrode placement may be difficult in adult females, obese individuals, and persons with chest-wall deformities. Even slight alterations of the position of these electrodes may significantly distort the appearance of the cardiac waveforms. Comparison of serial ECG recordings relies upon precise electrode placement.

OTHER PRACTICAL POINTS FOR RECORDING THE ECG

Care should be taken to ensure that technique is uniform from one ECG recording to another. The following points are important to consider when preparing to record an ECG:

1. Electrodes should be selected for maximum adhesiveness and minimum discomfort, electrical noise, and skin–electrode impedance. The standards for electrodes published by the American Association for Advancement of Medical Instrumentation[10] should be followed.
2. Effective contact between electrode and skin is essential. Sites with skin irritation or skeletal abnormalities should be avoided. The skin should be cleaned with only a "dry wipe." Poor electrode contact may produce instability of the baseline of the recording, termed *baseline wander*, when the instability occurs gradually, or baseline shift when the instability occurs abruptly (Fig. 2.9A).
3. Calibration of the ECG signal is typically 1 mV = 10 mm. When large QRS waveform amplitudes require that calibration be reduced to 1 mV = 5 mm, this should be noted to facilitate interpretation.
4. ECG paper speed is typically 25 mm/sec, and variations used for particular clinical purposes should be noted. A faster speed may be used to provide a clearer depiction of waveform morphology, and a slower speed may be used to provide visualization of a greater number of cardiac cycles in order to facilitate rhythm analysis.
5. Electrical artifacts in the ECG may be external or internal. External artifacts introduced by line current (50 or 60 Hz) may be minimized by straightening the lead wires so that they are aligned with the patient's body. Internal artifacts may result from muscle tremors, shivering, hiccups, or other factors, as illustrated in Figure 2.9B.
6. It is important that the patient be in the supine position during recording of the ECG. If another position is clinically required, notation of the altered position should be made. Lying on either side or elevation of the torso may change the position of the heart within the chest. A change in body position may have an effect on the accuracy of an ECG recording[11] similar to a change in electrode placement.

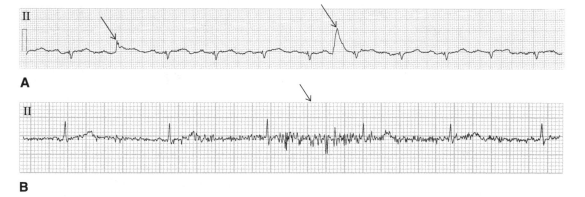

Figure 2.9. **A.** A "shifting baseline" is produced by slight body movements during recording of the long axis oriented lead II. *Arrows* indicate this movement during the second cycle, and between the sixth and seventh cycles. **B.** A "noisy baseline" produced by shivering is continuously present. An *arrow* indicates the area of maximal baseline deformity. The ECG shown in **A** is presented at half scale for illustrative purposes.

ALTERNATIVE LEAD PLACEMENT

Several reasons exist for selecting alternative sites for placement of ECG electrodes, as follows:

1. The standard sites are unavailable because of patient pathology (e.g., amputation or burns) or other impediments (e.g., bandages). In these instances, the electrodes should be positioned as closely as possible to the standard sites, and the alternative sites should be noted on the recording.

2. The standard electrode-placement sites are not in the optimal position to detect a particular cardiac waveform or abnormality (e.g., P waves obscured within T waves or *situs inversus dextrocardia*). Detection of P waves requires sufficient time between cardiac cycles to provide a baseline between the end of the T wave and the beginning of the QRS complex. In the presence of a rapid cardiac rate (*tachycardia*), alternative lead placement may reveal recognizable atrial activity (Fig. 2.10*A*). This may be accomplished by any of the following methods: (a) moving lead V1 up by one intercostal space above its standard site; (b) using this site as the positive pole and the *xiphoid process* of the sternum as the negative pole; or (c) recording from a *transesophageal* electrode.

When the congenital position of the heart is rightward (situs inversus dextrocardia), the right and left arm leads should be reversed (and the precordial leads should be recorded from rightward-oriented V leads progressing from V1R (standard lead V2) to V6R (Fig. 2.10*B*). *Right ventricular hypertrophy* and *infarction* may best be detected via an electrode in the V3R or V4R position. In infants, in whom the right ventricle is normally more prominent, standard lead V3 is often replaced by lead V4R.

Experimental studies have used multiple rows of electrodes on the anterior and posterior torso to identify specific cardiac abnormalities. This provides improved capability for diagnosis of clinical problems such as *left ventricular hypertrophy* or various locations of myocardial infarction.[12] The posterior thoracic recording leads V7 to V9 may provide added capability for identifying a posterior infarction.

3. The standard sites produce a recording obscured by artifacts (e.g., skeletal muscle potentials during ambulatory monitoring). When alternative sites are used, there should be careful notation on the recording.

Alternative Lead Placement for Continuous ECG Recording

Continuous monitoring of the cardiac electrical activity may be useful for evaluating abnormalities of cardiac *rhythm* or of myocardial blood flow. Monitoring may be performed in three different situations: (a) at the bedside; (b) during exercise stress testing; or (c) during routine ambulatory activity. Each situation may require particular alternative electrode placement because of Reasons 2 or 3 in the list given above.

Bedside

When monitoring for disturbances of cardiac rhythm, electrodes should be placed elsewhere than in the left parasternal area, to allow easy access for clinical examination of the heart and possible use of an external defibrillator. A modified lead, MCL_1, with the positive electrode in the same position as lead V1 and the negative electrode near the left shoulder, usually provides good visualization of atrial activity (Fig. 2.10*C*). Since using the original V1 site as the positive pole provides the optimal short-axis view of left versus right cardiac activity, as presented in Figures 1.13 and 1.14, lead MCL_1 may be useful for multiple cardiac diagnostic purposes.

When monitoring for evidence of cardiac ischemia, a complete set of 12 leads may be preferred for recording the ECG. Krucoff and coworkers described the usefulness of continuous ST-segment monitoring with 12 leads during various unstable coronary syndromes. Some of the major applications of this technique include detection of reoccluded coronary arteries after balloon angioplasty,[13] detection of *reperfusion* and *reocclusion* in acute myocardial infarction,[14,15] and surveillance during *unstable angina*.

A modification of the *Mason–Likar*[16] system has been developed for continuous ST-segment monitoring.

Exercise Stress Testing

The lead that is most useful during exercise stress testing has its positive electrode positioned at the V5 level. The negative electrode may be placed in a variety of distant positions. A second useful lead has an orientation similar to that of lead aVF, with its positive electrode on the left midaxillary line over the lowest rib.

Monitoring of all 12 ECG leads during exercise necessitates moving the limb electrodes from standard distal to more central positions. Alternative torso sites for the right and left arm and left leg electrodes are on bony prominences close to the bases of the respective limbs (Fig. 2.10D). Ideally, these sites would: (a) avoid skeletal muscle artifact; (b) provide stability for the recording electrodes; and (c) record waveforms similar to those from the limb sites. The Mason–Likar[16] designations of torso sites are commonly used for the alternative sites of electrode placement for ECG recording during exercise. The resultant recording, however, has some features that differ from the standard 12-lead recording.

Routine Ambulatory Activity

The method of continuous monitoring and recording of cardiac electrical activity is referred to as Holter monitoring[17] after its developer. Originally, only one lead was used. In monitoring for abnormalities of cardiac rhythm, the American Heart Association recommends use of a "V1-type" lead, with the positive electrode in the fourth right intercostal space 2.5 cm from the sternum and the negative electrode below the left clavicle. Currently, a second or even a third lead is added to facilitate interpretation and to assure recording of some information if one electrode is detached. These second or third leads are placed at the positions for lead V5 and modified lead aVF, as indicated for use in exercise stress testing (Fig. 2.10E).

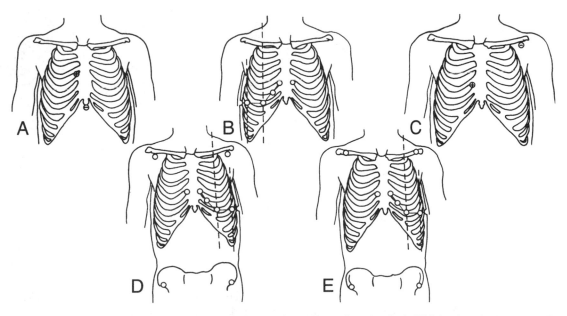

Figure 2.10. Locations of positive and negative poles of a single ECG lead are indicated for **A** and **C**. Locations of the electrodes for each of the precordial V leads are shown in **B**, **D**, and **E**. Torso locations of RA (right arm), LA (left arm), RL (right leg), and LL (left leg) positive electrodes are shown in **D** and **E**. The right midclavicular line is indicated in **B**. Both the left midclavicular and left anterior axillary lines are indicated in **D** and **E**.

DISPLAY OF THE 12 STANDARD ELECTROCARDIOGRAM LEADS

The 12-lead ECG is typically presented via a three-channel recording, with the two groups of frontal-plane leads preceding the two groups of transverse plane leads (Fig. 2.11*A*). The six precordial leads are presented in their orderly sequence (V1 through V6), but the six frontal-plane leads are typically presented in the groups in which they were historically developed (I, II, and III; then aVR, aVL, and aVF). These leads have been arranged in their "orderly sequence" by Cabrera[18]: aVL, I, -aVR, II, aVF, and III (Fig. 2.11*B*). Note that lead aVR is inverted to -aVR to provide the same long-axis orientation as lead II. The orderly sequence of frontal-plane leads followed by the transverse-plane leads provides a *panoramic display*[19] of cardiac electrical activity proceeding from left (aVL) to right (III), and then from right (V1) to left (V6). The Swedish version of the panoramic display is shown in Figure 2.11*C*. There is the disadvantage of lack of continuity between the two planes; however, there is also the advantage of vertical alignment allowing identification of the true times of the beginnings and endings of the individual ECG waveforms.

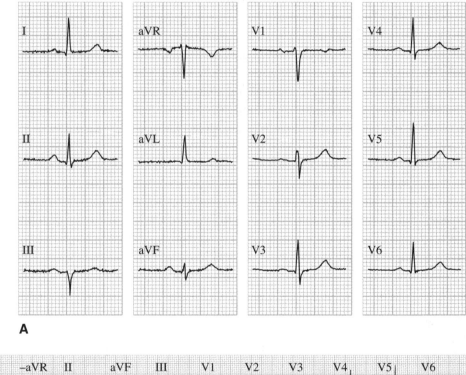

A

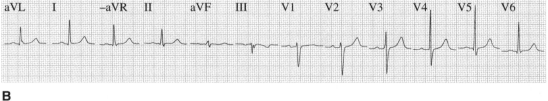

B

Figure 2.11. The 12 leads appear in four columns of three leads each (**A**). All 12 leads appear in a single horizontal display in **B**, and the six limb leads and the six precordial leads appear in parallel vertical displays recorded at double speed (50 mm/sec) in **C**.

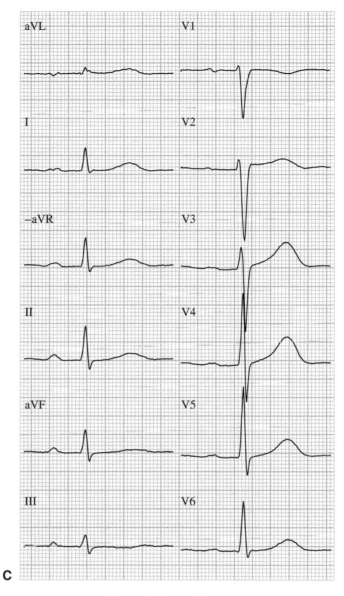

C

Figure 2.11. *(continued)*

GLOSSARY

aV lead: an augmented V lead (see below); it uses a modified central terminal with inputs from the electrode on the designated limb (R for right arm, L for left arm, and F for left foot) as its positive pole, and the average of the potentials from the leads on the other two limbs as its negative pole.

Angina: Angina pectoris, precordial pressure or pain caused by cardiac ischemia or lack of blood flow to the heart muscle.

Angioplasty: a procedure using a balloon-tipped arterial catheter to break up atherosclerotic plaques.

Anterior axillary line: a vertical line on the thorax at the level of the anterior aspect of the axilla, which is the area where the arm joins the body.

Artifact: an electrocardiographic waveform that arises from sources other than the myocardium.

Baseline wander: a back-and-forth movement of the isoelectric line or baseline, interfering with precise measurement of the various ECG waveforms; sometimes termed baseline shift when it is abrupt.

Central terminal: a terminal created by Wilson and colleagues that connects all three limb electrodes through a 5,000-Ω resistor so that it can serve as the negative pole for an exploring positive electrode to form a V lead.

Einthoven triangle: an equilateral triangle composed of limb leads I, II, and III that provides an orientation for electrical information from the frontal plane.

Electrocardiograph: a device used to record the electrocardiogram (ECG).

Frontal plane: a vertical plane of the body (also called the coronal plane) that is perpendicular to both the horizontal and sagittal planes.

Hypertrophy: an increase in muscle mass; it most commonly occurs in the ventricles when they are compensating for a pressure (systolic) overload.

Infarct: an area of necrosis in an organ, resulting from an obstruction in its blood supply.

Intercostal: situated between the ribs.

Ischemia: an insufficiency of blood flow to an organ that is so severe that it disrupts the function of the organ; in the heart, ischemia is often accompanied by precordial pain and diminished contraction.

Lead: a recording of the electrical potential difference between a positive and a negative body-surface electrode. The negative electrode can originate from a combination of two or three electrodes (see V lead and aV lead).

Mason-Likar: a system for alternative lead placement, used for recording from the limb leads while the patient is moving about or exercising; in this system the electrodes are moved from the limbs to the torso.

MCL_1: a modified lead V1 used to enhance visualization of atrial activity.

Midaxillary line: a vertical line on the thorax at the level of the midpoint of the axilla, which is the area where the arm joins the body.

Midclavicular line: a vertical line on the thorax at the level of the midpoint of the clavicle or collarbone.

Panoramic display: the typical ECG display of the precordial leads in their orderly sequence from right to left, with an innovative display of the frontal-plane leads from left to right (aVL, I, –aVR, II, aVF, and III). Limb lead aVR is inverted to obtain the same positive leftward orientation as the other five limb leads.

Precordial: situated on the thorax, directly overlying the heart.

Proximal: situated near the point of attachment or origin of a limb; the opposite of distal.

Reocclusion: a recurrence of a complete obstruction to blood flow.

Reperfusion: the restoration of blood circulation to an organ or tissue upon reopening of a complete obstruction to blood flow.

Rhythm: the pattern of recurrence of the cardiac cycle.

Situs inversus dextrocardia: an abnormal condition in which the heart is situated on the right side of the body and the great blood vessels of the right and left sides are reversed.

Sternum: the narrow, flat bone in the middle of the anterior thorax; breastbone.

Tachycardia: a rapid heart rate with a frequency above 100 beats/min.

Transverse plane: the horizontal plane of the body; it is perpendicular to both the frontal and sagittal planes.

V lead: an ECG lead that uses a central terminal with inputs from leads I, II, and III as its negative pole and an exploring electrode as its positive pole.

Xiphoid process: the lower end of the sternum; it has a triangular shape.

REFERENCES

1. Einthoven W, Fahr G, de Waart A. Uber die richtung und die manifeste grosse der potentialschwankungen im menschlichen herzen und uber den einfluss der herzlage auf die form des elektrokardiogramms. Pfluegers Arch 1913;150:275–315. (Translation: Hoff HE, Sekelj P. Am Heart J 1950;40:163–194.)

2. Wilson FN, Macloed AG, Barker PS. The interpretation of the initial deflections of the ventricular complex of the electrocardiogram. Am Heart J 1931;6:637–664.

3. Goldberger E. A simple, indifferent, electrocardiographic electrode of zero potential and a technique of obtaining augmented, unipolar, extremity leads. Am Heart J 1942;23:483–492.

4. Wilson FN, Johnston FD, Macloed AG, et al. Electrocardiograms that represent the potential variations of a single electrode. Am Heart J 1934;9:447–471.

5. Kossmann CE, Johnston FD. The precordial electrocardiogram. I. The potential variations of the precordium and of the extremities in normal subjects. Am Heart J 1935;10:925–941.

6. Joint recommendations of the American Heart Association and the Cardiac Society of Great Britain and Ireland. Standardization of precordial leads. Am Heart J 1938;15:107–108.

7. Committee of the American Heart Association for the Standardization of Precordial Leads. Supplementary report. Am Heart J 1938;15:235239.

8. Committee of the American Heart Association for the Standardization of Precordial Leads. Second supplementary report. JAMA 1943;121: 1349–1351.

9. Pahlm O, Haisty WK, Edenbrandt L, et al. Evaluation of changes in standard electrocardiographic QRS waveforms recorded from activity-compatible proximal limb lead positions. Am J Cardiol 1992;69:253–257.

10. A Report for Health Professionals by a Task Force of the Council on Clinical Cardiology, AHA. Instrumentation and practice standards for electrocardiographic monitoring in special care units. Circulation 1989;79:464–471.

11. Sutherland DJ, McPherson DD, Spencer CA, et al. Effects of posture and respiration on body surface electrocardiogram. Am J Cardiol 1983;52:595–600.

12. Kornreich F, Rautaharju PM, Warren J, et al. Identification of best electrocardiographic leads for diagnosing myocardial infarction by statistical analysis of body surface potential maps. Am J Cardiol 1985;56:852–856.

13. Krucoff MW, Parente AR, Bottner RK, et al. Stability of multilead ST segment "fingerprints" over time after percutaneous transluminal coronary angioplasty and its usefulness in detecting reocclusion. Am J Cardiol 1988;61:1232–1237.

14. Krucoff MW, Wagner NB, Pope JE, et al. The portable programmable microprocessor driven realtime 12 lead electrocardiographic monitor: a preliminary report of a new device for the noninvasive detection of successful reperfusion of silent coronary reocclussion. Am J Cardiol 1990;65:143–148.

15. Krucoff MW, Croll MA, Pope JE, et al. Continuously updated 12 lead ST segment recovery analysis for myocardial infarct artery patency assessment and its correlation with multiple simultaneous early angiographic observations. Am J Cardiol 1993;71:145–151.

16. Mason RE, Likar I. A new system of multiplelead exercise electrocardiography. Am Heart J 1966;71:196–205.

17. Holter NJ. New method for heart studies. Science 1961;134:1214–1220.

18. Cabrera E: Bases electrophysiologiques de L'electrocardiographie, ses applications clinique. Paris: Masson, 1948.

19. Anderson ST, Pahlm O, Selvester RH, et al. A panoramic display of the orderly sequenced twelve lead electrocardiogram. J Electrocardiogr 1994 27:347–352.

CHAPTER 3

Interpretation of the Normal Electrocardiogram

ELECTROCARDIOGRAPHIC FEATURES

Every electrocardiogram (ECG) has nine features that should be examined systematically:

1. Rate and regularity.
2. P-wave morphology.
3. PR interval.
4. QRS-complex morphology.
5. ST-segment morphology.
6. T-wave morphology.
7. U-wave morphology.
8. QTc interval.
9. Rhythm.

Rate, *regularity*, and *rhythm* are commonly grouped together. However, to accurately assess rhythm, it is necessary to consider not only rate and regularity, but also the various waveforms and intervals on the ECG.

Determination of cardiac rate and regularity requires understanding of the grid markings provided on the ECG paper (Fig. 3.1). The paper shows thin lines every 1 mm and thick lines every 5 mm. The thin lines therefore form small (1 mm) squares and the thick lines form large (5 mm) squares. These vertical lines facilitate measurements of time, such as the cardiac rate and the various intervals. At the usual paper speed of 25 mm/s, the thin lines occur at 0.04-s (40-msec) intervals and thick lines occur at 0.20-s (200-msec or ⅕-s) intervals. The horizontal lines facilitate measurements of waveform amplitudes. At the usual calibration of 10 mm/mV, the thin lines are at 0.1-mV increments and the thick lines are at 0.5-mV increments.

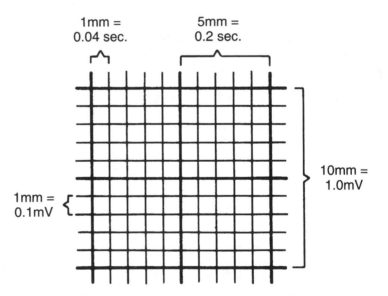

Figure 3.1. The time intervals indicated for the thick and thin *vertical grid lines* on the ECG paper are appropriate for the standard paper speed of 25 mm/sec; the amplitudes indicated for the thick and thin *horizontal grid lines* are appropriate for the standard gain of 10 mm/mV. Each small square is therefore 0.04 s × 0.1 mV, and each large square is 0.20 s × 0.5 mV.

Much of the information provided by the ECG is contained in the morphologies of the principal waveforms: the P wave, the QRS complex, and the T wave. It is helpful to develop a systematic approach to the analysis of these waveforms by:

1. Examining their contours.
2. Measuring their durations.

3. Measuring their maximal positive and negative amplitudes.
4. Estimating their axes in each of the two planes of the ECG recording.

The guidelines for measuring and estimating these four parameters for each of the three principal ECG waveforms are presented below. The definitions of the various waveforms and intervals have been presented in Chapter 1 ("Cardiac Electrical Activity") in the context of describing ECG recordings of base-to-apex and left-versus right-sided cardiac activity.

RATE AND REGULARITY

The cardiac rhythm is rarely precisely regular. Even when the cardiac electrical activity is initiated normally in the sinus node, the rate is affected by the autonomic nervous system. When the individual is at rest, minor variations in autonomic balance are produced by the phases of the respiratory cycle. A glance at the sequence of cardiac cycles is enough to determine whether the cardiac rate is essentially regular or irregular. Normally, there are the same numbers of P waves and QRS complexes and either of these may be used to determine cardiac rate and regularity. When, in the presence of certain abnormal cardiac rhythms, the numbers of P waves and QRS complexes are not the same, the atrial and ventricular rates and regularities must be determined separately.

If there is essential regularity in the cardiac rhythm, the cardiac rate can easily be determined by counting the number of large squares between cycles. Since there are 300 fifths of a second in a minute (5 × 60), it is necessary only to determine the number of fifths (0.2) of a second (large squares) between consecutive cycles and divide this number by 300 to obtain the cardiac rate. It is most convenient to select a prominent ECG waveform that begins on a thick line and then count the number of large squares before the same waveform recurs in the following cycle. When this interval is only one-fifth of a second (0.2 s), the cardiac rate would be 300 beats/min; if the interval is two-fifths of a second (0.4 s), the cardiac rate would be 150 beats/min; if the interval is three-fifths of a second (0.6 s), the cardiac rate would be 100 beats/min, and so forth.

When the cardiac rate is less than 100 beats/min, it is sufficient to consider only the large squares on the ECG paper. When the rate is greater than 100 beats/min (tachycardia), however, small differences in the observed rate may alter the assessment of the underlying cardiac rhythm, and the number of small squares must also be considered (Fig. 3.2). Since there are five small squares in each large square, the number of small squares between successive waveforms of the same type must be divided into 1,500 (6 squares = 250 beats/min, 7 squares = 214 beats/min, etc.). Rate determination is facilitated by the use of cardiac "rate rulers," which are easily obtained from representatives of pharmaceutical companies.

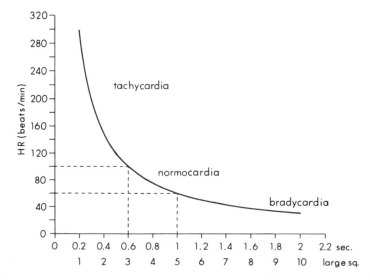

Figure 3.2. Use of time intervals between successive similar ECG waveforms to estimate the cardiac rate. This illustrates the importance of considering the small squares (0.04 s or 40 msec) rather than the large squares (0.2 s or 200 msec) for estimating rates in the tachycardia range, where small differences in the number of intervals between cardiac cycles result in large differences in the estimated rate.

If there is irregularity of the cardiac rate, the number of cycles over a particular interval of time should be counted to determine the average cardiac rate. Many electrocardiographic recordings conveniently provide markers at 3-s intervals. A simple and quick method for estimating cardiac rate is to count the number of cardiac cycles in 6 s and to multiply by 10.

P-WAVE MORPHOLOGY

At either slow or normal heart rates, the small, rounded P wave is clearly visible just before the taller, more peaked QRS complex. At more rapid rates, however, the P wave may merge with the preceding T wave and become difficult to identify. Four steps should be taken to define the morphology of the P wave, as follows:

1. Examine the contour of the wave. The P-wave contour is normally smooth, and is either entirely positive or entirely negative (Fig. 1.9) (monophasic) in all leads except V1. In the short-axis view provided by lead V1, which best distinguishes left- versus right-sided cardiac activity, the divergence of right- and left-atrial activation may produce a diphasic P wave (Fig. 1.14). The contributions of right- and left-atrial activation to the beginning, middle, and end of the P wave are indicated in Figure 3.3.

2. Measure the duration of the wave. The P-wave duration is normally less than 0.12 s.

3. Measure the maximal amplitude of the wave. The maximal P-wave amplitude is normally no more than 0.2 mV in the frontal-plane leads and no more than 0.1 mV in the transverse-plane leads.

4. Estimate the axis of the wave in each of the two planes of the ECG recording. The P wave normally appears entirely upright on leftward and inferiorly oriented leads such as I, II, aVF, and V4 to V6. It is negative in aVR because of the rightward orientation of that lead, and it is variable in the other standard leads. The direction of the P wave, or its axis in the frontal plane, should be determined according to the method for determining the axis of an ECG waveform presented in the section below, on the morphology of the QRS complex. The normal limits of the P-wave axis are 0 degrees and +75 degrees.[1]

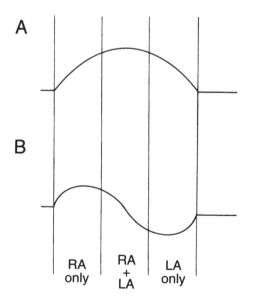

Figure 3.3. Typical appearance of a normal P wave in a long-axis lead such as II **(A)** and a short-axis lead such as V1 **(B)**. The P-wave duration is divided into thirds (*vertical lines*) to indicate the relative times of activation of the right (*RA*) and left (*LA*) atria.

THE PR INTERVAL

The PR interval measures the time required for an electrical impulse to travel from the atrial myocardium adjacent to the sinoatrial (SA) node to the ventricular myocardium adjacent to the fibers of the Purkinje network (Fig. 1.12). This duration is normally from 0.10 to 0.21 s. A major portion of the PR interval reflects the slow conduction of an impulse through the AV node, which is controlled by the balance between the sympathetic and parasympathetic divisions of the autonomic nervous system. Therefore, the PR interval varies with the heart rate, being shorter at faster rates when the sympathetic component predominates, and vice versa. The PR interval tends to increase with age[2]:

In childhood	0.10–0.12 s
In adolescence	0.12–0.16 s
In adulthood	0.14–0.21 s

MORPHOLOGY OF THE QRS COMPLEX

The following steps should be taken to determine the morphology of the QRS complex:

1. Examine the contour of the complex. The QRS complex is composed of higher-frequency signals than are the P and T waves, thereby causing its contour to be peaked rather than rounded. Positive and negative components of the P and T waves are simply termed *positive* and *negative deflections*, whereas those of the QRS complex are assigned specific labels, such as "Q wave" (Fig. 1.10).

   (a) Q waves. In some leads (V1, V2, and V3), the presence of any Q wave should be considered abnormal, whereas in all other leads (except rightward-oriented leads III and aVR), a "normal" Q wave would be very small. The "upper limit of normal" for such Q waves in each lead is indicated in Table 3.1 and is illustrated in Figure 3.4.[3]

Table 3.1. Normal Q Wave Duration Limits

Limb Leads		Precordial Leads	
Lead	Upper Limit	Lead	Upper Limit
I	<0.03 sec	V1	Any Q
II	<0.03 sec	V2	Any Q
III	None	V3	Any Q
aVR	None	V4	<0.02 sec
aVL	<0.03 sec	V5	<0.03 sec
aVF	<0.03 sec	V6	<0.03 sec

Modified from Wagner GS, Freye CJ, Palmeri ST, et al. Evaluation of a QRS scoring system for estimating myocardial infarct size. I. Specificity and observer agreement. Circulation 1982;65:345.

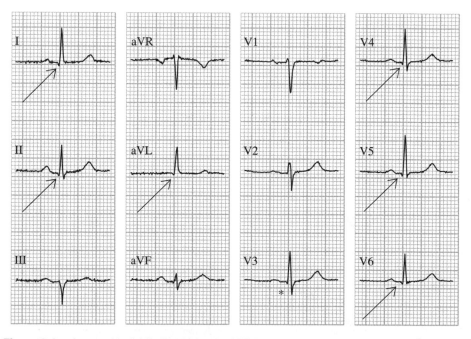

Figure 3.4. A normal individual's 12-standard ECG leads are presented in the classical format of four columns consisting of three leads each. *Arrows* indicate the small Q waves that may normally occur in leads *I, II, aVL, V4, V5*, and *V6*. The *asterisk* in lead V3 indicates the minute Q wave that may rarely occur normally.

The absence of small Q waves in leads V5 and V6 should be considered abnormal. A Q wave of any size is normal in leads III and aVR because of their rightward orientations (Fig. 2.4). Q waves may be enlarged by conditions such as local loss of myocardial tissue (infarction), enlargement (hypertrophy or dilatation) of the ventricular myocardium, or abnormalities of ventricular conduction.

(b) R waves. Since the precordial leads provide a panoramic view of the cardiac electrical activity progressing from the thinner right ventricle across the thicker left ventricle, the positive R wave normally increases in amplitude and duration from lead V1 to lead V4 or V5 (Fig. 3.5). Reversal of this sequence, with larger R waves in leads V1 and V2, can be produced by right-ventricular enlargement, and accentuation of this sequence, with larger R waves in leads V5 and V6, can be produced by left-ventricular enlargement. Loss of normal R-wave progression from lead V1 to lead V4 may indicate loss of left-ventricular myocardium, as occurs with myocardial infarction (Chapter 10: "Myocardial Infarction").

(c) S waves. The S wave also has a normal sequence of progression in the precordial leads. It should be large in V1, larger in V2, and then progressively smaller from V3 through V6 (Fig. 3.5). As with the R wave, this sequence could be altered by enlargement of one of the ventricles or myocardial infarction.

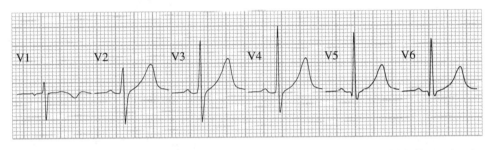

Figure 3.5. The typical panoramic display of the six precordial leads of the ECG, illustrating the normal progression and regression of R- and S-wave amplitudes.

2. Measure the duration of the QRS complex. The duration of the QRS complex is termed the QRS interval, and it normally ranges from 0.07 s to 0.11 s (Fig. 1.12). The duration of the complex tends to be slightly longer in males than in females. The QRS interval is measured from the beginning of the first-appearing Q or R wave to the end of the last-appearing R, S, R', or S' wave. Figure 3.6 illustrates the use of three simultaneously recorded leads to identify the true beginning and end of the QRS complex. Such multilead comparison is necessary, since either the beginning or the end of the QRS complex may be isoelectric (neither positive nor negative) in a particular lead, causing an apparently shorter QRS duration. This isoelectric appearance occurs whenever the summation of ventricular electrical forces is perpendicular to the involved lead. The onset of the QRS complex is usually quite apparent in all leads, but its ending at the junction with the ST segment is often indistinct, particularly in the precordial leads. The QRS interval has no lower limit that indicates abnormality. Prolongation of the QRS interval may be caused by left-ventricular enlargement, an abnormality in intraventricular impulse conduction, or a ventricular site of origin of the cardiac impulse.

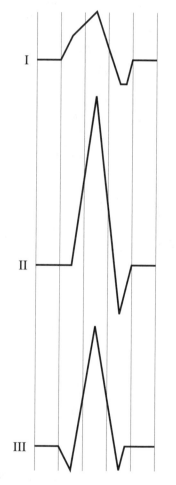

Figure 3.6. Magnified schematic diagram of QRS complexes recorded simultaneously via limb leads *I*, *II*, and *III*, presented on a grid of 0.04-s time lines. Only lead I reveals the true QRS duration (0.12 s). An isoelectric period of approximately 0.02 s is apparent in lead II at the beginning of the QRS complex, and an isoelectric period of approximately 0.01 s is apparent in lead III at the end of the QRS complex.

The duration from the beginning of the earliest-appearing Q or R wave to the peak of the R wave in several of the precordial leads has been termed the *intrinsicoid deflection* (Fig. 3.7). Electrical activation of the myocardium begins at the endocardial insertions of the Purkinje network. The end of the intrinsicoid deflection represents the time at which the electrical impulse arrives at the epicardial surface located beneath the recording electrode. The deflection is called an "intrinsic" deflection when the electrode is on the epicardial surface, and an "intrinsicoid" deflection when the electrode is on the body surface.[4] The intrinsicoid deflection for the thinner-walled right ventricle is measured in leads V1 or V2 (upper limit: 0.035 s), and for the left ventricle is measured in leads V5 or V6 (upper limit: 0.045 s). The intrinsicoid deflection time is prolonged either by hypertrophy of the ventricle or by intraventricular conduction delay.

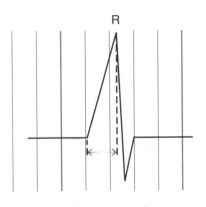

Figure 3.7. Magnified schematic of a QRS complex presented on a grid of standard ECG time lines. The length of the *arrow* indicates the duration (0.05 s) of the prolonged intrinsicoid deflection as measured from the beginning of the QRS complex to the peak of the R wave.

3. Measure the maximal amplitude of the QRS complex. The amplitude of the overall QRS complex has wide normal limits. It varies with age; increasing until about age 30 and then gradually decreasing. The amplitude is generally larger in males than in females. Overall QRS amplitude is measured between the peaks of the tallest positive and negative waveforms in the complex. It is difficult to set an arbitrary upper limit for normal voltage of the QRS complex; amplitudes as high as 3.0 mV are occasionally seen in normal individuals. Factors that contribute to higher amplitudes include youth, physical fitness, slender body build, intraventricular conduction abnormalities, and ventricular enlargement.

An abnormally low QRS amplitude occurs when the overall amplitude is no more than 0.5 mV in any of the limb leads and no more than 1.0 mV in any of the precordial leads. The QRS amplitude is decreased by any condition that increases the distance between the myocardium and the recording electrode, such as a thick chest wall or various intrathoracic conditions that decrease the electrical signal that reaches the electrode.

4. Estimate the axis of the QRS complex in each of the two planes of the ECG recording. The QRS axis represents the average direction of the total force produced by right-ventricular and left-ventricular depolarization. Although the Purkinje network facilitates the spread of the depolarization wavefront from the apex to the base of the ventricles (Chapter 1: "Cardiac Electrical Activity"), the QRS axis is normally in the positive direction in the frontal-plane leads (except aVR) because of the endocardial-to-epicardial spread of depolarization in the thicker-walled left ventricle.

In the frontal plane, the full 360-degree circumference of the hexaxial reference system is provided by the positive and negative poles of the six limb leads (Fig. 2.4), and in the transverse plane it is provided by the positive and negative poles of the six precordial leads (Fig. 2.7).

Identification of the frontal-plane axis of the QRS complex would be easier if the six leads were displayed in their orderly sequence (Fig. 2.11*B*) than it is in the typical display. A simple method for identifying the frontal-plane axis of the QRS complex with the limb leads in orderly sequence is illustrated in Figure 3.8.[5]

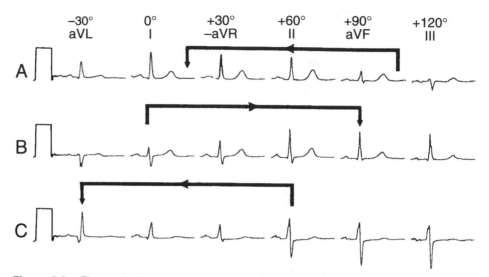

Figure 3.8. The *vertical line without an arrow* indicates the location of the frontal-plane QRS transitional lead. Note that there is no truly transitional lead in **A**, indicating that the QRS transition is located between leads aVF and III. The *long horizontal line* contains an *arrow* indicating movement to 90 degrees away from the transitional lead in the direction of the tallest R wave. The *vertical line with an arrow* indicates the location of the axis: +15 degrees in **A**; +90 degrees in **B**; and −30 degrees in **C**.

When the typical frontal-plane ECG display is used, a three-step method is required for determining the overall axis of the QRS complex.

1. Identify the *transitional lead* (the lead perpendicular to the waveform axis) by locating the lead in which the QRS complex has the most nearly equal positive and negative components. These positive and negative components may vary from miniscule to quite prominent.
2. Identify the lead that is oriented perpendicular to the transitional lead by using the hexaxial reference system (Fig. 3.9, top left).
3. Consider the predominant direction of the QRS complex in the lead identified in Step 2. If the direction is positive, the axis of is the same as the positive pole of that lead. If the direction is negative, the axis is the same as the negative pole of the lead. Note that the positive poles of each lead are labeled with the lead name in Figure 3.9.

The frontal-plane axis of the QRS complex is normally directed leftward and either slightly superiorly or inferiorly, in the region between −30 degrees and +90 degrees (Fig. 3.9, top right). Therefore, the QRS complex is normally predominantly positive in both leads I and II (Fig. 3.9*A*). However, if the QRS complex is negative in lead I but positive in lead II, its axis is deviated rightward, to the region between +90 degrees and ±180 degrees (*right axis deviation* [RAD]) (Fig. 3.9*B*). If the QRS complex is positive in lead I but negative in lead II, its axis is deviated leftward, to the region between −30 degrees and −120 degrees (*left axis deviation* [LAD]) (Fig. 3.9*C* and *D*). Right-ventricular enlargement may produce right-axis deviation and left-ventricular enlargement may produce left-axis deviation of the QRS complex. The axis of the QRS complex is rarely directed completely opposite to its normal direction (−90 to ±180 degrees) with a predominantly negative QRS orientation in both leads I and II (*extreme axis deviation* [EAD]) (Fig. 3.9*E*).

Using the foregoing method for determining the direction of the axis of the QRS complex in the frontal plane permits no more than a "rounding" of the direction to the nearest multiple of 30 degrees. Although automated ECG analysis provides axis designation to the nearest degree, the manual method described here is sufficient for clinical purposes.

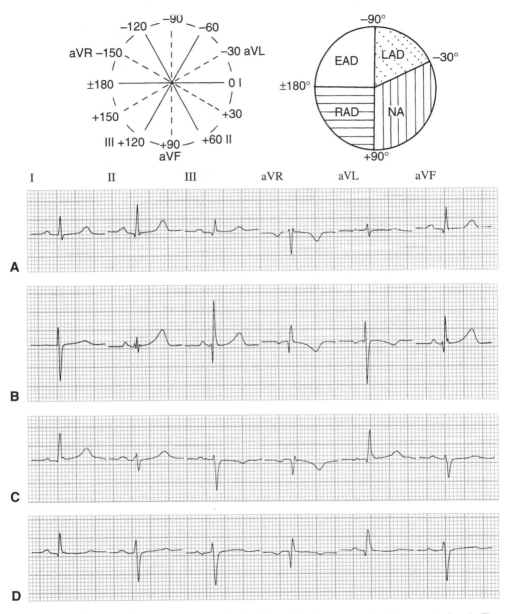

Figure 3.9. At the **top left**, the frontal-plane hexaxial reference system is presented as in Figure 2.4, and at the **top right** the sectors indicating the various designations of the frontal-plane QRS axis in adults are identified: normal axis (*NA*), right-axis deviation (*RAD*), left-axis deviation (*LAD*), and extreme axis deviation (*EAD*). At the **bottom**, examples of various frontal plane QRS axes are shown: **A**. +60 degrees; **B**. +150 degrees; **C**. −30 degrees; **D**. −60 degrees; and **E**. −120 degrees.

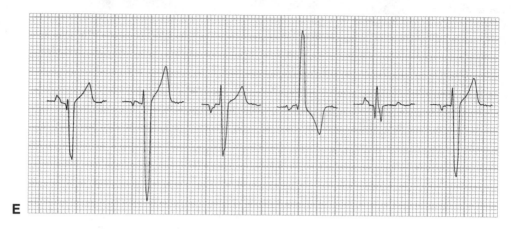

E

Figure 3.9. *(continued)*

The normal frontal-plane axis of the QRS complex is rightward in the neonate, moves to a vertical position during childhood, and then moves to a more leftward position during adulthood.[7] In normal adults, the electrical axis of the QRS complex is almost parallel to the anatomic base-to-apex axis of the heart, in the direction of lead II. However, these axes are more vertical in thin individuals and more horizontal in heavy individuals. This same normal growth-dependent rightward-to-leftward movement of the QRS axis that is seen in the frontal plane is also apparent in the transverse plane, but the transverse plane shows the anterior-to-posterior movement of the axis that is not visible in the frontal plane. In the adult, the transitional lead is usually V3 or V4, and the lead oriented perpendicular to this transitional lead would therefore be lead V6 or V1, respectively. Since the normal predominant direction of the QRS complex is positive in lead V6 and negative in lead V1, the axis of the QRS complex in the transverse plane in the adult is typically between −30 degrees and −60 degrees.

MORPHOLOGY OF THE ST SEGMENT

The ST segment represents the period during which the ventricular myocardium remains in an activated or depolarized state (Fig. 1.12). At its junction with the QRS complex (J point), the ST segment typically forms a nearly 90-degree angle with the up-slope of the S wave, and then proceeds nearly horizontally until it curves gently into the T wave. The length of the ST segment is influenced by factors that alter the duration of ventricular activation. Points along the ST segment are designated with reference to the number of milliseconds beyond the J point, such as "J + 20," "J + 40," and "J + 60."

The first section of the ST segment is normally located at the same horizontal level as the baseline formed by the PR segment discussed earlier and the TP segment that fills the space between electrical cardiac cycles (Fig. 3.10A). Slight upsloping, downsloping, or horizontal depression of the ST segment may occur as a normal variant (Fig. 3.10B). Another normal variant of the ST segment appears when there is early repolarization in epicardial areas within the ventricles.[8] This causes displacement of the ST segment by as much as 0.1 mV in the direction of the ensuing T wave (Fig. 3.10C).

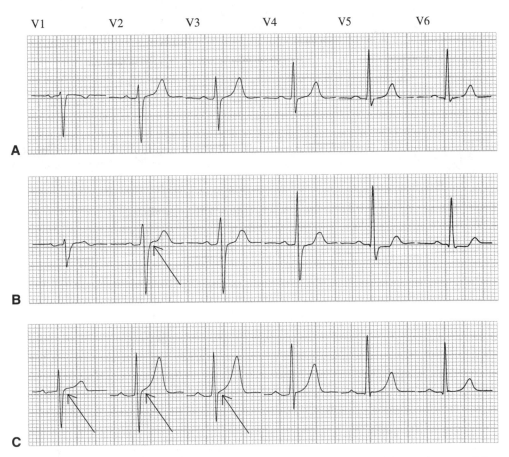

Figure 3.10. The six precordial leads are presented from a 25-year-old normal woman **(A)**, a 48-year-old man with acute chest pain of noncardiac origin **(B)**, a 54-year-old woman with acute chest pain of noncardiac origin **(C)**, a 20-year-old normal man **(D)**, and a 63-year-old man with aortic valve disease **(E)**. *Arrows* indicate the ST-segment deviations in **B** through **E**.

Occasionally, the ST segment in young males may show even greater elevation in leads V2 and V3 (Fig. 3.10D).[8] The appearance of the ST segment may also be altered when there is an abnormally prolonged QRS complex (Fig. 3.10E).

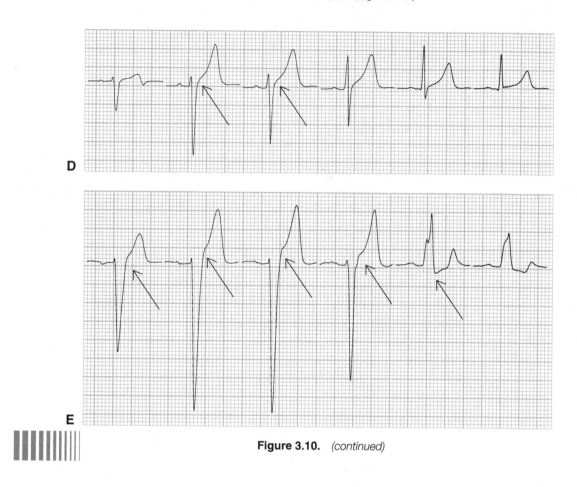

D

E

Figure 3.10. *(continued)*

T-WAVE MORPHOLOGY

The steps taken in examining the morphology of the T wave are to:

1. Examine the contour of the wave. Both the shape and axis of the normal T wave resemble those of the P wave (Figs. 1.9 and 1.14). The waveforms in both cases are smooth and rounded, and are positively directed in all leads except aVR, where they are negative, and V1, where they are biphasic (initially positive and terminally negative). Slight "peaking" of the T wave may occur as a normal variant, and "notching" of the T wave is common in children.

2. Measure the duration of the wave. The duration of the T wave itself is not usually measured, but is instead included in the QT interval discussed below.

3. Measure the maximal amplitude of the wave. The amplitude of the T wave, like that of the QRS complex, has wide normal limits. It tends to diminish with age and is larger in males than in females. T-wave amplitude tends to vary with QRS amplitude, and should always be greater than that of the U wave if the latter is present. T waves do not normally exceed 0.5 mV in any limb lead or 1.5 mV in any precordial lead. In females, the upper limits of T-wave amplitude are about two-thirds of these values. The T-wave amplitude tends to be lower at the extremes of the panoramic views (Fig. 2.11B) of both the frontal and transverse planes: the amplitude of the wave at these extremes does not normally exceed 0.3 mV in leads aVL and III or 0.5 mV in leads V1 and V6.[9]

4. Estimate the axis of the wave in each of the two ECG planes. The axis of the T wave should be evaluated in relation to that of the QRS complex. The rationale for the similar directions of the waveforms of these two ECG features, despite their representing the opposite myocardial electrical events of activation and recovery, has been presented in Chapter 1 ("Cardiac Electrical Activity"). The methods presented earlier for determining the axis of the QRS complex in the two ECG planes should be applied for determining the axis of the T wave. The term *QRS–T angle* is used to indicate the number of degrees between the axes of the QRS complex and the T wave in the frontal and transverse planes.[10]

The axis of the T wave in the frontal plane tends to remain constant throughout life, while the axis of the QRS complex moves from a vertical toward a horizontal position, as shown in the top of Figure 3.11.[7] Therefore, during childhood, the T-wave axis is more horizontal than that of the QRS complex, but during adulthood the T-wave axis becomes more vertical than that of the QRS complex. Despite these changes, the QRS-T angle in the frontal plane does not normally exceed 45 degrees.[10]

In the normal young child, the T-wave axis in the transverse plane may be so posterior that the T waves may be negative in even the most leftward precordial leads V5 and V6 (Fig 3.11, bottom). During childhood, the T-wave axis moves anteriorly, toward the positive pole of lead V5, and the QRS axis moves posteriorly, toward the negative pole of lead V1, where these two axes typically remain throughout life. The QRS-T angle in the transverse plane normally does not exceed 60 degrees in the adult.[10]

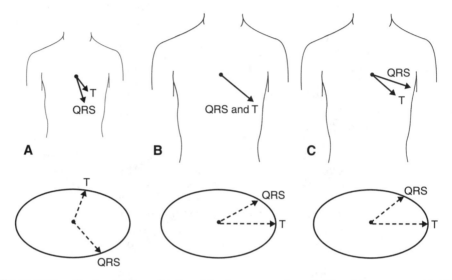

Figure 3.11. The frontal plane **(top)** and the transverse plane **(bottom)** for a young child **(A)**, a young adult **(B)**, and an elderly adult **(C)**. *Arrows* indicate directions of the QRS and T axes in *solid lines* in the frontal plane and *dashed lines* for the transverse plane at each age.

U-WAVE MORPHOLOGY

The U wave is normally either absent from the ECG or present as a small, rounded wave following the T wave (Figs. 1.9 and 1.12). It is normally oriented in the same direction as the T wave, has approximately 10% of the amplitude of the latter, and is usually most prominent in leads V2 or V3. The U wave is larger at slower heart rates, and both the U wave and the T wave diminish in size and merge with the following P wave at faster heart rates. The U wave is usually clearly separated from the T wave, with the *TU junction* occurring along the baseline of the ECG. However, there may be fusion of the T and U waves, making measurement of the QT interval more difficult. The source of the U wave is uncertain, but recent studies suggest that it is generated by "M cells" located in the midmyocardial regions of the left ventricle.[11,12]

QTc INTERVAL

The QT interval measures the duration of electrical activation and recovery of the ventricular myocardium, and varies inversely with the cardiac rate. To assure complete recovery from one cardiac cycle before the next cycle begins, the duration of recovery must decrease as the rate of activation increases. Therefore, the "normality" of the QT interval can be determined only by correcting for the cardiac rate. The corrected QT interval (*QTc interval*) rather than the measured QT interval is included in routine ECG analysis. Bazett developed the following formula for performing this correction[13]: QTc = QT/$\sqrt{\text{RR}}$ interval (in seconds).

The modification of Bazett's formula by Hodges and coworkers, as follows, corrects more completely for high and low heart rates: QTc = QT + 0.00175 (ventricular rate − 60).[14,15]

The upper limit of the duration of the QTc interval is approximately 0.46 s (460 ms). The QTc interval is slightly longer in females than in males, and increases slightly with age. Adjustment of the duration of electrical recovery to the rate of electrical activation does not occur immediately, but requires several cardiac cycles. Thus, an accurate measurement of the QTc interval can be made only after a series of regular, equal cardiac cycles.

The diagnostic value of the QTc interval is seriously limited by the difficulty of identifying the completion of ventricular recovery. The reasons for this difficulty are:

1. There is commonly a variation in the QT interval among the various leads. This "T-wave dispersion" occurs when the terminal portion of the T wave is isoelectric in some of the leads[16] (Fig. 3.12). The longest QT interval measured in multiple leads should therefore be considered the true QT interval.

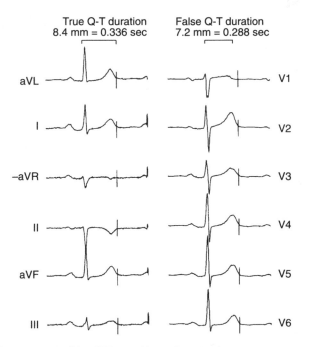

Figure 3.12. Measurement of the QT interval is confounded in lead V1 by the presence of a terminal isoelectric period of the T wave, suggesting an abnormally short QT interval. *Vertical lines* on the panoramically displayed limb and precordial leads indicate the true ending of the T wave. The longest interval should be considered the true QT interval.

2. The U wave may merge with the T wave, creating a TU junction that is not on the baseline of the ECG. In this instance, the onset of the U wave should be considered the approximate end of the QT interval.
3. At faster heart rates the P wave may merge with the T wave, creating a *TP junction*, which is not on the baseline. In this instance, the onset of the P wave should be considered the approximate end of the QT interval.

CARDIAC RHYTHM

Assessment of the final electrocardiographic feature named at the beginning of this chapter, the cardiac rhythm, requires consideration of all eight other electrocardiographic features. Certain irregularities of cardiac rate and regularity, P-wave morphology, and the PR interval may in themselves indicate abnormalities in cardiac rhythm, and certain irregularities of the remaining five electrocardiographic features may indicate the potential for development of abnormalities in cardiac rhythm.

Cardiac Rate and Regularity

The normal cardiac rhythm is called *sinus rhythm* because it is produced by electrical impulses formed within the SA node. The rate of sinus rhythm is normally between 60 and 100 beats/min during wakefulness and at rest. When it is below 60 beats/min, the rhythm is called *sinus bradycardia*, and when it is above 100 beats/min it is called *sinus tachycardia*. However, the designation of "normal" requires consideration of the level of activity of the individual: sinus bradycardia with a rate as low as 40 beats/min may be normal during sleep, and sinus tachycardia with a rate as rapid as 200 beats/min may be normal during exercise. Indeed, a rate of 90 beats/min would be "abnormal" during either sleep or vigorous exercise. Sinus rates in the bradycardic range may occur normally during wakefulness, especially in well-trained athletes whose heart rates may be in the range of 30 beats/min at rest, and which are often below 60 beats/min even with moderate exertion.

As indicated earlier, normal sinus rhythm is essentially but not absolutely regular because of continual variation of the balance between the sympathetic and parasympathetic divisions of the autonomic nervous system. Loss of this normal *heart-rate variability* may be associated with significant underlying autonomic or cardiac abnormalities.[17] The term *sinus arrhythmia* is used to indicate the normal variation in cardiac rate that cycles with the phases of respiration: the sinus rate accelerates with inspiration and slows with expiration (Fig. 3.13). Occasionally, sinus arrhythmia produces such marked irregularity that it can be confused with clinically important arrhythmias.

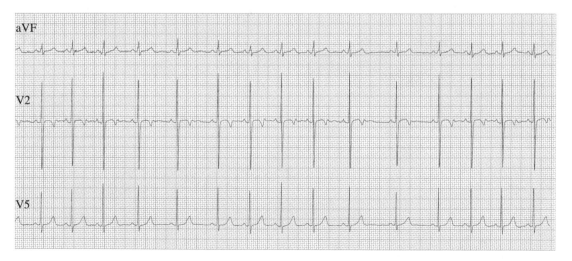

Figure 3.13. A 10-s rhythm recording made with three relatively orthogonal leads: superior–inferior (*aVF*), anterior–posterior (*V2*), and right–left (*V5*) from a healthy 15-year-old individual with symptoms of "palpitations."

P-Wave Morphology

The normal frontal-plane axis of the P wave was discussed earlier, in the section on P-wave morphology. Alteration of this axis to either less than +30 degrees or more than +75 degrees may indicate that the cardiac rhythm is being initiated from a site low in the right atrium, in the AV node, or in the left atrium.

PR Interval

The normal relationship between the P wave and QRS complex (termed the "PR interval") is presented schematically in Figure 3.14A, and various abnormal relationships between the P wave and QRS complex are illustrated in Figure 3.14B–F. An abnormal P-wave axis is often accompanied by an abnormally short PR interval, since the site of impulse formation has moved from the SA node to a position closer to the atrioventricular (AV) node (Fig. 3.14B). However, a short PR interval in the presence of a normal P-wave axis (Fig 3.14C) suggests either an abnormally rapid conduction pathway within the AV node or the presence of an abnormal bundle of cardiac muscle connecting the atria to the Bundle of His (an unusual source of *ventricular preexcitation* [discussed in Chapter 6: "Ventricular Preexcitation"]). This is not in itself an abnormality of the cardiac rhythm; however, the pathway either within or bypassing the AV node that is responsible for the preexcitation creates the potential for electrical *reactivation* or *reentry* into the atria, thereby producing a tachyarrhythmia.

An abnormally long PR interval in the presence of a normal P-wave axis indicates delay of impulse transmission at some point along the normal pathway between the atrial and ventricular myocardium (Fig. 3.14D). When a prolonged PR interval is accompanied by an abnormal P-wave contour, it should be considered that the P wave may actually be associated with the preceding rather than with the following QRS complex, owing to reverse activation from the ventricles to the atria (Fig. 3.14E). This would occur if the cardiac impulse originated from the ventricles rather than the atria. In this

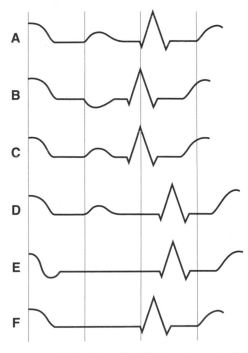

Figure 3.14. The normal P to QRS relationship **(A)** is contrasted with various abnormal relationships **(B–F)**. Each example begins with the completion of a T wave and ends with the initiation of the T wave of the following cardiac cycle. The vertical time lines are at 0.2-s intervals. The PR interval in **(A)** is therefore 0.2 s, which is near the upper limit of normal.

case, the P wave might only be identified as a distortion of the T wave. When the PR interval cannot be determined because of the absence of any visible P wave, there is obvious abnormality of the cardiac rhythm (Fig. 3.14*F*).

Morphology of the QRS Complex

Figure 3.14*A* is presented again as Fig. 3.15*A* for reference to a typical, normally appearing QRS complex with Q, R, and S waves present. Various causes of abnormal QRS-complex morphology are presented in Figure 3.15*B*, *C*, and *D*.

A normal P-wave axis with an abnormally short PR interval is accompanied by a normal morphology of the QRS complex when there is no AV-nodal bypass directly into the ventricular myocardium (Fig. 3.14*C*). When such a bypass directly enters the ventricular myocardium it creates abnormality in the morphology of the QRS complex (Fig. 3.15*B*). This ventricular "preexcitation" eliminates the isoelectric PR segment and creates a fusion between the P wave and the QRS complex. The initial Q or R wave begins slowly (in what is termed a "delta wave"), prolonging the duration of the QRS complex.

Abnormally slow impulse conduction within the normal intraventricular conduction pathways also produces abnormalities of QRS-complex morphology (Fig. 3.15*C*). The cardiac rhythm remains normal when the conduction abnormality is confined to either the right or left bundle branch. However, if the process responsible for the slow conduction spreads to the other bundle branch, the serious rhythm abnormality of partial or even total failure of AV conduction could suddenly occur.

An abnormally prolonged QRS duration in the absence of a preceding P wave suggests that the cardiac rhythm is originating from the ventricles rather than from the atria (Fig. 3.15*D*).

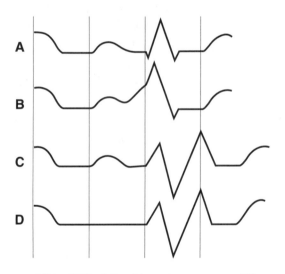

Figure 3.15. The normal P-to-QRS relationship and appearances **(A)** are contrasted with various conditions that produce obvious abnormalities **(B–D)**. The format is the same as in Figure 3.14. Each example begins and ends during a T wave.

ST Segment, T Wave, U Wave, and QTc Interval

Marked elevation of the ST segment (Fig. 3.16*B*), an increase or decrease in T-wave amplitude (Fig. 3.16*C* and *E*), prolongation of the QTc interval (Fig. 3.16*D*), or an increase in U-wave amplitude (Fig. 3.16*E*) may be indications of underlying cardiac conditions that may produce serious abnormalities of cardiac rhythm (Fig. 3.16). These are discussed in Chapters 9 (Fig. 3.16*B* and C), 11 (Fig. 3.16*C*, *D* and *E*), and 17 (Fig. 3.16*B* to *E*).

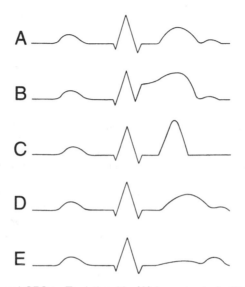

Figure 3.16. The normal QRS-to-T relationship **(A)** is contrasted with various abnormalities that may be associated with cardiac arrhythmias **(B–E)**. Each example begins with the completion of a TP segment and ends with the initiation of the following TP segment.

GLOSSARY

Autonomic nervous system: the nervous system that spontaneously controls involuntary bodily functions; it innervates glands, smooth-muscle tissue, blood vessels, and the heart.

Axis: direction of an ECG waveform in the frontal or horizontal plane, measured in degrees.

Bradycardia: a slow heart rate, of less than 60 beats/min.

Deflections: ECG waveforms moving either upward (positive deflection) or downward (negative deflection) with respect to the baseline.

Extreme axis deviation: deviation of the frontal-plane QRS axis from normal, with the axis located between −90 degrees and ±180 degrees.

Fusion: merging together of waveforms (i.e., P and T waves).

Intrinsicoid deflection: the time interval between the beginning of the QRS complex and the peak of the R wave; this represents the time required for the electrical impulse to travel from the endocardial to the epicardial surfaces of the ventricular myocardium.

Heart-rate variability: the normal range of variability of heart rates observed while an individual is in the resting state.

Left-axis deviation: deviation of the frontal-plane QRS axis from normal, with the axis located between −30 degrees and −90 degrees.

QRS–T angle: the number of degrees between the QRS complex and T-wave axes in the frontal and horizontal planes.

QTc interval: the corrected QT interval; it represents the duration of activation and recovery of the ventricular myocardium; the correction is applied by using a formula that takes into consideration the ventricular rate.

Rate: a measure of the frequency of occurrence of cardiac cycles; it is expressed in beats per minute.

Reentry or reactivation: passage of the cardiac electrical impulse for a second time or even greater number of times through a structure such as the AV node or the atrial or ventricular myocardium, as the result of a conduction abnormality in that area of the heart. Normally the cardiac electrical impulse, after its initiation in specialized pacemaking cells, spreads through each area of the heart only once.

Regularity: an expression for the consistency of the cardiac rate over a period of time.

Right-axis deviation: deviation of the frontal plane QRS axis from normal, with the axis located between +90 degrees and ±180 degrees.

Sinus arrhythmia: the normal variation in sinus rhythm that occurs during the inspiratory and expiratory phases of respiration.

Sinus rhythm: the normal cardiac rhythm originating via impulse formation in the sinoatrial or sinus node.

Tachycardia: a rapid heart rate of more than 100 beats/min.

Transitional lead: the lead in which the positive and negative components of an ECG waveform are of almost equal amplitude, indicating that that lead is perpendicular to the direction of the waveform.

TP junction: the merging point of the T and P waves that occurs at faster heart rates.

TU junction: the point of merging of the T and U waves; it is sometimes on and sometimes off of the isoelectric line.

Ventricular preexcitation: an event that occurs when a cardiac activating impulse bypasses the AV node and Purkinje system due to an abnormal bundle of muscle fibers connecting the atria and ventricles. Normally the electrical impulse must spread through the slowly conducting AV node and rapidly conducting Purkinje system to travel from the atrial to the ventricular myocardium.

REFERENCES

1. Grant RP. Clinical electrocardiography: the spatial vector approach. New York: McGraw–Hill, 1957.
2. Beckwith JR. Grant's clinical electrocardiography. New York: McGraw–Hill, 1970:50.
3. Wagner GS, Freye CJ, Palmeri ST, et al. Evaluation of a QRS scoring system for estimating myocardial infarct size. I. Specificity and observer agreement. Circulation 1982;65:342–347.
4. Beckwith JR. Basic electrocardiography and vectorcardiography. New York: Raven Press, 1982:46.
5. Anderson ST, Pahlm O, Selvester RH, et al. A panoramic display of the orderly sequenced 12 lead electrocardiogram. J Electrocardiol 1994;27;347–352.
6. Macfarlane PW, Lawrie TDV, eds. Comprehensive electrocardiology. vol III. New York: Pergamon Press, 1989:1458.
7. Macfarlane PW, Lawrie TDV, eds. Comprehensive electrocardiology. vol III. New York: Pergamon Press, 1989:1459.
8. Surawicz B. STT abnormalities. In: Macfarlane PW, Lawrie TDV, eds. Comprehensive electrocardiology. vol I. New York: Pergamon Press, 1989:46–47.
9. Macfarlane PW, Lawrie TDV, eds. Comprehensive electrocardiology. vol III. New York: Pergamon Press, 1989:1446–1457.
10. Beckwith JR. Grant's clinical electrocardiography. New York: McGraw–Hill, 1970:59–63.
11. Lepeschkin E. The U wave of the electrocardiogram. AHA Modern Concepts of Cardiovascular Disease. 1969;38:39–45.
12. Hoffman BF, Cranefield PF. Electrophysiology of the heart. New York: McGraw–Hill, 1960:202.

13. Bazett HC. An analysis of the time relations of electrocardiograms. Heart 1920;7:353—370.
14. Hodges M, Salerno D, Erlien D. Bazett's QT correction reviewed. Evidence that a linear QT correction for heart is better. J Am Coll Cardiol 1983;1:69 (abst).
15. Macfarlane PW, Lawrie TDV. The normal electrocardiogram and vectorcardiogram. In: Macfarlane PW, Lawrie TDV, eds. Comprehensive electrocardiology. Vol. I. New York: Pergamon Press, 1989:451–452.
16. Day CP, McComb JM, Campbell RW. QT dispersion in sinus beats and ventricular extrasystoles in normal hearts. Br Heart J 1992;67:39–41.
17. Kleiger RE, Miller JP, Bigger JT, et al. The MultiCenter PostInfarction Research Group. Decreased heart rate variability and its association with increased mortality after acute myocardial infarction. Am J Cardiol 1987; 59:256–262.

II

ABNORMAL WAVE MORPHOLOGY

CHAPTER 4

Chamber Enlargement

ATRIAL ENLARGEMENT

Cardiac-chamber enlargement may occur because of either an increase in the volume of blood within the chamber or an increase in the resistance to blood flow out of it. The former condition is termed *volume overload* or *diastolic overload* and the latter condition is termed *pressure overload* or *systolic overload*.[1] The increase in blood volume causes *dilation* of the chamber, and the increase in resistance causes thickening of the myocardial wall of the chamber (*hypertrophy*). The thinner-walled atrial chambers generally respond to both of these overloads with characteristic changes in the electrocardiogram (ECG). The usual terms for enlargement of the atria are *right-atrial enlargement* (*RAE*) and *left-atrial enlargement* (*LAE*). Indeed, "overload" rather than "enlargement" might be a more accurate general term for the ECG changes seen with enlargement, because electrical effects may occur before measurable dilation or hypertrophy of the affected chamber (as can be seen by echocardiography).

The ECG evaluation of RAE and LAE is facilitated by the differing times of initiation of activation of the two atria and by the differing directions of the spread of activation in each. As indicated in Figure 2.5, the optimal lead for differentiating left versus right cardiac activity is V1, with its positive electrode in the fourth intercostal space at the right sternal border (Fig. 2.6). Right-atrial activation begins first. It proceeds from the sinoatrial (SA) node in an inferior and anterior direction, and produces the initial deflection of the P wave, which has a positive direction in all leads except aVR (Fig. 4.1*A*). Left-atrial activation begins later. It proceeds from high in the interatrial septum in a left, inferior, and posterior direction, and produces the final deflection of the P wave, which is positive in long-axis lead II but negative in short-axis lead V1. Therefore, RAE is char-

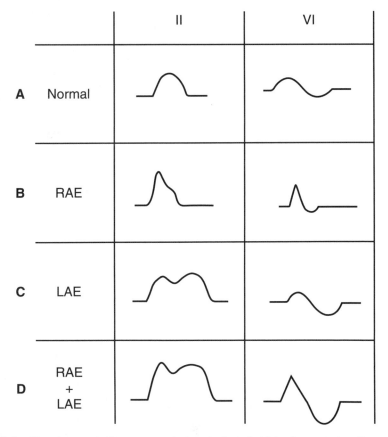

Figure 4.1. The changes in P-wave morphology typical of atrial enlargement as they appear in leads II and V1. **A.** Normal. **B.** Right-atrial enlargement (*RAE*). **C.** Left-atrial enlargement (*LAE*). **D.** Biatrial enlargement (*RAE + LAE*).

acterized by an increase in the initial deflection (Figs. 4.1*B* and 4.2*A*) and LAE by an increase in the final deflection of the P wave (Figs. 4.1*C* and 4.2*B*). In most of the other standard leads, both the right- and left-atrial components of the P wave appear as similarly directed deflections. An increase in both the initial and final aspects of the P wave suggests biatrial enlargement (Figs. 4.1*D* and 4.2*C*).

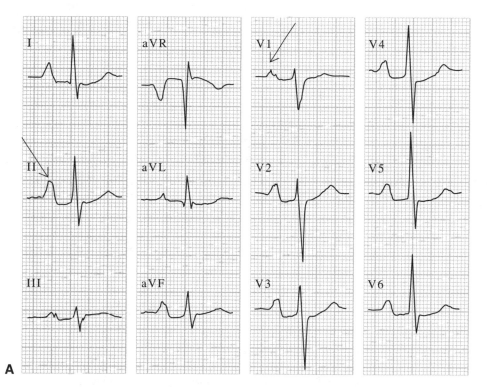

Figure 4.2.   Twelve-lead ECGs from a 23-year-old intravenous drug addict with tricuspid valve disease **(A)**, a 68-year-old man with aortic valve disease **(B)**, and a 42-year-old woman with combined mitral and aortic valve disease **(C)**. *Arrows* indicate the characteristic P-wave changes of atrial enlargement, and *asterisks* those of left-atrial enlargement. Note the prolonged PR interval (0.28 s) in **A**.

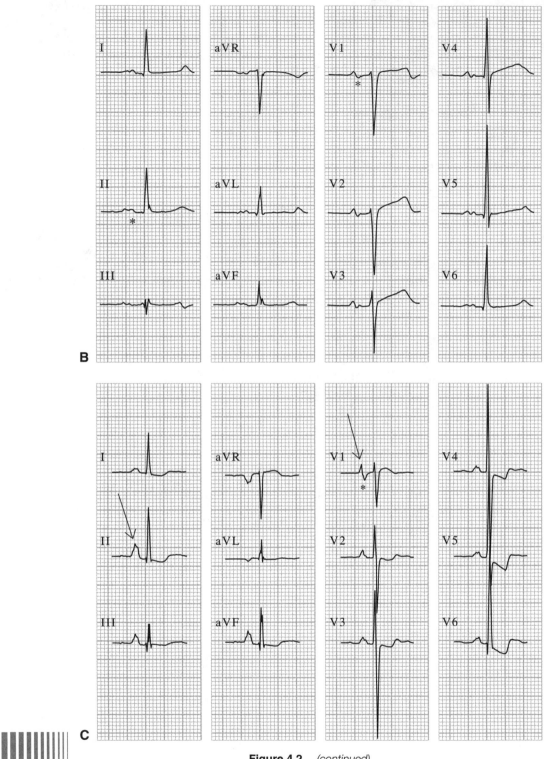

Figure 4.2. *(continued).*

SYSTEMATIC APPROACH TO THE EVALUATION OF ATRIAL ENLARGEMENT

The systematic approach to waveform analysis introduced in Chapter 3 ("Interpretation of the Normal Electrocardiogram") can be applied to the evaluation of atrial enlargement (Fig. 4.1):

1. Examine the Contour of the P Wave.

The smooth, rounded contour of the P wave is changed by RAE, which gives the wave a peaked appearance; and by LAE, which causes a notch in the middle of the wave, followed by a second "hump." In leads such as II, the P waves of RAE have an "A-like" appearance (termed *P pulmonale*), and the changes of LAE have an "M-like" appearance (termed *P mitrale*).

2. Measure the Duration of the P Wave.

RAE does not affect the duration of the P wave. LAE prolongs the total P-wave duration to >0.12 s. It also prolongs the duration of the terminal, negatively directed portion of the P wave in lead V1 to >0.04 s.

3. Measure the Maximal Amplitude of the P Wave.

RAE increases the maximal amplitude of the P wave to >0.20 mV in leads II and aVF, and to >0.10 mV in leads V1 and V2 . Usually, LAE does not increase the overall amplitude of the P wave, but increases only the amplitude of the terminal, negatively directed portion of the wave in lead V1 to >0.10 mV.

4. Estimate the Axes of the P Wave in the Two Electrocardiographic Planes.

RAE may cause a slight rightward shift and LAE may cause a slight leftward shift in the P-wave axis in the frontal plane. However, the axis usually remains within the normal limits of 0 degrees to +75 degrees.

With extreme RAE, the P wave may be inverted in lead V1, creating the illusion of LAE. With extreme LAE, the P-wave amplitude may increase and the terminal portion of the wave may become negative in leads II, III, and aVF. Biatrial enlargement produces characteristics of RAE and LAE, as illustrated in Figures 4.1*D* and 4.2*C*.

Munuswamy and colleagues,[2] using echocardiography as the standard for determining LAE, have evaluated the percentage of patients with truly positive and truly negative ECG criteria for LAE (Table 4.1). They found that the most *sensitive* criterion for LAE is an increased duration (>0.04 s) of the terminal, negative portion of the P wave in lead V1, whereas the most *specific* criterion for LAE is a wide, notched P wave that resembles the P wave seen in the case of an intraatrial block.

Table 4.1. Echocardiographic Evaluation of ECG Criteria for LAE[a]

ECG Criteria	% True Positive[b]	% True Negative[c]
Duration of terminal negative P wave deflection in lead V1 > 0.04 sec	83	80
Amplitude of terminal negative P wave deflection in lead V1 > 0.10 mV	60	93
Duration between peaks of P wave notches > 0.04 sec	15	100
Maximal P wave duration > 0.11 sec	33	88
Ratio of P wave duration to PR segment duration > 1:1.6	31	64

[a] Modified from Alpert MA, Martin RH. Munuswamy K, et al., Sensitivity and specificity of commonly used electrocardiographic criteria for left atrial enlargement determined by M-mode echocardiography. Am J Cardiol 1984;53:829.
[b] Percentage of patients with LAE by echocardiogram who meet the ECG criterion for LAE.
[c] Percentage of patients without LAE by echocardiogram who do not meet the ECG criterion for LAE.

VENTRICULAR ENLARGEMENT

 The thick-walled ventricles dilate in response to receiving excess volume of blood during diastole, and they become hypertrophied in response to exerting excess pressure in ejecting the blood during systole (Fig. 4.3). Enlargement of the right or left ventricle is commonly accompanied by enlargement of its corresponding atrium. Therefore, ECG findings that meet the criteria for atrial enlargement should be considered suggestive of ventricular enlargement.

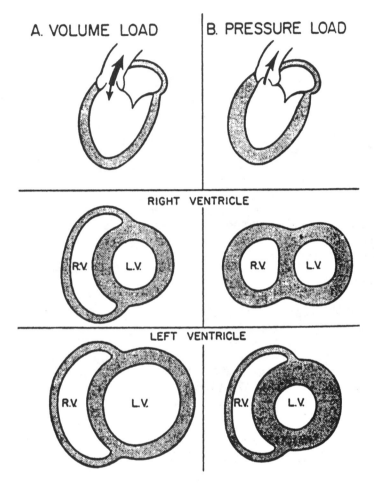

Figure 4.3. The changes in the sizes of the right-ventricular (*RV*) and left-ventricular (*LV*) myocardium produced by increases in volume overload caused by regurgitation of some of the already ejected blood (*thick upward arrow*) back through a leaking outflow valve (*thin downward arrow*) **(A)**; and pressure overload caused by obstruction to ejection (*thin upward arrow*) through a narrowed outflow valve **(B)**. (From Rushmer RF. Cardiac compensation, hypertrophy, myopathy and congestive heart failure. In: Rushmer RF, ed. Cardiovascular dynamics. 4th ed. Philadelphia: WB Saunders, 1976:538.)

Figure 4.4 illustrates the typical changes in the QRS waveforms that occur with enlargement of the right, left, and both ventricles. Lead I is selected instead of lead II for detecting these changes because predominance of its negative QRS waveforms indicates that the cardiac electrical axis is shifted to the right. In the absence of either right- or left-ventricular enlargement, a predominantly positive QRS complex appears in lead I and a predominantly negative QRS complex appears in lead V1 (Fig 4.4*A*). These QRS complexes increase in amplitude but do not change in direction with left-ventricular enlargement (Fig. 4.4*B*). With right-ventricular enlargement, however, the directions of the overall QRS waveform reverse; to predominantly negative in lead I and predominantly positive in lead V1 (Fig. 4.4C). With combined right- and left-ventricular enlargement, a hybrid of these waveform abnormalities results (Fig. 4.4D).

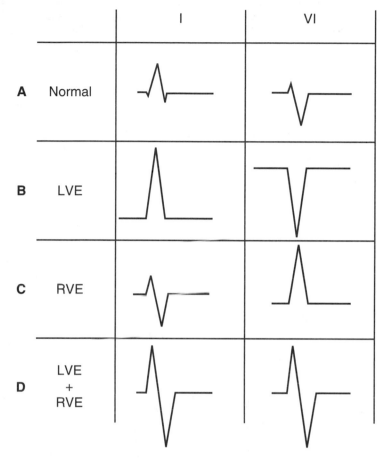

Figure 4.4. The changes in the QRS complex typical of ventricular enlargement as they appear in leads I and V1. **A.** Normal. **B.** Left-ventricular enlargement (*LVE*). **C.** Right-ventricular enlargement (*RVE*). **D.** Biventricular enlargement (*LVE + RVE*).

RIGHT-VENTRICULAR DILATION

The right ventricle dilates either during compensation for volume overload or after its hypertrophy eventually fails to compensate for pressure overload. Because of this dilation, the right ventricle takes longer to activate than is normally the case. Instead of completing its activation during the midportion of the QRS complex (Chapter 1: "Cardiac Electrical Activity"), the dilated right ventricle contributes anterior and rightward forces during the time of completion of left-ventricular activation. Thus, the frontal-plane QRS axis shifts rightward and an RSR′ pattern appears in leads V1 and V2, with an appearance similar to that in *incomplete right-bundle-branch block* (*RBBB*), which will be discussed in Chapter 5, "Intraventricular Conduction Abnormalities." The duration of the QRS complex may become so prolonged that the ECG changes occurring in right-ventricular dilation mimic those in *complete RBBB*. These ECG changes may appear during the early or compensatory phase of volume overload, or during the advanced or failing phase of pressure overload[3] (Fig. 5.4).

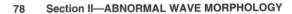

RIGHT-VENTRICULAR HYPERTROPHY

The right ventricle hypertrophies because of compensation for pressure overload. The final third of the QRS complex is normally produced solely by activation of the thicker-walled left ventricle and interventricular septum. As the right ventricle hypertrophies, it provides an increasing contribution to the early portion of the QRS complex, and also begins to contribute to the later portion of the complex.

Lead V1, with its left-right orientation, provides the optimal view of the competition between the two ventricles for electrical predominance. As shown in Figure 4.4A, the normal QRS complex in the adult is predominantly negative in lead V1, with a small R wave followed by a prominent S wave. When the right ventricle hypertrophies in response to pressure overload, this negative predominance may be lost, producing a prominent R wave and a small S wave (Fig. 4.4C). In mild right-ventricular hypertrophy (RVH) the left ventricle retains predominance, and there is either no ECG change or the QRS axis moves rightward (Fig. 4.5A). Note the S>R amplitude in lead I, indicating that the frontal-plane axis is slightly greater than +90 degrees, meeting the threshold presented in Chapter 3 for right-axis deviation (RAD). With moderate RVH, the initial QRS forces are predominately anterior (with an increased R wave in lead V1), and the terminal QRS forces may or may not be predominately rightward (Figure 4.5B). These changes could also be indicative of posterior myocardial infarction as presented in Chapter 10, "Myocardial Infarction." With severe right-ventricular hypertrophy the QRS complex typically becomes predominantly negative in lead I and positive in lead V1, and the delayed repolarization of the right-ventricular myocardium may produce negativity of the ST segment, and a T wave pattern indicative of so-called right ventricular *strain* in leads such as V1 to V3 (Fig. 4.5C).[4]

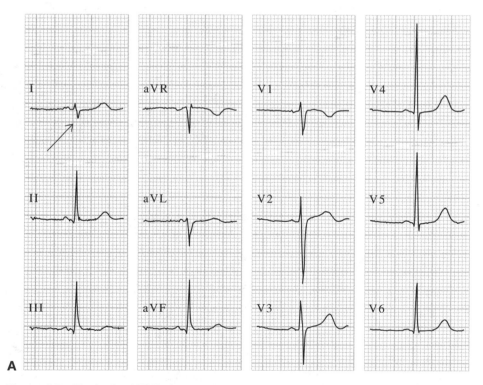

Figure 4.5. Twelve-lead ECGs from a 53-year-old woman with chronic obstructive lung disease **(A)**, a 59-year-old man with severe chronic obstructive lung disease **(B)**, and an 18-year-old man with congenital heart disease and pulmonary hypertension **(C)**. *Arrows* indicate the changes of RVH in the QRS waveforms, and an *asterisk* in **C** indicates the ST- and T-wave changes of RV strain.

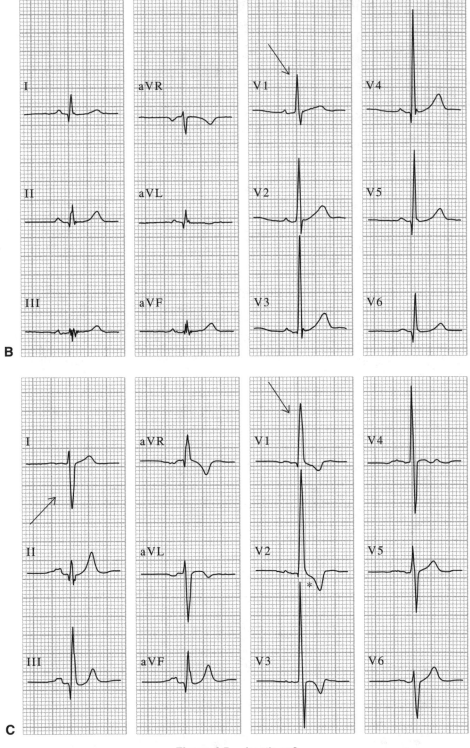

Figure 4.5. *(continued).*

In the neonate, the right ventricle is more hypertrophied than the left because there is greater resistance in the pulmonary circulation than in the systemic circulation during fetal development (Fig. 4.6). Right-sided resistance is greatly diminished when the lungs fill with air, and left-sided resistance is greatly increased when the placenta is removed.[5] From this time onward, the ECG evidence of right-ventricular predominance is gradually lost, as the left ventricle becomes hypertrophied in relation to the right. Therefore, hypertrophy, like dilation, may be a compensatory rather than a pathologic condition.[6] A pressure overload of the right ventricle may recur in later years because of increased resistance to blood flow through the pulmonary valve, the pulmonary circulation, or the left side of the heart.

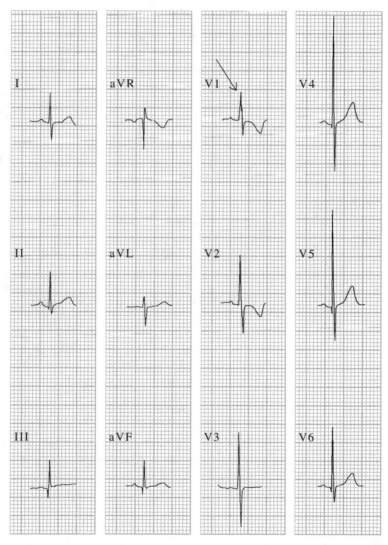

Figure 4.6.   Twelve-lead ECG from a 1-month-old healthy girl. An *arrow* shows the QRS waveforms in lead V1 that indicate the normal RV predominance at this early stage of development.

LEFT-VENTRICULAR DILATION

The left ventricle dilates for the same reasons indicated previously for the right ventricle. The longer time required for the spread of an electrical impulse across the dilated left ventricle may produce an ECG pattern similar to that of *incomplete left-bundle branch-block* (*LBBB*), which will be discussed in Chapter 5 "Intraventricular Conduction Abnormalities." The duration of the QRS complex may become so prolonged that the ECG changes in left-ventricular dilation mimic those in complete LBBB.

Dilation enlarges the surface area of the left ventricle and moves the myocardium closer to the precordial electrodes, which increases the amplitudes of leftward and posteriorly directed QRS waveforms[7] (Fig. 4.7). The S-wave amplitudes are increased in leads V2 and V3, and the R-wave amplitudes are increased in leads I, aVL, V5, and V6, as illustrated in Figure 4.4B. The T-wave amplitudes may also be increased in the same direction as the amplitudes of the QRS complex (Fig. 4.7A), or the T waves may be directed away from the QRS complex, indicating left-ventricular "strain" (Fig. 4.7B). Figure 4.7A illustrates ECG changes indicating mild to moderate left-ventricular dilation, while Figure 4.7B shows more severe changes, including abnormally prominent Q waves in many leads and left-ventricular strain.

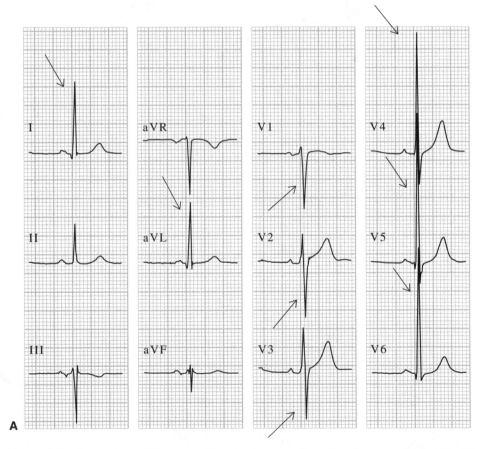

Figure 4.7. Twelve-lead ECGs from a 67-year-old man with aortic valve regurgitation **(A)** and a 74-year-old woman just prior to aortic valve replacement for severe regurgitation with congestive heart failure **(B)**. *Arrows* indicate the increased leftward and posterior QRS waveforms typical of left-ventricular hypertrophy. Note in **B** the additional ST-segment changes and T-wave changes of left-ventricular strain (*asterisks*).

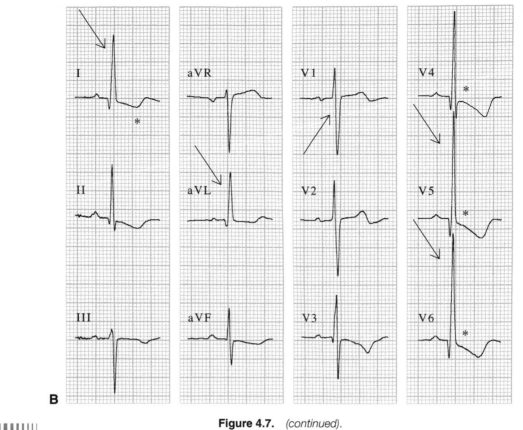

Figure 4.7. *(continued).*

LEFT-VENTRICULAR HYPERTROPHY

As discussed earlier, the left ventricle normally becomes hypertrophied relative to the right ventricle after the neonatal period. Abnormal hypertrophy, which occurs in response to a pressure overload, produces exaggeration of the normal ECG pattern of left-ventricular predominance. Like dilation, hypertrophy enlarges the surface area of the left ventricle, which increases the voltages of leftward and posteriorly directed QRS waveforms, thereby causing similar shifts in the frontal- and transverse-plane axes.

With left-ventricular hypertrophy (LVH), a longer period is required for spread of electrical activation from the endocardial to the epicardial surfaces of the hypertrophied myocardium, prolonging the intrinsicoid deflection (Fig. 3.7). Thus, a longer time is required for total left-ventricular activation. Since the left ventricle normally produces the final portion of the QRS complex, an interventricular conduction delay mimicking incomplete or even complete LBBB may occur with LVH as with left-ventricular dilation (Fig. 4.8A).

Pressure overload causes sustained delayed repolarization of the left ventricle, producing a negative ST segment and T wave in leads with leftward orientation (i.e., V5–V6); this condition is termed *left ventricular strain* (Fig. 4.8B).[8] The epicardial cells no longer repolarize early, reversing the spread of recovery so that it proceeds from endocardium to epicardium. The mechanism responsible for the strain is uncertain, but it is related to the increased pressure (overload) in the left-ventricular cavity. The development of strain has been shown to correlate with increasing left-ventricular mass as determined with echocardiography.[9]

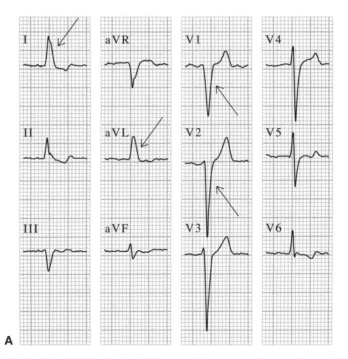

Figure 4.8. Twelve-lead ECGs from a 75-year-old woman with symptoms of heart failure caused by longstanding hypertension **(A)** and a 70-year-old man with severe aortic valve stenosis just prior to surgical replacement **(B)**. *Arrows* indicate the intraventricular conduction delay in **A** and the ST-segment depression and T-wave inversion in **B**.

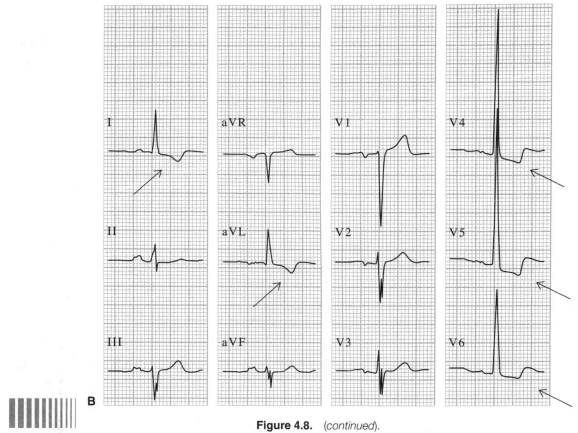

Figure 4.8. (*continued*).

COMBINED RIGHT- AND LEFT-VENTRICULAR HYPERTROPHY

 Enlargement of both ventricles is suggested if any of the following combinations of ECG changes are present:

1. High-voltage, biphasic RS complexes in the midprecordial leads, which is seen in many congenital lesions and is perhaps most common in ventricular septal defect (Fig. 4.9A).

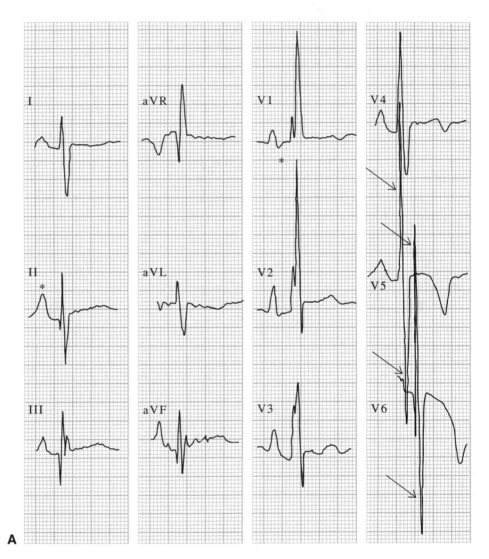

A

Figure 4.9. Twelve-lead ECGs from a 60-year-old woman with aortic insufficiency and left-ventricular failure **(A)**, a 23-year-old man with mitral stenosis and insufficiency **(B)**, a 40-year-old man with both systemic and pulmonary hypertension **(C)**, and a 22-year-old man with a ventricular septal defect **(D)**. *Arrows* indicate the high-voltage biphasic RS complexes in **A**, S>R in lead I, prominent R in lead V1, and increased S in lead V3 in **B** and **C**, and prominent R in the precordial leads over both the right and left ventricles in **D**. *Asterisks* indicate the typical P-wave abnormalities of RAE in **A**, **B**, and **C** and left-atrial enlargement in **A** and **B**. Note that waveforms for lead V6, shown in **A**, are displaced rightward only for illustrative purposes.

2. Voltage criteria for LVH in the precordial leads combined with right-axis deviation in the limb leads (Fig. 4.9B).
3. A low-amplitude S wave in lead V1 combined with a very deep S wave in lead V2 (Fig. 4.9C).
4. Criteria for LVH in the left precordial leads combined with prominent R waves in the right precordial leads (Fig. 4.9D).
5. LAE as the sole criterion for LVH, combined with any criterion suggestive of RVH.

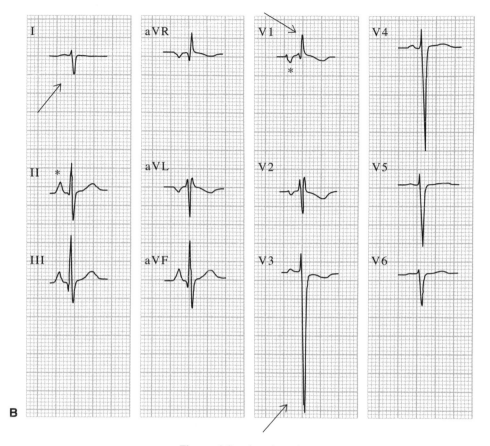

Figure 4.9. *(continued).*

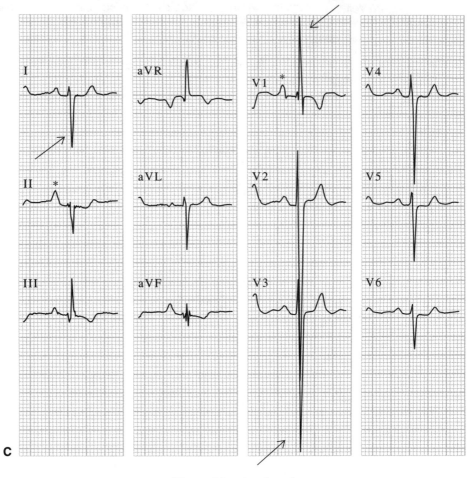

Figure 4.9. *(continued).*

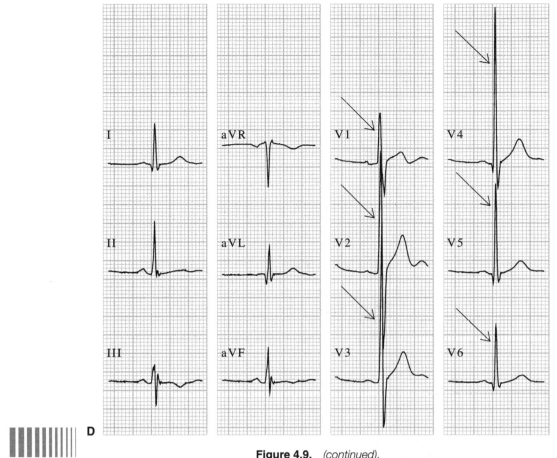

Figure 4.9. *(continued).*

SYSTEMATIC APPROACH TO THE EVALUATION OF VENTRICULAR ENLARGEMENT

Although the two varieties of right- and left-ventricular enlargement—dilation and hypertrophy—have somewhat different effects on ECG waveforms, as discussed earlier, no specific sets of criteria for dilation versus hypertrophy have been developed. The term "enlargement" has currently been accepted with regard to the atria, but the term "hypertrophy" is still used instead of "enlargement" with regard to the ventricles. Therefore, the systematic approach to waveform analysis introduced in Chapter 3 is here applied to "ventricular hypertrophy." Steps in this approach are to:

1. Examine the Contour of the QRS Complex.

Prolongation of the intrinsicoid deflection by the hypertrophied ventricular myocardium diminishes the slope of the initial waveforms of the QRS complex. As activation of the ventricular myocardium spreads, the smooth contour of the mid-QRS waveforms may be disrupted by indentations or notches (Fig. 4.9A). The terminal portions of the prolonged QRS complexes have low-frequency, smooth waveforms.

The contour of the ECG baseline may be altered. Ventricular hypertrophy shifts the J point off the horizontal baseline formed by the PR and TP segments, and causes the ST segment to slope in the direction of the T wave (Figs. 4.5C and 4.8B). When this occurs in the rightward precordial leads, it is referred to as right-ventricular strain, and in the left precordial leads it is referred to as left-ventricular strain.

2. Measure the Duration of the QRS Complex.

Hypertrophy of the left ventricle may cause prolongation of the QRS complex beyond its normal limit of 0.07 to 0.10 s, but hypertrophy of the right ventricle usually does not prolong the duration of the QRS complex. RVH can cause slight prolongation of the QRS complex when there is marked right-ventricular dilation. However, hypertrophy of the left ventricle, even without dilation, may prolong the duration of the QRS complex to 0.13 or 0.14 s. When complete LBBB is also present, the duration of the QRS complex may even extend to 0.20 s.

3. Measure the Maximal Amplitude of the QRS Complex.

The amplitude of the QRS complex is normally maximal in the left posterior direction. This is accentuated by LVH and opposed by RVH. All criteria for LVH contain thresholds for maximal left-posterior waveform amplitudes. The Cornell criteria[10] and the Romhilt–Estes criteria[11] consider both frontal- and transverse-plane leads, but the Sokolow–Lyon criteria[12] consider only transverse-plane leads.

The Sokolow–Lyon criteria for RVH contain thresholds for rightward and anterior amplitudes in the transverse-plane leads.[13] The Butler–Leggett[14] criteria require that the combination of maximal anterior and maximal rightward amplitudes exceeds the maximal leftward posterior amplitude by a threshold voltage difference.

4. Estimate the Axes of the QRS Complex in the Two Electrocardiographic Planes.

RVH shifts the frontal-plane QRS axis rightward, to a vertical or rightward position, and shifts the transverse-plane QRS axis anteriorly (Fig. 4.5C). LVH shifts the frontal-plane QRS axis only slightly leftward, but shifts the transverse-plane QRS axis markedly posteriorly (Fig. 4.2C).

RVH shifts the direction of both the ST segment and the T wave away from the right ventricle, opposite to the shift that such hypertrophy produces in the QRS complex. Typically, in rightward leads such as V1, the QRS complex would be abnormally positive, while the ST segment and T wave would be abnormally negative (Fig. 4.5C). LVH shifts the ST segment and T wave away from the left ventricle, in the direction opposite to the shift it produces in the QRS complex. Therefore, in leftward leads such as aVL and V5, the QRS complex would be abnormally positive, and the ST segment and T wave would be abnormally negative (Fig. 4.8B).

Three sets of criteria for LVH (Tables 4.2, 4.3 and 4.4) and two of criteria for RVH (Tables 4.5 and 4.6) are presented. As stated earlier, there is no distinction between dilation and hypertrophy.

Table 4.2. Romhilt–Estes Scoring System for LVH[a,b]

1. R or S in any limb lead ≥ 2.0 mV
   or S in lead V1 or V2
   or R in lead V5 or V6 ≥ 3.0 mV
	3 points

2. Left ventricular strain
   ST segment and T wave in opposite direction to QRS complex
   without digitalis
   with digitalis
	
	3 points
	1 point

3. Left atrial enlargement
   Terminal negativity of the P wave in lead V1 is ≥ 0.10 mV in depth and ≥ 0.04
   sec in duration
	
	3 points

4. Left axis deviation ≥ −30 degrees	2 points
5. QRS duration ≥ 0.09 s	1 point
6. Intrinsicoid detection in lead V5 or V6 ≥ 0.05 s	1 point
Total	13 points

[a] Modified from Romhilt DW, Bove KE, Norris RJ, et al. A critical appraisal of the electrocardiographic criteria for the diagnosis of left ventricular hypertrophy. Circulation 1969;40:185.
[b] LVH, 5 points; probable LVH, 4 points.

Table 4.3. Sokolow–Lyon Criteria for LVH[a]

S wave in lead V1 + R wave in lead V5 or V6 > 3.50 mV
or
R wave in lead V5 or V6 > 2.60 mV

[a] Modified from Sokolow M, Lyon TP. The ventricular complex in left ventricular hypertrophy as obtained by unipolar precordial and limb leads. Am Heart J 1949;37:161.

Table 4.4. Cornell Voltage Criteria for LVH[a]

Females	R wave in lead aVL + S wave in lead V3 > 2.00 mV
Males	R wave in lead aVL + S wave in lead V3 > 2.80 mV

[a] Modified from Casale PN, Devereux RB, Alonso DR, et al. Improved sex-specific criteria of left ventricular hypertrophy for clinical and computer interpretation of electrocardiograms: validation with autopsy findings. Circulation 1987;75:565.

Table 4.5. Butler–Leggett Formula for RVH[a]

Directions	Anterior	Rightward	Posterior–leftward
Amplitude	Tallest R or R' in lead V1 or V2	Deepest S in lead 1 or V6	S in lead V1
RVH formula	A + R − PL ≥ 0.70 mV		

[a] Modified from Butler PM, Leggett SI, Howe CM, et al. Identification of electrocardiographic criteria for diagnosis of right ventricular hypertrophy due to mitral stenosis. Am J Cardiol 1986;57:640.

Table 4.6. Sokolow–Lyon Criteria for RVH[a]

R wave in lead V1 + S wave in lead V5 or V6 ≥ 1.10 mV

[a] Modified from Sokolow M, Lyon TP. The ventricular complex in right ventricular hypertrophy as obtained by unipolar precordial and limb leads. Am Heart J 1949;38:273–294.

TYPICAL ELECTROCARDIOGRAPHIC CHANGES IN SELECTED CONGENITAL HEART DISEASES

Certain rare congenital heart diseases cause ventricular enlargement, and are associated with typical combinations of abnormalities on the ECG. These diseases and the resulting ECG abnormalities are as follows:

1. An anomalous left coronary artery originating from the pulmonary artery. This produces Q waves, elevation of the ST segment, and T-wave inversion in leads I, aVL, V4, V5, and V6.

2. Dextrocardia with situs inversus. This causes inversion of P waves, QRS complexes, and T waves in conventionally recorded lead 1. Mirror-image electrode positions should be used routinely in these individuals.

3. Ostium primum atrial septal defect (common AV canal). This causes marked left-axis deviation of the QRS complex in the frontal plane, with the typical appearance of left anterior fascicular block (Chapter 5: "Intraventricular Conduction Abnormalities"). The RBBB and other changes described above for right-ventricular dilation also occur with the ostium primum defect.

4. Ebstein's Anomaly.[15] This is reflected by the finding of extremely tall P waves indicative of RAE without evidence of right-ventricular involvement. There is also a slowed initial aspect of the QRS-complex of ventricular preexcitation (Chapter 6, "Ventricular Preexcitation"). The QRS complex is positive in lead V1, appearing as in the case of an atypical RBBB. There is also generally low QRS voltage.

5. Ventricular septal defect and patent ductus arteriosus. This produces combined RVH and LVH, and is characterized by high-voltage, biphasic QRS complexes in the midprecordial leads, as discussed earlier in the section on biventricular hypertrophy. Frequently, there are also prominent Q waves in the left precordial leads or in inferiorly oriented limb leads.

A more detailed discussion of the foregoing abnormalities has been published.[16]

GLOSSARY

Biatrial enlargement (BAE): enlargement of both the right and left atria.

Complete bundle-branch block: total failure of conduction in the right or left bundle branch; defined by a QRS duration >0.12 s with RBBB and >0.14 s with LBBB.

Dilation: stretching of the myocardium beyond its normal dimensions.

Enlargement: dilation or hypertrophy of a cardiac chamber.

Hypertrophy: (noun) An increase in bulk of a cardiac chamber, caused by the thickening of myocardial fibers. (verb) To increase in bulk.

Incomplete bundle-branch block: partial failure of conduction in the right or left bundle branch; defined by a QRS-complex duration of 0.10 to 0.11 s with RBBB and of 0.11 to 0.13 s with LBBB.

Intraatrial block: a conduction delay within the atria.

Left-atrial enlargement (LAE): dilation of the left atrium to accommodate an increase in blood volume or resistance to outflow.

Left bundle-branch block (LBBB): partial or complete failure of conduction in the left bundle branch of the ventricular Purkinje system.

Left ventricular strain: LVH accompanied by delayed repolarization, causing negativity of the ST segment and T wave.

P mitrale: appearance of the P wave in left atrial enlargement; named for its common occurrence in mitral valve disease.

P pulmonale: appearance of the P wave in RAE; named for its common occurrence in chronic pulmonary disease.

Pressure or systolic overload: a condition in which a ventricle is forced to pump against an increased resistance during systole.

Right-atrial enlargement (RAE): dilation of the right atrium to accommodate an increase in blood volume or resistance to outflow.

Right bundle-branch block (RBBB): partial or complete failure of conduction in the right branch of the ventricular Purkinje system.

Sensitive: a term referring to the ability (sensitivity) of a test to indicate the presence of a condition (i.e., if the test is positive in every subject with the condition, it attains 100% sensitivity).

Specific: a term referring to the ability (specificity) of a test to indicate the absence of a condition (i.e., if the test is negative in every control subject without the condition, it attains 100% specificity).

Strain: an ECG pattern characteristic of marked hypertrophy, and is reflected by ST-segment and T-wave changes in addition to changes in the QRS complex.

Volume or diastolic overload: a condition in which a ventricle becomes filled with an increased amount of blood during diastole.

REFERENCES

1. Rushmer RF, ed. Cardiac compensation, hypertrophy, myopathy and congestive heart failure. In: Cardiovascular dynamics. Philadelphia: WB Saunders, 1976; 532–565.
2. Munuswamy K, Alpert MA, Martin RH, et al. Sensitivity and specificity of commonly used electrocardiographic criteria for left atrial enlargement determined by M-mode echocardiography. Am J Cardiol 1984; 53:829.
3. Walker IC, Scott RC, Helm RA. Right ventricular hypertrophy; II. Correlation of electrocardiographic right ventricular hypertrophy with the anatomic findings. Circulation 1955;11:215.
4. Cabrera E, Monroy JR. Systolic and diastolic loading of the heart. II. Electrocardiographic data. Am Heart J 1952;43:669.
5. Rushmer RF, ed. Cardiovascular dynamics. Philadelphia: WB Saunders, 1991;452–456.
6. Rushmer RF, ed. Cardiac compensation, hypertrophy, myopathy and congestive heart failure. In: Cardiovascular dynamics. Philadelphia: WB Saunders, 1976; 532–565.
7. Cabrera E, Monroy JR. Systolic and diastolic loading of the heart. II. Electrocardiographic data. Am Heart J 1952;43:661.
8. Devereux RB, Reichek N. Repolarization abnormalities of left ventricular hypertrophy. J Electrocardiol 1982; 15:47.
9. Palmeiri V, Dahlof B, DeQuattro V, etc al. Reliability of echocardiographic assessment of left ventricular structure and function: the PRESERVE study. Prospective randomized study evaluating regression of ventricular hypertrophy. J Am Coll Cardiol 1999;34: 1625–1632.
10. Casale PN, Devereux RB, Alonso DR, et al. Improved sex-specific criteria of left ventricular hypertrophy for clinical and computer interpretation of electrocardiograms: validation with autopsy findings. Circulation 1987;75:565.
11. Romhilt DW, Bove KE, Norris RJ, Conyers E, Conradi S, Rowlands DT, Scott RC. A critical appraisal of the electrocardiographic criteria for the diagnosis of left ventricular hypertrophy. Circulation 1969;40:185.
12. Sokolow M, Lyon TP. The ventricular complex in left ventricular hypertrophy as obtained by unipolar precordial and limb leads. Am Heart J 1949;37:161.

13. Sokolow M, Lyon TP. The ventricular complex in right ventricular hypertrophy as obtained by unipolar precordial and limb leads. Am Heart J 1949;38:273–294.
14. Butler PM, Leggett SI, Howe CM, et al. Identification of electrocardiographic criteria for diagnosis of right ventricular hypertrophy due to mitral stenosis. Am J Cardiol 1986;57:639–643.
15. Schiebler GL, Adams P Jr, Anderson RC. The Wolff—Parkinson—White syndrome in infants and children. Pediatrics 1959;24:585.
16. Liebman J, Plonsey R, Rudy Y, eds. Pediatric and fundamental electrocardiography. Boston: Martinus Nijhoff, 1987.

CHAPTER 5

Intraventricular Conduction Abnormalities

NORMAL CONDUCTION

Many cardiac conditions cause electrical impulses to be conducted abnormally through the ventricular myocardium, producing changes in QRS complexes and T waves. Therefore, it is important to understand the conditions required to facilitate normal intraventricular impulse conduction. These are as follows

1. The left and right ventricles are not in an enlarged state that would prolong the time required for their activation and recovery (Chapter 4, "Chamber Enlargement").
2. Myocardial ischemia or infarction is not present or is of insufficient magnitude to disrupt the spread of the activation and recovery waves (Chapter 7, "Myocardial Ischemia and Infarction").
3. There is rapid impulse conduction through the right- and left-ventricular Purkinje networks so that the endocardial surfaces are activated almost simultaneously (as discussed later in this chapter).

4. There are no accessory pathways for conduction from the atria to the ventricles (Chapter 6, "Ventricular Preexcitation").

BUNDLE-BRANCH AND FASCICULAR BLOCK

 Since the activation of the ventricular Purkinje system is not represented on the surface electrocardiogram (ECG) (Fig. 1.9), abnormalities of its conduction must be detected indirectly by their effects on myocardial activation and recovery. The most specific changes indicative of such abnormalities occur within the QRS complex. A conduction disturbance within the right bundle branch (RBB), left bundle branch (LBB), left bundle *fascicles*, or between the Purkinje fibers and the adjacent myocardium may alter the QRS complex and T wave (Fig. 5.1). A conduction disturbance in the common bundle (Bundle of His) has similar effects on the entire distal Purkinje system, and therefore does not alter the appearance of the QRS complex or T wave.

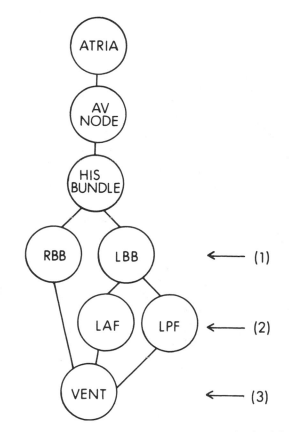

Figure 5.1. LAF and LPF indicate the left anterior and left posterior fascicles, respectively. (*1*), (*2*), and (*3*) indicate the locations at which intraventricular conduction abnormalities can produce alterations of the QRS complex and T wave. (Modified from Wagner GS, Waugh RA, Ramo BW. Cardiac arrhythmias. New York: Churchill Livingstone, 1983;18.)

Block of an entire bundle branch requires that its ventricle be activated by myocardial spread of electrical activity from the other ventricle, with prolongation of the overall QRS complex. Block of the entire RBB is termed complete right bundle-branch block (RBBB), while block of the entire LBB is termed complete left bundle-branch block (LBBB). In both of these conditions, the ventricles are activated successively instead of simultaneously. The other conditions in which the ventricles are activated successively occur when one ventricle is preexcited via an accessory atrioventricular (AV) pathway (Chapter 6, "Ventricular Preexcitation") and when there are independent ventricular rhythms (Chapters 13 and 17). Under these conditions, there is a fundamental similarity in the distortions of the ECG waveforms: the duration of the QRS complex is prolonged and the ST segment slopes into the T wave in the direction away from the ventricle in which the abnormality is located (Fig. 5.2).

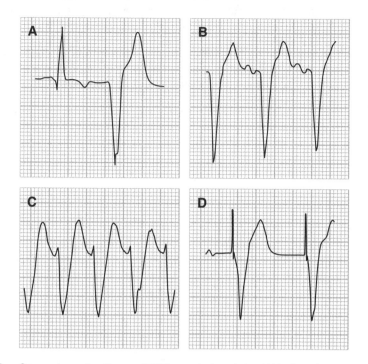

Figure 5.2. Comparison of patterns of QRS morphology in lead V1 when the two ventricles are activated successively rather than simultaneously: **A.** A ventricular beat. **B.** Bundle branch block. **C.** Ventricular tachycardia. **D.** Artificially paced ventricular rhythm.

A ventricular conduction delay with only slight prolongation of the QRS complex could be termed incomplete RBBB or incomplete LBBB. However, it is important to remember from Chapter 4 ("Chamber Enlargement") that enlargement of the right ventricle may produce a distortion of the QRS complex that mimics incomplete RBBB (Fig. 4.9B), whereas enlargement of the left ventricle may produce a prolongation of the QRS complex that mimics incomplete LBBB (Fig. 4.8A). Since the LBB has multiple fascicles, another form of incomplete LBBB could be produced by a disturbance in one of its major fascicles.

The ventricular Purkinje system is considered trifascicular. It consists of the RBB and the anterior and posterior portions of the LBB. The proximal RBB is small and compact, and may therefore be considered either a bundle branch or a fascicle. The proximal LBB is also compact, but is too large to be considered a fascicle. It remains compact for 1 to 2 cm and then fans into its two fascicles.[1] As Demoulin and Kulbertus have shown in humans,[2] there are multiple anatomic variations in these fascicles among individuals. Based on their anatomic locations, the two fascicles are termed the left-anterior fascicle (LAF) and left-posterior fascicle (LPF), as seen in Figure 5.3. The LAF of the LBB courses toward the anterior-superior papillary muscle, and the LPF of the LBB courses toward the posterior-inferior papillary muscle. There are also Purkinje fibers that emerge from the very proximal LBB that proceed along the surface of the interventricular septum and initiate left-to-right spread of activation through the interventricular septum.

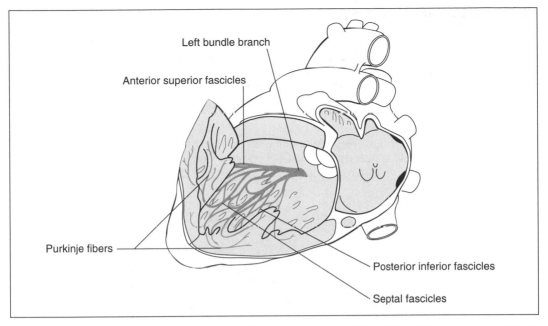

Left bundle branch

Anterior superior fascicles

Purkinje fibers

Posterior inferior fascicles

Septal fascicles

Figure 5.3. The left ventricle has been opened to reveal the LBB and its fascicles as originally presented in Figure 1.7C. Note that the anterior and posterior fascicles of the LBB are also designated superior and inferior, respectively, because these terms indicate their true anatomic positions. (From Netter FH. The Ciba collection of medical illustrations. vol 5. Heart. Summit, NJ: Ciba–Geigy, 1978:13.)

Rosenbaum and coworkers described the concept of blocks in the fascicles of the LBB, which they termed *left anterior and left posterior hemiblock*.[3] However, these two kinds of block are more appropriately termed left anterior fascicular block (LAFB) and left posterior fascicular block (LPFB). Isolated LAFB, LPFB, or RBBB is considered *unifascicular* block. Complete LBBB or combinations of RBBB with LAFB or with LPFB are *bifascicular blocks*, and the combination of RBBB with both LAFB and LPFB is considered *trifascicular block*.

UNIFASCICULAR BLOCKS

The term "unifascicular block" is used when there is ECG evidence of blockage of only the RBB, LAF, or LPF. Isolated RBBB or LAFB occur commonly, while isolated LPFB is rare. Rosenbaum and coworkers identified only 30 patients with LPFB, as compared with 900 patients with LAFB.[3]

Right Bundle-Branch Block

Since the right ventricle contributes minimally to the normal QRS complex, RBBB produces little distortion of the QRS complex during the time required for left-ventricular activation. Figure 5.4 illustrates the minimal distortion of the early portion and

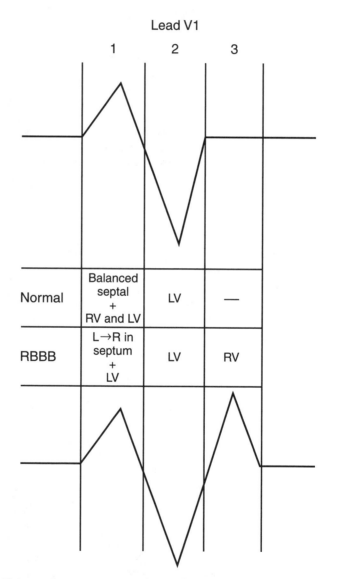

Figure 5.4. The contributions from activation of the interventricular septum and the right and left ventricular free walls to the appearance of the QRS complex in lead V1, with normal intraventricular conduction **(top)** and with RBBB **(bottom)**. The numbers refer to the first, second, and third sequential 0.04-s periods of time. Only two 0.04-s periods are required for normal conduction, but a third is required when RBBB is present.

marked distortion of the late portion of the QRS complex that typically occurs with RBBB. The minimal contribution of the normal right-ventricular myocardium is completely subtracted from the early portion of the QRS complex and then added later, when the right ventricle is activated via the spread of impulses from the left ventricle. This produces a late prominent positive wave in lead V1 termed R′, because it follows the earlier positive R wave produced by the normal left-to-right spread of activation through the interventricular septum (Fig. 5.4 and Table 5.1).

Table 5.1. Criteria for Right Bundle Branch Block

Lead V1	Late intrinsicoid, M-shaped QRS (RSR′); sometimes wide R or qR
Lead V6	Early intrinsicoid, wide S wave
Lead I	Wide S wave

RBBB has many variations in its ECG appearance, as illustrated by the examples in Figure 5.5A to C. In Figure 5.5A, the RBBB is considered "incomplete" because the duration of the QRS complex is only 0.10 s; but in Figure 5.5B and C, the RBBB is considered "complete" because the duration of the QRS complex is ≥ 0.12 s.

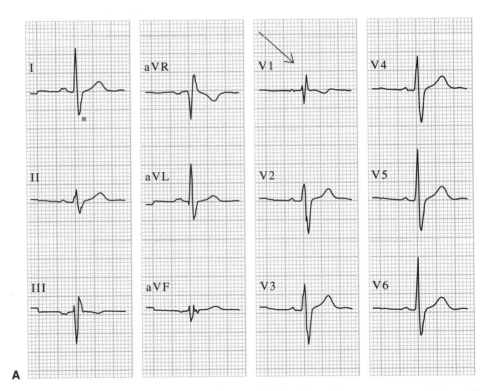

A

Figure 5.5. Twelve-lead ECGs from a 17-year-old girl with an ostium secundum atrial septal defect **(A)**, an 81-year-old woman with fibrosis of the RBB **(B)**, and an 82-year-old man with fibrosis of both the RBB and the anterior fascicle of the LBB **(C)**. *Arrows* in **A**, **B**, and **C** indicate the prominent terminal R′ wave in V1, and *asterisks* in **A** and **C** indicate the rightward and leftward axis shifts, respectively.

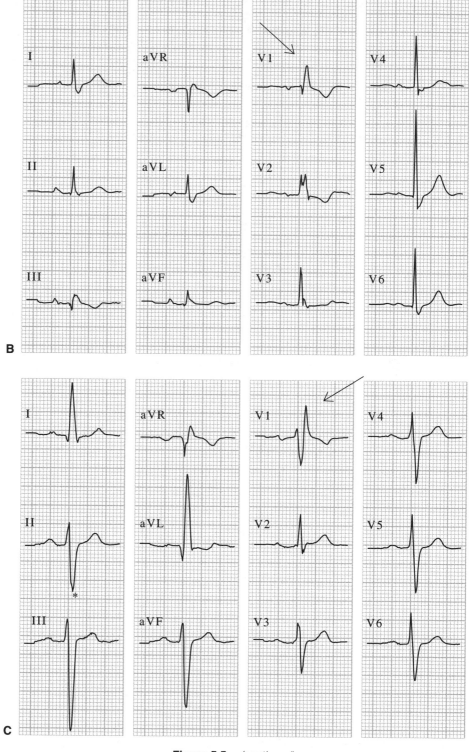

Figure 5.5. *(continued)*.

Left-Fascicular Blocks

Normal activation of the left-ventricular free wall spreads simultaneously from two sites (near the insertions of the papillary muscles of the mitral valve). Wavefronts of activation spread from these endocardial sites to the overlying epicardium. Since the wavefronts travel in opposite directions, they neutralize each other's influence on the ECG in a phenomenon called *cancellation*. When block in either the LAF or LPF is present, activation of the free wall proceeds from one site instead of two. Since the cancellation is removed, the waveforms of the QRS complex change, as described below (Fig. 5.6 and Tables 5.2 and 5.3).

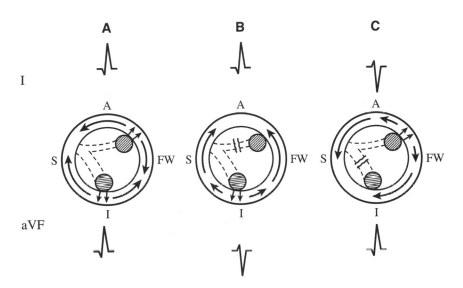

Figure 5.6. Schematic left ventricle viewed from its apex upward toward its base. The interventricular septum (*S*), left-ventricular free wall (*FW*), and anterior (*A*) and inferior (*I*) regions of the left ventricle are indicated. The typical appearances of the QRS complexes in leads I **(top)** and aVF **(bottom)** are presented for normal **(A)**, LAFB **(B)**, and LPFB left-ventricular activation **(C)**. *Dashed lines* within the inner circles represent the fascicles; the two *wavy lines* crossing a fascicle indicate the sites of block. *Small crosshatched circles* represent the papillary muscles; *outer rings* represent the endocardial and epicardial surface of the left ventricular myocardium. *Arrows* within the outer rings indicate the directions of the wavefronts of activation as they spread from the unblocked fascicles through the myocardium.

Table 5.2. Criteria for Left Anterior Fascicular Block

1. Left axis deviation (usually ≥ -60 degrees)
2. Small Q in leads I and aVL, small R in II, III and aVF
3. Usually normal QRS duration
4. Late intrinsicoid deflection in aVL (>0.045 s)
5. Increased QRS voltage in limb leads

Table 5.3. Criteria for Left Posterior Fascicular Block

1. Right axis deviation (usually $\geq +120$ degrees)
2. Small R in leads I and aVL, small Q in II, III and aVF
3. Usually normal QRS duration
4. Late intrinsicoid deflection in aVF (>0.045 s)
5. Increased QRS voltage in limb leads
6. No evidence for right ventricular hypertrophy

Left Anterior Fascicular Block. If the LAF of the LBB is blocked (Fig. 5.6B), the initial activation of the left-ventricular free wall occurs via the LPF. Activation spreading from endocardium to the epicardium in this region is directed inferiorly and rightward. Since the block in the LAF has removed the initial superior and leftward activation, a Q wave appears in leads that have their positive electrodes in a superior / leftward position (i.e., lead I) and an R wave appears in leads that have their positive electrodes in an inferior / rightward position (i.e., lead aVF). Following this initial period, the activation wave spreads over the remainder of the left-ventricular free wall in a superior / leftward direction, producing a prominent R wave in lead I and a prominent S wave in lead aVF. This change in the left-ventricular activation sequence produces a leftward shift of the axis of the QRS complex to at least −45 degrees. The overall duration of the QRS complex may be normal (Fig. 5.7A) or prolonged by 0.01 to 0.04 s (Fig. 5.7B).[4]

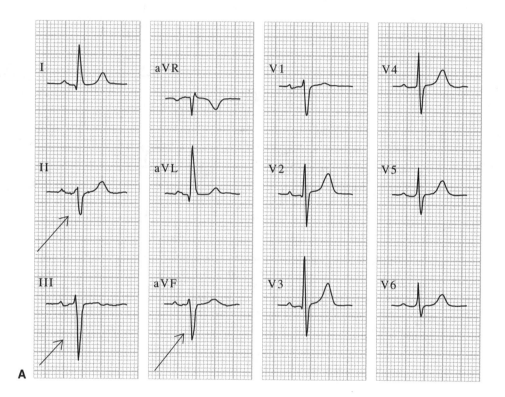

Figure 5.7. Twelve-lead ECGs from a 53-year-old woman with no medical problems **(A)** and a 75-year-old man with a long history of poorly treated hypertension **(B)**. *Arrows* indicate the deep S waves in leads II, III, and aVF that reflect extreme left axis deviation.

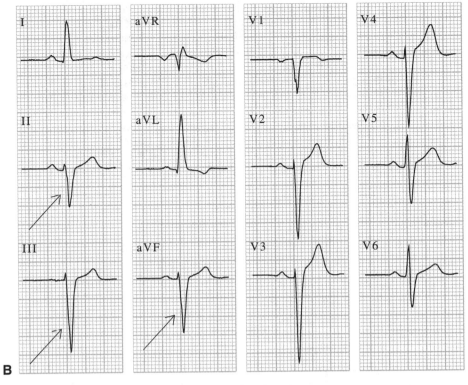

Figure 5.7. (*continued*).

Left Posterior Fascicular Block.   If the LPF of the LBB is blocked (Fig. 5.6*C*), the situation is reversed from that in LAF block, and the initial activation of the left-ventricular free wall occurs via the LAF. Activation spreading from the endocardium to the epicardium in this region is directed superiorly and leftward. Since the block in the LPF has removed the initial inferior and rightward activation, a Q wave appears in leads with their positive electrodes in an inferior/rightward position (i.e., lead aVF) and an R wave appears in leads with their positive electrodes in a superior/leftward direction (i.e., lead I). Following this initial period, the activation spreads over the remainder of the left-ventricular free wall in an inferior/rightward direction, producing a prominent R wave in lead aVF and a prominent S wave in lead I. This change in the left-ventricular activation sequence produces a rightward shift of the axis of the QRS complex to at least +90 degrees.[5] The duration of the QRS complex may be normal or slightly prolonged (Fig. 5.8).

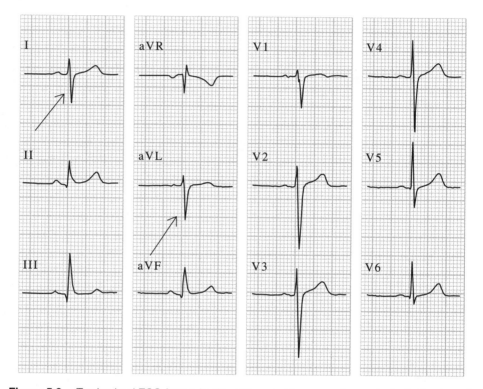

Figure 5.8.   Twelve-lead ECG from a healthy 77-year-old woman. *Arrows* indicate the deep S waves in leads I and aVL typical of both LPFB and RVH.

The consideration that LPFB may be present requires that there be no evidence of right-ventricular hypertrophy (RVH) from either the precordial leads (Fig. 5.8) or from other clinical data. However, even the absence of RVH does not allow diagnosis of LPFB, because RVH can produce the same pattern as LPFB in the limb leads, and RVH is much more common than is LPFB.

BIFASCICULAR BLOCKS

The term "bifascicular block" is used when there is ECG evidence of involvement of any two of the RBBB, LAF, or LPF. Such evidence may appear at different times or may coexist on the same ECG. Bifascicular block is sometimes applied to complete LBBB, and is commonly applied to the combination of RBBB with either LAFB or LPFB. The term "bilateral bundle-branch block" is also appropriate when RBBB and either LAFB or LPFB are present.[6] When there is bifascicular block, the duration of the QRS complex is prolonged to at least 0.12 s.

Left Bundle-Branch Block

Figure 5.9 illustrates the marked distortion of the entire QRS complex produced by LBBB. Complete LBBB may be caused by disease in either the main left bundle branch

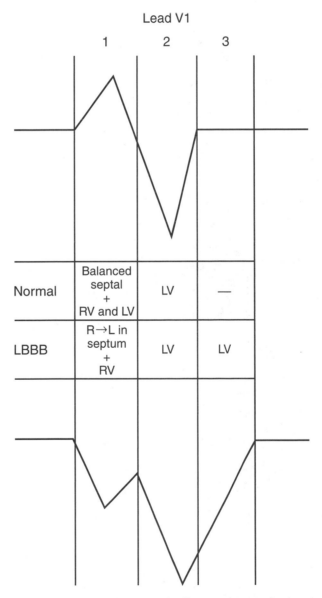

Figure 5.9. The format of Figure 5.4 is repeated to illustrate the contributions from activation of the various aspects of the ventricular myocardium to the appearances of the QRS complex in lead V1 with LBBB.

(LBB) (*predivisional*) or in both of its fascicles (*postdivisional*). When the impulse cannot progress along the LBB, electrical activation must first occur in the right ventricle and then travel through the interventricular septum to the left ventricle.

Normally, the interventricular septum is activated from left to right, producing an initial R wave in the right precordial leads and a Q wave in leads I, aVL, and the left precordial leads. When complete LBBB is present, however, the septum is activated from right to left. This produces Q waves in the right precordial leads and eliminates the normal Q waves in the leftward-oriented leads. The activation of the left ventricle then proceeds sequentially from the interventricular septum, to the adjacent anterior and inferior walls, and then to the posterior-lateral free wall. This sequence of ventricular activation in complete LBBB tends to produce monophasic QRS complexes, with QS complexes in lead V1 and R waves in leads I, aVL, and V6 (Table 5.4).

Table 5.4. Criteria for Left Bundle Branch Block

Lead V1	QS or rS
Lead V6	Late intrinsicoid, no Q waves, monophasic R
Lead I	Monophasic R wave, no Q

LBBB has many variations in its ECG appearance, as illustrated by the examples in Figure 5.10A to C. Figure 5.10A shows the typical appearance of complete LBBB. In Figure 5.10B the extreme LAD indicates that conduction is even slower in the LAF than in the LPF, and only minimal R waves are seen in leads V1 through V4. In Figure 5.10C the aberration of a markedly prolonged QRS complex is present, suggesting the coexistence of left-ventricular hypertrophy (LVH).

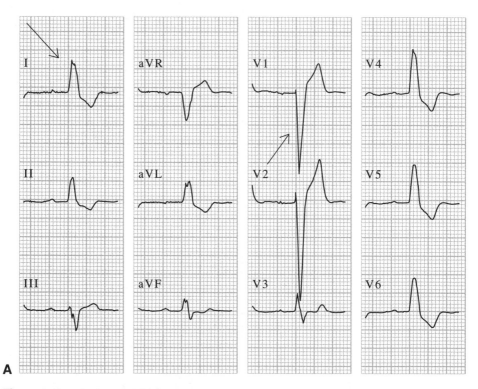

A

Figure 5.10. Twelve-lead ECGs from an 82-year-old woman with no medical problems **(A)**, a 71-year-old man with chronic heart failure **(B)**, and a 74-year-old man with a long history of hypertension **(C)**. *Arrows* in **A** and **C** indicate the typical characteristics of LBBB in leads I and V1, and *arrows* in **B** indicate the deep S waves in leads II, III, and aVF and decreased R waves in leads V2–V4.

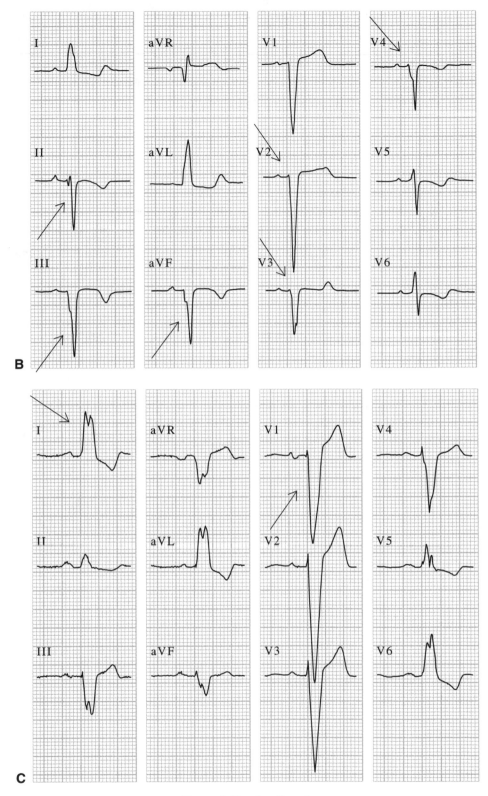

Figure 5.10. *(continued).*

Right Bundle-Branch Block with Left Anterior Fascicular Block

Just as LAFB appears as a unifascicular block much more commonly than does LPFB, it more commonly accompanies RBBB as a bifascicular block. The diagnosis of LAFB plus RBBB is made by observing the late prominent R or R′ wave in precordial lead V1 of RBBB, and the initial R waves and prominent S waves in limb leads II, III, and aVF of LAFB. The duration of the QRS complex should be at least 0.12 s and the frontal-plane axis of the complex should be between −45 degrees and −120 degrees (Fig. 5.11). In Figure 5.11*A* only LAFB is present, while in Figure 5.11*B* the presence of RBBB indicates that a second fascicle has been blocked.

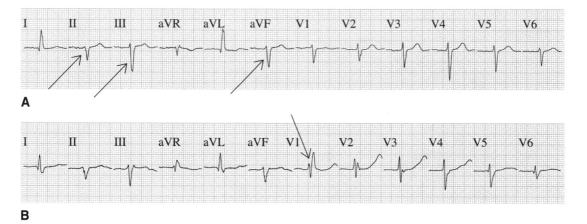

Figure 5.11. Twelve-lead ECGs from a 1-year previous **(A)** and a current **(B)** evaluation of a 73-year-old woman with no medical problems and no other evidence of heart disease. *Arrows* indicate the deep S waves in II, III, and aVF that are characteristic of LAFB in **A**, and a prominent R′ wave characteristic of RBBB in V1 in **B**.

Right Bundle-Branch Block with Left Posterior Fascicular Block

The example of bifascicular block consisting of RBBB with LPFB rarely occurs. Even when changes in the ECG are entirely typical of this combination, the diagnosis should be considered only if there is no clinical evidence of RVH. The diagnosis of RBBB with LPFB should be considered when precordial lead V1 shows changes typical of RBBB and limb leads I and aVL show the initial R waves and prominent S waves typical of LPFB. The duration of the QRS complex should be at least 0.12 s and the frontal-plane axis of the complex should be at least +90 degrees (Fig. 5.12).[7]

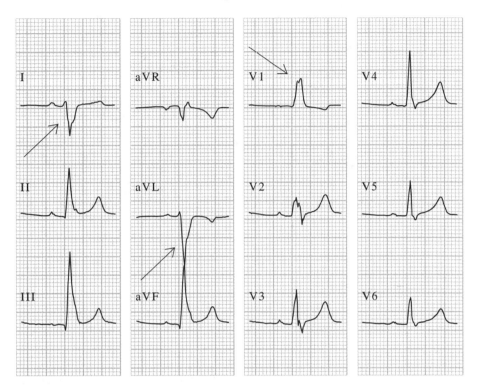

Figure 5.12. Twelve-lead ECG from an 82-year-old woman with no complaints and no other evidence of heart disease. *Arrows* indicate the prominant S waves in I and aVL and RR' complex in V1.

SYSTEMATIC APPROACH TO THE ANALYSIS OF BUNDLE-BRANCH AND FASCICULAR BLOCKS

The following steps should be taken in analyzing bundle-branch and fascicular blocks:

1. Examine the contour of the QRS complex.

RBBB and LBBB have opposite effects on the contour of the QRS complex. RBBB adds a new waveform directed toward the right ventricle following the completion of slightly altered waveforms directed toward the left ventricle (Fig. 5.4). Therefore, the QRS complex in RBBB tends to have a triphasic appearance. In lead V1, which is optimal for visualizing right- versus left-sided conduction delay, the QRS in RBBB has the appearance of "rabbit ears" (Figs. 5.5). Typically, the "first ear" (R wave) is shorter than the "second ear" (R′ wave). (Although the term "rabbit ears" in this context refers to a triphasic QRS, it can also refer to two peaks found in monophasic QRS complexes.) When RBBB is accompanied by block in one of the LBB fascicles, the positive deflection in lead V1 is often monophasic, as in Figure 5.12.

In LBBB, a sequential spread of activation through the interventricular septum and left-ventricular free wall replaces the normal, competing and simultaneous spread of activation through these areas. As a result, the QRS complex tends to have a monophasic appearance that is notched rather than smooth.

Although LBBB and LVH have many ECG similarities, they also show marked differences. Whereas the normal Q waves over the left ventricle may be present or even exaggerated in LVH, they are absent in LBBB. When the LBB is completely blocked, the septum is entirely activated from its right side. Figure 5.13 illustrates the appearance of incomplete (Fig 5.13*B*) and complete (Fig. 5.13*C*) LBBB in a patient with LVH (Fig. 5.13*A*).

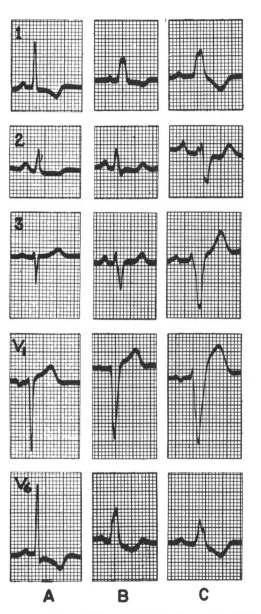

Figure 5.13. The five representative ECG leads illustrate the evolving ECG changes in a patient with severe hypertension as the LVH is complicated by LBBB. **A**. Age 60 years. **B**. Age 63 years. **C**. Age 67 years.

2. Measure the Duration of the QRS Complex.

Complete RBBB increases the duration of the QRS complex by 0.03 to 0.04 s, and complete LBBB increases the duration of the complex by 0.04 to 0.05 s. Block within the LAF or LPF of the LBB usually prolongs the duration of the QRS complex by only 0.01 to 0.02 s (Figs. 5.7B and 5.8).[4]

3. Measure the Maximal Amplitude of the QRS Complex.

Bundle-branch block (BBB) produces QRS waveforms with lower voltage and more definite notching than those that occur with ventricular hypertrophy. However, the amplitude of the QRS complex does increase in LBBB because of the relatively unopposed spread of activation over the left ventricle.

One general rule for differentiating between LBBB and LVH is that the greater the amplitude of the QRS complex, the more likely is LVH to be the cause of this. Similarly, the more prolonged is the duration of the QRS complex, the more likely is LBBB to be the cause of this effect. Klein and colleagues[8] have suggested that in the presence of LBBB, either of the following criteria are associated with LVH:

A. S wave in V2 + R wave in V6 > 45 mm.
B. Evidence of left-atrial enlargement with a QRS-complex duration > 0.16 s.

4. Estimate the Direction of the QRS Complex in the Two Planes of the ECG.

Since complete RBBB and complete LBBB alter conduction to entire ventricles, they might not be expected to produce much net alteration of the frontal-plane QRS axis. However, Rosenbaum studied patients with intermittent LBBB in which blocked and unblocked complexes could be examined side by side.[4] LBBB was often observed to produce a significant left-axis shift and sometimes even a right axis shift. The axis was unchanged in only a minority of patients.

However, block in either the LAF or LPF of the LBB alone produces marked axis deviation. The initial 0.20 s of the QRS complex is directed away from the blocked fascicles, and the middle and late portions are directed toward the blocked fascicles, causing the overall direction of the QRS complex to be shifted toward the site of the block (Figs. 5.7 and 5.8).[5] When block in either of these LBB fascicles is accompanied by RBBB, an even later waveform is added to the QRS complex, thereby further prolonging its duration. The direction of this final waveform in the frontal plane is in the vicinity of 180 degrees, as a result of the RBBB (Fig. 5.5C).[5]

In BBB, the T wave is usually directed opposite to the later portion of the QRS complex (e.g., in Figure 5.14A, the T wave in lead I is inverted and the later part of the QRS complex is upright; in Figure 5.14B the T wave is upright and the later part of the QRS complex is negative). This opposite polarity is the natural result of the depolarization–repolarization disturbance produced by the BBB, and is therefore termed *secondary*. Indeed, if the direction of the T wave is similar to that of the terminal part of the QRS complex (Fig. 5.14C), it should be considered abnormal. Such T-wave changes are primary and imply myocardial disease. The diagnosis of myocardial infarction in the presence of BBB is considered in Chapter 10 ("Myocardial Infarction").

One method of determining the clinical significance of T-wave changes in BBB is to measure the angle between the axis of the T wave and that of the terminal part of the QRS complex. Obviously, if the two are oppositely directed (as they are with secondary T-wave changes), the angle between them will be wide and may approach 180 degrees. It has been proposed that if this angle is less than 110 degrees, myocardial disease is present. In Figure 5.14B, the angle is about 150 degrees, whereas in Figure 5.14C it is only a few degrees.

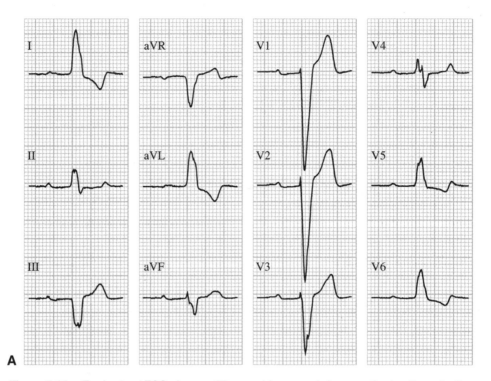

A

Figure 5.14. Twelve-lead ECGs from an 89-year-old woman during a routine health evaluation **(A)**, a 45-year-old pilot during an annual health evaluation **(B)**, and a 64-year-old woman on the first day after coronary bypass surgery **(C)**. *Arrows* indicate the concordant directions of the terminal QRS complex and of the T wave in leads V2–V4 in **C**.

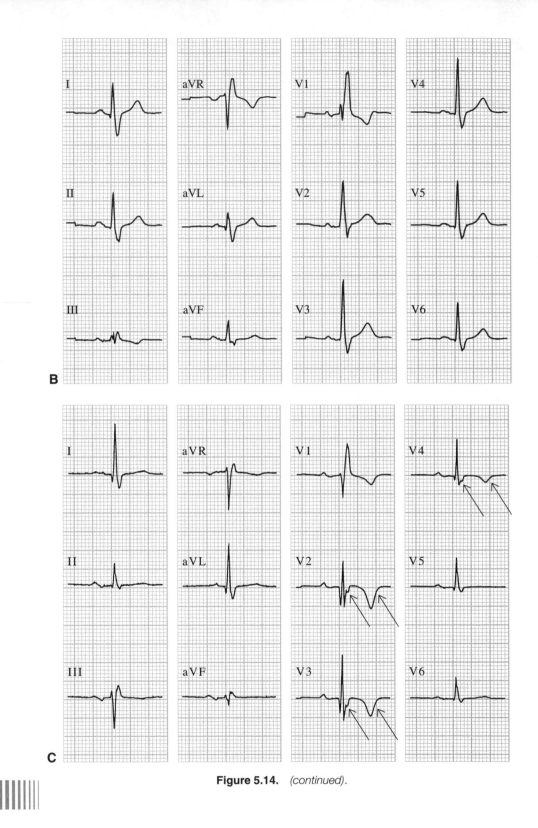

Figure 5.14. *(continued).*

CLINICAL PERSPECTIVE ON INTRAVENTRICULAR CONDUCTION DISTURBANCES

Both RBBB and LBBB are often seen in apparently normal individuals.[9] The cause of this is fibrosis of the Purkinje fibers, which has been described as Lenegre's disease[10] or Lev's disease.[11] The process of Purkinje fibrosis progresses slowly: a 10-year follow-up study of healthy aviators with BBB revealed no incidence of complete AV block, syncope, or sudden death.[12] The pathologic process may be accelerated by systemic hypertension: it preceded the appearance of BBB in 60% of the individuals in the Framingham study. The mean age of onset of the BBB was 61 years.[13]

Insight into the long-term prognosis for individuals with chronic BBB but no other evidence of cardiac disease comes from studies of the ECG changes preceding the development of transient or permanent complete AV block. Friedberg and associates have documented the common presence of some combination of bundle-branch or fascicular block immediately before onset of the AV block. The most common combination was RBBB with LAFB.[14]

The combined results of these studies suggest that Lenegre's or Lev's disease is a slowly developing process of fibrosis of the Purkinje fibers that has the ultimate potential of causing complete AV block because of bilateral bundle-branch involvement. Since the Purkinje cells lack the physiologic capacity of the AV-nodal cells to conduct at varying speeds, a sudden progression from no AV block to complete AV block may occur.[15] When this does occur, ventricular activation can result only from impulse formation within a Purkinje cell beyond the site of the block. Several clinical conditions may result, including syncope and sudden death.

Bundle-branch or fascicular block may also be the result of other serious cardiac diseases. In Central and South America, Chagas disease, produced by infection with *Trypanosoma cruzi*, is almost endemic and is a common cause of RBBB with LAFB.[16] As indicated in Chapter 4, RBBB is commonly produced by the distention of the right ventricle that occurs with volume overloading. Transient RBBB may be produced during right-heart catheterization, as illustrated in Figure 5.15.

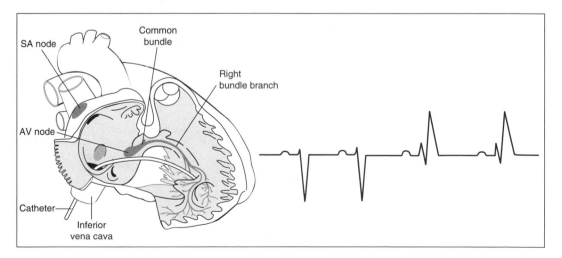

Figure 5.15. RBBB is induced by trauma to the RBB. A catheter has been advanced from the leg via the inferior vena cava, and its tip lies against the right ventricular endocardium in the vicinity of the RBB. The resultant RBBB is illustrated in the third and fourth beats of the schematic lead V1 ECG recording. (Modified from Netter FH. The CIBA collection of medical illustrations. vol 5. Heart. Summit, NJ: CIBA–Geigy, 1978:13.)

Any combination of the bundle branches or proximal fascicles may be blocked during an episode of myocardial cell death in a patient with coronary atherosclerosis. These structures receive their blood supply via the proximal septal perforating branch of the left anterior descending coronary artery (Fig. 5.16). Therefore, the bundle branches and their proximal fascicles become involved when there is an occlusion in either the left main coronary artery or the origin of its anterior descending branch. Individuals who survive to reach the hospital after occlusion of such a major coronary artery may have any combination of bundle-branch or fascicular blocks complicating extensive myocardial infarction. Since the acute and long-term mortality rates in these patients are very high, they do not represent a significant portion of the overall population of individuals with chronic bundle-branch and fascicular block.[17]

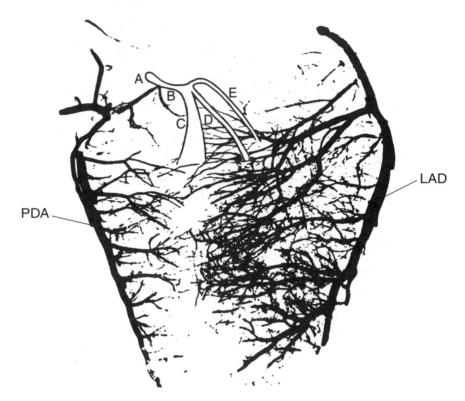

Figure 5.16. The proximal portion of specialized conduction system is shown in relation to its blood supply from a right anterior oblique view: *A*, AV node; *B*, Common bundle; *C*, LPF; *D*, LAF; *E*; RBB. Note the lengths of the septal perforating branches of the left anterior descending (*LAD*) coronary artery in contrast to those of the posterior descending artery (*PDA*). (From Rotman M, Wagner GS, Wallace AG. Bradyarrhythmias in acute myocardial infarction. Circulation 1972;45:703–722, with permission. Copyright 1972 American Heart Association.)

Intermittent BBB (prolonged QRS complexes present at some times but not at others) usually represents a transition stage before permanent block is established. Figure 5.17A and B show examples of the sudden onsets of LBBB and RBBB, respectively.

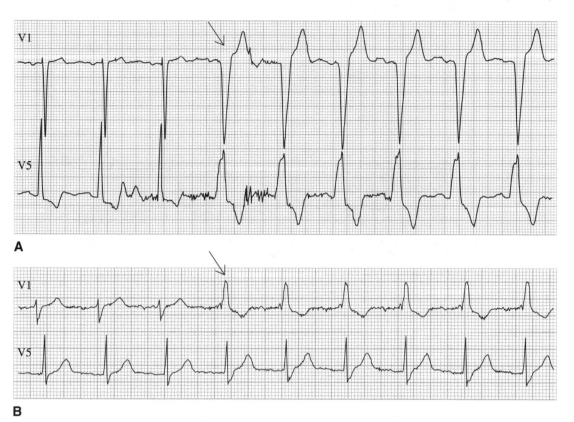

A

B

Figure 5.17. Precordial leads V1 and V5 are shown from a 62-year-old woman during routine ECG monitoring after uncomplicated abdominal surgery **(A)** and a 54-year-old man during 24-hour ECG monitoring for a complaint of dizziness **(B)**. *Arrows* indicate the onsets in the V1 leads of typically appearing LBBB in **A** and RBBB in **B**.

At times, intermittent BBB is determined by the heart rate. As the rate accelerates, the RR interval shortens and the descending impulse finds one of the bundle branches still in its refractory period (Fig. 5.18). With this *tachycardia-dependent BBB*, slowing of the heart rate allows descending impulses to arrive after the refractory period of the entire conduction system, and normal conduction is resumed.

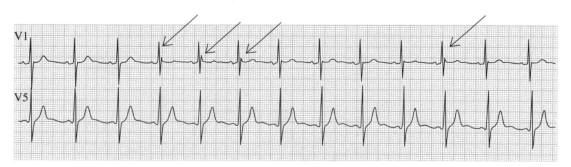

Figure 5.18. Precordial leads V1 and V5 during routine ECG monitoring of a 47-year-old woman after breast cancer surgery. *Arrows* indicate the appearance of incomplete RBBB following the shorter cycle intervals.

A rarer form of intermittent BBB, which develops only when the cardiac cycle length-ens rather than shortens (Fig. 5.19), is termed *bradycardia-dependent BBB*. Intermittent BBB is a form of intermittent aberrant conduction of electrical impulses through the ventricular myocardium.

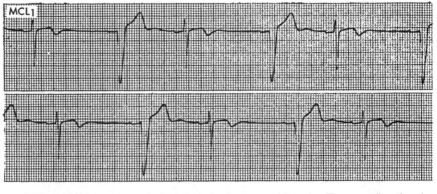

Figure 5.19.   All beats are conducted sinus beats grouped in pairs. Those ending the shorter cycles are conducted normally, while those ending the longer cycles are conducted with LBBB.

GLOSSARY

Atherosclerosis: a thickening of the inner arterial wall caused by the deposition of fatty substances.

AV block: a block in the cardiac conduction system that causes a disruption of atrial-to-ventricular electrical conduction.

Bifascicular block: an intraventricular conduction abnormality involving any two of: the RBB, the anterior division of the LBB, and the posterior division of the LBB.

Bilateral bundle-branch block: an intraventricular conduction abnormality involving both the right and left bundle branches, as indicated either by the presence of some conducted beats with RBBB and others with LBBB, or by AV block located distal to the common bundle.

Bradycardia-dependent BBB: RBBB or LBBB that is intermittent, appearing only with a slowing of the atrial rate.

Cancellation: Elimination of an abnormality produced by a particular cardiac problem by a similar abnormality in another part of the heart or by a different abnormality in the same part of the heart, since the ECG waveforms represent the summation of the wavefronts of activation and recovery within the heart.

Chagas disease: a tropical disease caused by the flagellate organism *Trypanosoma cruzi*, which is marked by prolonged high fever, edema, and enlargement of the spleen, liver, and lymph nodes, and is complicated by cardiac involvement.

Fascicle: a group of Purkinje fibers too small to be called a "branch."

Fibrosis: a condition in which Purkinje fibers are transformed into nonconducting interstitial fibrous tissue.

Left anterior fascicular block: a conduction abnormality in the anterior fascicle of the LBB.

Left posterior fascicular block: to a conduction abnormality in the posterior fascicle of the LBB.

Lenegre's (Lev's) disease: both Lenegre and Lev described variations of fibrosis of the intraventricular Purkinje fibers in the absence of other significant cardiac disease.

Predivisional and postdivisional: terms referring to block within the LBB either "pre-" or proximal to its division into fascicles, or "post-" and involving both the anterior and posterior fascicles.

Primary and secondary T-wave changes: in the presence of RBBB or LBBB, the term "primary T-wave changes" refers to abnormal T waves that are directed similarly to the latter portion of the QRS complex, and "secondary T-wave changes" refers to normal T waves that are directed opposite to the latter portion of the QRS complex.

Refractory period: the period following electrical activation during which a cardiac cell cannot be reactivated.

RR interval: the period between successive QRS complexes.

Septal Q wave: a normal, initially negative QRS waveform that appears in leftward-oriented ECG leads because of earliest activation of the interventricular septum via the septal fascicles of the LBB.

Syncope: a brief loss of consciousness associated with transient lack of cerebral blood flow.

Tachycardia-dependent BBB: RBBB or LBBB that is intermittent, appearing only with an acceleration of the atrial rate.

Trifascicular block: an intraventricular conduction abnormality involving the RBB and both the anterior and posterior fascicles of the LBB.

Unifascicular block: an intraventricular conduction abnormality involving only one of the three principal fascicles of the intraventricular Purkinje system.

REFERENCES

1. Wellens HJJ, Lie KI, Janse MJ, eds. The conduction system of the heart: structure, function and clinical implications. The Hague: Martinus Nijhoff, 1978:287–295.
2. Demoulin JC, Kulbertus HE. Histopathological examination of the concept of left hemiblock. Br Heart J 1972;34:807–814.
3. Rosenbaum MB, Elizari MV, Lazzari JO. The hemiblocks. Oldsmar, FL: Tampa Tracings, 1970.
4. Rosenbaum MB. Types of left bundle branch block and their clinical significance. J Electrocardiol 1969;2:197–206.
5. Eriksson P, Hansson PO, Eriksson H, Dellborg M. Bundle-branch block in a general male population: the study of men born in 1913. Circulation 1998;98:2494–2500.
6. Hindman MC, Wagner GS, JaRo M, et al. The clinical significance of bundle branch block complicating acute myocardial infarction. II. Indications for temporary and permanent pacemaker insertion. Circulation 1978;58:689–699.
7. Willems JL, Robles De Medina EO, Bernard R, et al. Criteria for intraventricular-conduction disturbances and preexcitation. J Am Coll Cardiol 1985;5:1261–1275.
8. Klein RC, Vera Z, DeMaria AN, et al. Electrocardiographic diagnosis of left ventricular hypertrophy in the presence of left bundle branch block. Am Heart J 1984;108:502–506.
9. Hiss RG, Lamb LE. Electrocardiographic findings in 122,043 individuals. Circulation 1962;25:947.

10. Lenegre J. Etiology and pathology of bilateral bundle branch block in relation to complete heart block. Progr Cardiovasc Dis 1964;6:409.
11. Lev M. Anatomic basis for atrioventricular block. Am J Med 1964;37:742.
12. Rotman M, Triebwasser JH. A clinical and follow-up study of right and left bundle branch block. Circulation 1975;51:477–484.
13. Schneider JF, Thomas HE, McNamara PM, et al. Clinical-electrocardiographic correlates of newly acquired left bundle branch block: the Framingham study. Am J Cardiol 1985;55:1332–1338.
14. Lasser RP, Haft JI, Friedberg CK. Relationship of right bundle-branch block and marked left axis deviation (with left parietal or peri-infarction block) to complete heart block and syncope. Circulation 1968; 47:429–437.
15. Pick A, Langendorf R. Interpretation of complex arrhythmias. Philadelphia: Lea & Febiger, 1979: 314–317.
16. Acquatella H, Catalioti F, Comez-Mancebo JR, et al. Long term control of Chagas disease in Venezuela: effects on serologic findings, electrocardiographic abnormalities and clinical outcome. Circulation 1987;76:556–562.
17. Hindman MC, Wagner GS, JaRo M, et al. The clinical significance of bundle branch block complicating acute myocardial infarction. I. Clinical characteristics, hospital mortality, and one-year follow-up. Circulation 1978;58: 679–688.

CHAPTER 6

Ventricular Preexcitation

HISTORICAL PERSPECTIVE

In the normal heart, there are no muscular connections between the atria and ventricles. In 1893, Kent described the rare occurrence of such connections, but wrongly assumed that they represented pathways of normal conduction.[1] Mines suggested in 1914 that this accessory atrioventricular (AV) connection (*Bundle of Kent*) might cause tachyarrhythmias. In 1930, Wolff and White in Boston and Parkinson in London reported their combined series of 11 patients with bizarre ventricular complexes and short PR intervals.[2] Then, in 1944, Segers introduced the triad of short PR interval, pre-excitation of the ventricles characterized by a prolonged upstroke of the QRS complex (*delta wave*), and tachyarrhythmia that characterize the *Wolff–Parkinson–White (WPW) syndrome*.

CLINICAL PERSPECTIVE

Ventricular preexcitation refers to a congenital cardiac abnormality in which a part of the ventricular myocardium receives electrical activation from the atria before the arrival of an impulse via the normal AV conduction system (Fig. 6.1). AV myocardial bundles commonly exist during fetal life, but then disappear by the time of birth.[3] When even a single myocardial connection persists, there is the potential for ventricular preexcitation. In some individuals, evidence of preexcitation may not appear until late in life, while in others with lifelong evidence of ventricular preexcitation on the electrocardiogram (ECG), the WPW syndrome may not occur until late in life. Conversely, infants with the WPW syndrome may outgrow any or all evidence of this abnormality within a few years.[4]

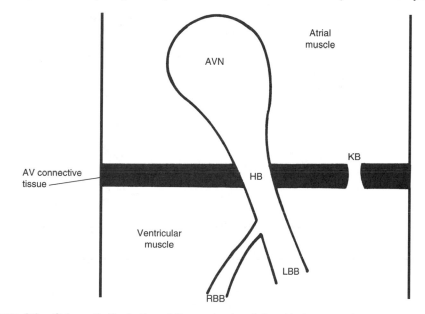

Figure 6.1. Schematic illustration of the anatomic relationship between the normal AV conduction system and the accessory AV conduction pathway provided by the Bundle of Kent. The *solid bar* represents the nonconducting structures (including the coronary arteries and veins, valves, and fibrous and fatty connective tissue) that prevent conduction of electrical impulses from the atrial myocardium to the ventricular myocardium. (*AVN*, AV node; *HB*, His bundle; *RBB*, right bundle branch; *KB*, Kent bundle; *LBB*, left bundle branch.)

Figure 6.2 illustrates the contrast between the alteration of the PR and QRS intervals that results from bundle-branch block (BBB) and from ventricular preexcitation. Right or left BBB (Fig. 6.2A) does not alter the PR interval, but prolongs the QRS complex by delaying activation of one of the ventricles. Ventricular preexcitation (Fig. 6.2B) shortens the PR interval and produces a "delta wave" in the initial part of the QRS complex. The total time from the beginning of the P wave to the end of the QRS complex

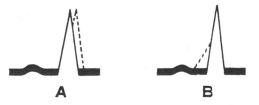

A   **B**

Figure 6.2. The two types of altered or "aberrant" conduction from the atria to the ventricles. The *dashed line* in **A** represents late activation of the ventricle served by the blocked bundle branch, and the *dashed line* in **B** represents the early activation of the ventricle connected with the atria via an accessory muscle bundle.

remains the same as in the normal condition because conduction via the abnormal pathway does not interfere with conduction via the normal AV conduction system. Therefore, before the entire ventricular myocardium can be activated by progression of the preexcitation wave front, electrical impulses from the normal conducting system arrive to activate the remainder of the ventricular myocardium.

Figure 6.3A illustrates the normal cardiac anatomy that permits AV conduction only via the AV node (the open channel at the crest of the interventricular septum). Thus, there is normally delay in the activation of the ventricular myorcardium (PR segment), as noted in the ECG recording shown in the figure. When the congenital abnormality responsible for the WPW syndrome is present (Fig. 6.3B) the ventricular myocardium is activated from two sources: (a) via the preexcitation pathway (the open channel between the right atrium and right ventricle); and (b) via the normal AV conduction pathway. The resultant abnormal QRS complex (termed a *fusion beat*) is composed of the abnormal preexcitation wave and normal mid- and terminal QRS waveforms.

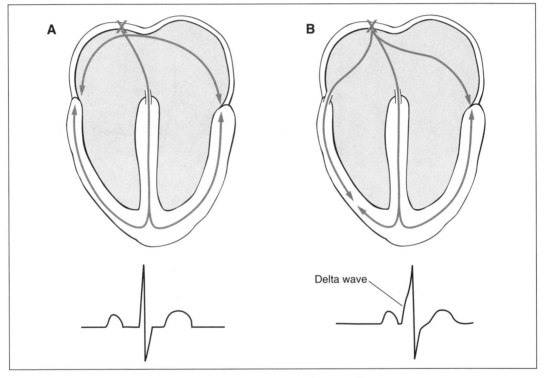

Figure 6.3. Relationship between an anatomic Bundle of Kent and physiologic preexcitation of the ventricular myocardium **(top)**, and the typical ECG changes of ventricular preexcitation **(bottom)**. Normal condition is presented **(A)** for contrast with the abnormal condition **(B)**. (Modified from Wagner GS, Waugh RA, Ramo BW. Cardiac arrhythmias. New York: Churchill Livingstone, 1983:13.)

The ECG of an individual with ventricular preexcitation is abnormal in several ways:

1. In the presence of a normal sinus rhythm, the PR interval is abnormally short and the duration of the QRS complex is abnormally prolonged. Ventricular preexcitation produces a prolonged upstroke of the QRS complex, which has been termed a delta wave (Fig. 6.4).

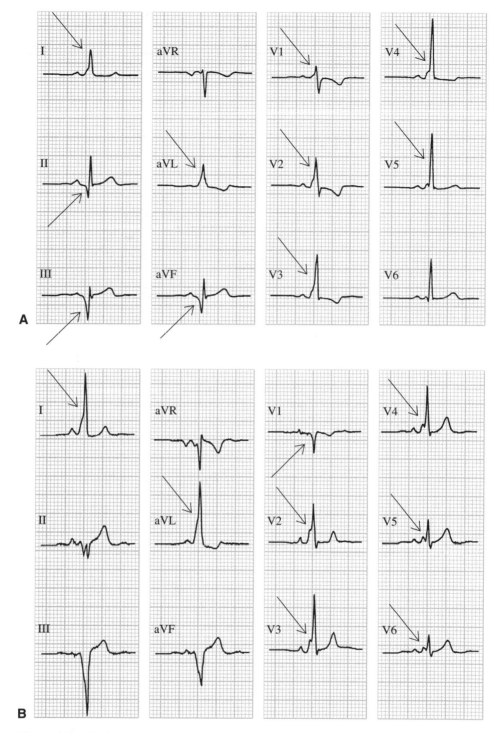

Figure 6.4. Twelve-lead ECG of an 18-year-old woman with a history of frequent episodes of "heart fluttering" **(A)** and a 34-year-old man without cardiac symptoms **(B)**. *Arrows* indicate the positive delta waves in many leads and the negative delta waves in leads II, III, and aVF in **A** and in lead V1 in **B**.

2. In the presence of an atrial tachyarrhythmia, such as atrial flutter/fibrillation (Chapter 15, "Reentrant Atrial Tachycardias—The Atrial Flutter/Fibrillation Spectrum"), the ventricular rate also becomes rapid. The ventricles are no longer "protected" by the slowly conducting AV node (Fig. 6.5).

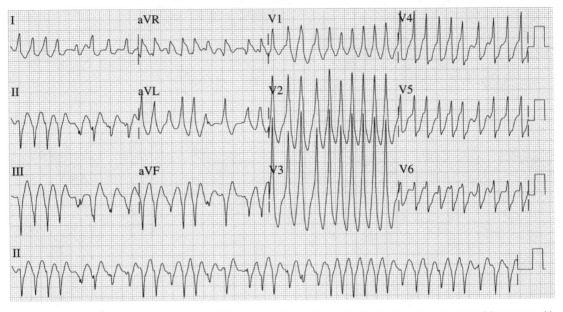

Figure 6.5. Twelve-lead ECG recording and lead II rhythm strip of a 24-year-old woman with ventricular preexcitation during atrial fibrillation. The irregularities of both the ventricular rate and QRS-complex morphology are apparent, especially on the 10-s lead II rhythm strip at the bottom.

3. The abnormal AV muscular connection completes a circuit by providing a pathway for electrical reactivation of the atria from the ventricles. This circuit provides a continuous loop for the electrical activating current, which may result in a single premature beat or a prolonged, regular, rapid atrial and ventricular rate called a *tachyarrhythmia* (Fig. 6.6). In Figure 6.6*B*, an atrial premature beat has occurred which sends a wave of depolarization through the atria and toward the Bundle of Kent. Because this beat originated in such close proximity to the Bundle of Kent, the bundle has not had sufficient time to repolarize. As a result, the premature wave of depolarization cannot continue through this accessory AV conduction pathway to preexcite the ventricles. However, the premature wave is able to progress to the ventricles via the normal AV conduction pathway in the AV node and interventricular septum. This depolarization wave then travels through the ventricles, and since it does not collide with an opposing wave (as occurs with ventricular preexcitation in Figure 6.6*A*), it reenters the atrium through the Bundle of Kent, creating a retrograde atrial excitation (Fig. 6*C*).

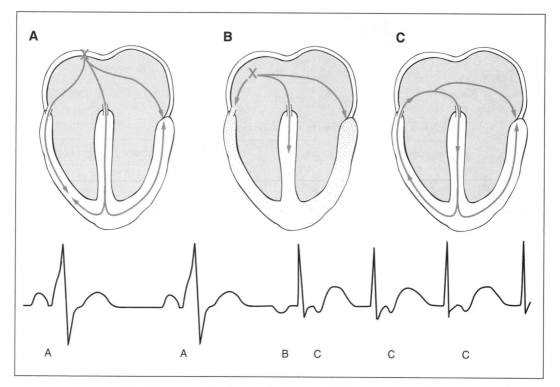

Figure 6.6. The schematic diagram from Figure 6.3 is reproduced with the normal example omitted. Typical ventricular preexcitation appears again in **A**. In **B**, the *x* indicates the site of origin of the atrial premature beat and the *stippling* in the ventricular myocardium indicates persistent refractoriness as a result of the previous excitation. In **C**, the *completed circle* includes the right atrium, AV node, His bundle, RBB, right ventricle, and Bundle of Kent. (Modified from Wagner GS, Waugh RA, Ramo BW. Cardiac arrhythmias. New York: Churchill Livingstone, 1983:13.)

The influence of ventricular preexcitation on the ventricular rate during atrial flutter/fibrillation and on tachyarrhythmias induced by an accessory pathway is discussed in Chapters 15 ("Reentrant Atrial Tachycardias—The Atrial Flutter/Fibrillation Spectrum") and 16 ("Reentrant Junctional Tachyarrhythmias"), respectively.

The combination of a PR interval of duration <0.12 s, a delta wave at the beginning of the QRS complex, and a rapid, regular tachyarrhythmia has been termed the Wolff–Parkinson–White (WPW) syndrome. The PR interval is short because the descending electrical impulse bypasses the normal AV-nodal conduction delay. The delta wave is produced by slow intramyocardial conduction that results when the descending impulse, instead of being delivered to the ventricular myocardium via the normal conduction system, is delivered directly into the ventricular myocardium via an abnormal or "anomalous" muscle bundle. The duration of the QRS complex is prolonged because it begins "too early," in contrast to the situations presented in Chapters 4 ("Chamber Enlargement") and 5 ("Intraventricular Conduction Abnormalities"), in which the duration of the QRS complex is prolonged because it ends too late. The ventricles are activated successively rather than simultaneously: the preexcited ventricle is activated via the Bundle of Kent, and the other ventricle is then activated via the normal AV node and His-Purkinje system (Fig. 6.3).

Various terms have been applied to the abnormal anatomic structure and resulting abnormal electrophysiologic function responsible for the WPW syndrome (Table 6.1).

Table 6.1. Structure and Function Terms

Anatomic Structure	Electrophysiologic Function
Myocardial bundle	Ventricular preexcitation
Bundle of Kent	Accessory AV conduction pathway
Bypass tract	AV nodal bypass pathway

ELECTROCARDIOGRAPHIC DIAGNOSIS OF VENTRICULAR PREEXCITATION

Typically, with ventricular preexcitation, the PR interval is less than 0.12 s in duration and the QRS complex is greater than 0.10 s. However, the PR interval is not always abnormally short (Fig. 6.7A) and the QRS complex is not always abnormally prolonged (Fig. 6.7B). Conduction through the Bundle of Kent may be relatively slow, or the Bundle of Kent may directly enter the His bundle. Among almost 600 patients with documented ventricular preexcitation, 25% had PR intervals of 0.12 s or longer and 25% had a QRS-complex duration of 0.10 s or shorter.[5]

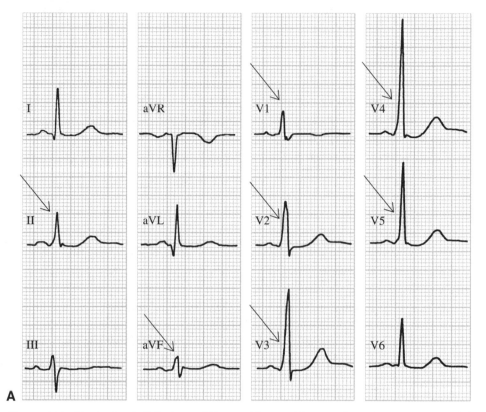

Figure 6.7. Twelve-lead ECGs from a 57-year-old man without cardiac-related symptoms **(A)** and a 41-year-old woman with recurrent episodes of weakness and who sensed a rapid heart rate **(B)**. *Arrows* in **A** indicate abnormally slow onset of the QRS complex following a normal PR interval (0.16 s) and *arrows* in **B** indicate an abnormally short PR interval preceding a QRS complex of normal duration (0.08 s).

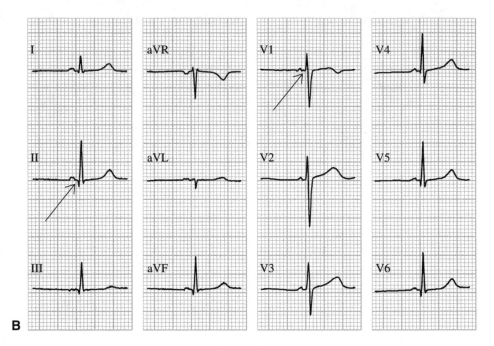

Figure 6.7. *(continued)*.

When ventricular preexcitation is suspected in a patient with tachyarrhythmias but no ECG evidence preexcitation, the following diagnostic procedures may be helpful:

1. Pace the atria electronically at increasingly rapid rates to induce conduction via any existing accessory pathway.
2. Produce vagal nerve stimulation to impair normal conduction through the AV node so as to induce conduction via any existing accessory pathway.
3. Infuse digoxin intravenously for the same purpose as in Procedure 2.

Ventricular preexcitation may mimic a number of other cardiac abnormalities. When there is a wide, positive QRS complex in leads V1 and V2, it may simulate right bundle-branch block (RBBB), right-ventricular hypertrophy (RVH), or a posterior myocardial infarction. When there is a wide, negative QRS complex in lead V1 or V2, preexcitation may be mistaken for left bundle-branch block (LBBB) (Fig. 6.8A) or left-ventricular hypertrophy (LVH). A negative delta wave, producing Q waves in the appropriate leads, may imitate anterior, lateral, or inferior infarction. As will be discussed in Chapter 10 ("Myocardial Infarction"), the prominent Q waves in leads aVF and V1 in Figure 6.8B could be mistaken for inferior or anterior infarction, respectively. Similarly, the deep, wide Q wave in lead aVF and broad initial R wave in lead V1 in Figure 6.8C could be mistaken for inferior or posterior infarction, respectively.

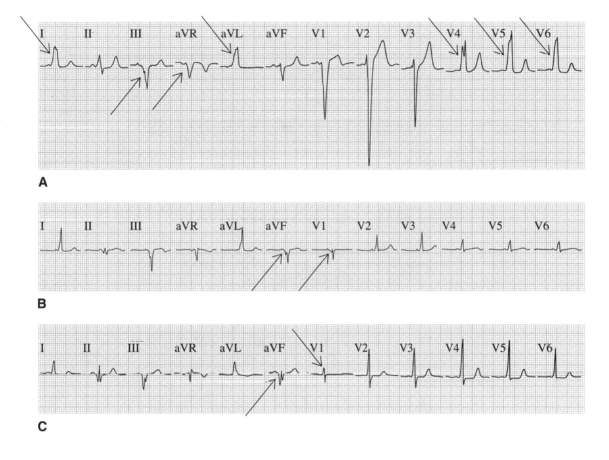

Figure 6.8. Twelve-lead ECGs from a 40-year-old woman admitted to a hospital emergency department for symptoms of dizziness **(A)**, a 46-year-old woman admitted to a coronary care unit with chest pain but no clinical confirmation of a myocardial infarction **(B)**, and a 31-year-old male medical resident without cardiac symptoms but an incorrect diagnosis of myocardial infarction by computerized interpretation of a routine ECG **(C)**. *Arrows* in **A** indicate delta waves producing QRS complexes mimicking LBBB, and *arrows* in **B** and **C** indicate delta waves producing QRS complexes mimicking myocardial infarction.

ELECTROCARDIOGRAPHIC LOCALIZATION OF THE PATHWAY OF VENTRICULAR PREEXCITATION

Many attempts have been made to determine the myocardial location of ventricular preexcitation according to the direction of the delta waves in the various ECG leads. Rosenbaum and colleagues[6] divided patients into two groups (Group A and Group B) on the basis of the direction of the "main deflection of the QRS complex" in transverse-plane leads V1 and V2 (Table 6.2).

Table 6.2. Relationship Between Pathway Location and ECG Changes

ECG Appearance	Location of Abnormal Pathway
Group A: QRS mainly positive in leads V1 and V2	LA-LV
Group B: QRS mainly negative in leads V1 and V2	RA-RV

Other classification systems consider the direction only of the abnormal delta wave in attempting to better localize the pathway of ventricular preexcitation. Since curative surgical and catheter ablation techniques for eliminating it have become available, more precise localization of the accessory pathway is clinically important,[7] and many additional ECG criteria have therefore been proposed for achieving this. However, precise localization of an accessory AV pathway is made difficult by several factors, including minor degrees of preexcitation, the presence of more than one accessory pathway, distortions of the QRS complex caused by superimposed myocardial infarction, or ventricular hypertrophy. Nevertheless, Milstein and his associates[8] devised the algorithm presented in Figure 6.9 that enabled them to correctly identify the location of 90% of more than 140 accessory pathways.

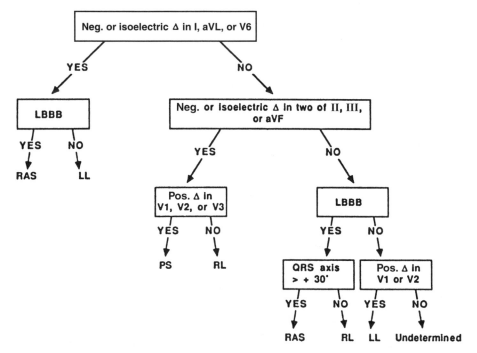

Figure 6.9.   Milstein's algorithm for localization of accessory pathways. Note: For purposes of this schema, *LBBB* indicates a positive QRS complex in lead I with a duration of at least 0.09 s and with rS complexes in leads V1 and V2. (*RAS*, right anteroseptal; *LL*, left lateral; *PS*, posteroseptal; *RL*, right lateral.) (Modified from Milstein S, Sharma AD, Guiraudon GM, et al. An algorithm for the electrocardiographic localization of accessory pathways in the Wolff-Parkinson-White syndrome. Pacing Clin Electrophysiol 1987;10:555–563.)

Although accessory pathways may be found anywhere in the connective tissue between the atria and ventricles, nearly all are found in three general locations (Fig. 6.10), as follows

1. Left laterally, between the left-atrial and left-ventricular free walls (50%).
2. Posteriorly, between the atrial and ventricular septa (30%).
3. Right laterally or anteriorly, between the right atrial and right ventricular free walls (20%).

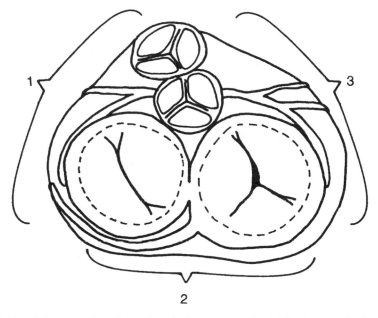

Figure 6.10.   Schematic view (from above) of a cross-section of the heart at the junction between the atria and the ventricles. The ventricular outflow aortic and pulmonary valves are located anteriorly, and the ventricular inflow mitral (bicuspid) and tricuspid valves are located posteriorly. The three general locations of Bundles of Kent are: *1*, LA-LV free wall; *2*, posterior septal; and *3*, the right anteroseptal and right lateral locations of Milstein and colleagues combined as RA-RV free wall. (Modified from Tonkin AM, Wagner GS, Gallagher JJ, et al. Initial forces of ventricular depolarization in the Wolff-Parkinson-White syndrome. Analysis based upon localization of the accessory pathway by epicardial mapping. Circulation 1975;52:1031.)

Tonkin and associates presented a simple method for localizing accessory pathways to one of the foregoing areas on the basis of the direction of the delta wave (Table 6.3).[9] They considered a point 20 ms after the onset of the delta wave in the QRS complex as their reference.

Table 6.3.   Consideration of Delta Wave at QRS Onset + 0.02 s

Direction of Preexcitation	Location of Pathway	Incidence Correct
Rightward	LA-LV free wall	10 of 10
Leftward and superior	Posterior septal	9 of 10
Leftward and inferior	RA-RV free wall	6 of 7

ABLATION OF ACCESSORY PATHWAYS

   Figures 6.11A and 6.12A illustrate the typical ECG appearances of preexcitation of the right ventricular free wall and the interventricular septum, respectively. Successful ablation of the accessory pathways (Figs. 6.11B and 6.12B) revealed the underlying presence of normal QRS complexes.

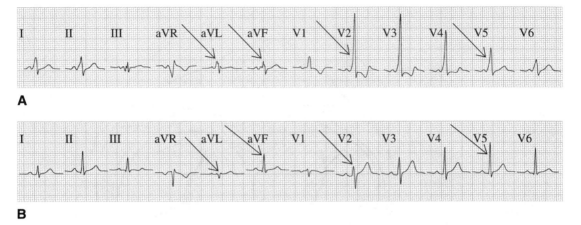

Figure 6.11. Serial 12-lead ECGs from a 44-year-old woman with a history of recurrent symptoms of dizziness and shortness of breath just before **(A)** and 1 week after **(B)** catheter-induced radio-frequency ablation of her Bundle of Kent. *Arrows* indicate delta waves in **A** and a normal appearance of the QRS complex in **B**.

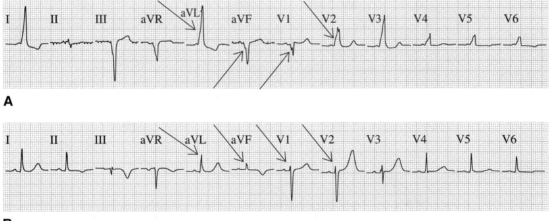

Figure 6.12. Serial 12-lead ECGs from a 28-year-old woman with recurrent episodes of rapid heart beat 1 day before **(A)** and 1 day after **(B)** catheter-induced radio-frequency ablation of her Bundle of Kent. *Arrows* indicate delta waves in **A** and a normal appearance of the QRS complex in **B**.

GLOSSARY

Bundle of Kent: a congenital abnormality in which a bundle of myocardial fibers connects the atria and the ventricles.

Delta wave: a slowing of the initial aspect of the QRS complex caused by premature excitation (preexcitation) of the ventricles via a Bundle of Kent.

Fusion beat: activation of the ventricles by two different wave fronts, resulting in an abnormal appearance of the QRS complexes on the ECG.

Preexcitation: premature activation of the ventricular myocardium via an abnormal AV pathway called a Bundle of Kent.

Tachyarrhythmia: an abnormal cardiac rhythm with a ventricular rate ≥ 100 beats/min.

Woff–Parkinson–White syndrome: the clinical combination of a short PR interval, an increased duration of the QRS complex caused by an initial slow deflection (delta wave), and supraventricular tachyarrhythmias.

REFERENCES

1. Kent AFS. Researches on the structure and function of the mammalian heart. J Physiol 1893;14:233.
2. Wolff L. Syndrome of short P-R interval with abnormal QRS complexes and paroxysmal tachycardia (Wolff-Parkinson-White syndrome). Circulation 1954;10:282.
3. Becker AE, Anderson RH, Durrer D, et al. The anatomical substrates of Wolff-Parkinson-White syndrome. Circulation 1978;57:870–879.
4. Giardina ACV, Ehlers KH, Engle MA. Wolff-Parkinson-White syndrome in infants and children: a long term follow up study. Br Heart J 1972;34:839–846.
5. Goudevenos JA, Katsouras CS, Graeklas G, et al. Ventricular pre-excitation in the general population: a study on the mode of presentation and clinical course. Heart 2000;83:29–34.
6. Rosenbaum FF, Hecht HH, Wilson FN, et al. Potential variations of thorax and esophagus in anomalous atrioventricular excitation (Wolff-Parkinson-White syndrome). Am Heart J 1945;29:281–326.
7. Gallagher JJ, Gilbert M, Svenson RH, et al. Wolff-Parkinson-White syndrome: the problem, evaluation, and surgical correction. Circulation 1975;51:767–785.
8. Milstein S, Sharma AD, Guiraudon GM, et al. An algorithm for the electrocardiographic localization of accessory pathways in the Wolff-Parkinson-White syndrome. Pace 1987;10:555–563.
9. Tonkin AM, Wagner GS, Gallagher JJ, et al. Initial forces of ventricular depolarization in the Wolff-Parkinson-White syndrome: analysis based upon localization of the accessory pathway by epicardial mapping. Circulation 1975;52:1030–1036.

CHAPTER 7

Myocardial Ischemia and Infarction

INTRODUCTION TO ISCHEMIA AND INFARCTION

The energy required to maintain the cardiac cycle is generated by a process known as aerobic metabolism, in which oxygen is required for energy production. Oxygen and essential nutrients are received by the cells of the myocardium from the blood supplied by the coronary arteries (*myocardial perfusion*). If the blood supply to the myocardium becomes insufficient, an energy deficiency occurs. To compensate for diminished aerobic metabolism, the myocardial cells must use a different metabolic process, *anaerobic metabolism*, in which oxygen is not required. In this process, the cells use their reserve supply of glucose stored in glycogen molecules to generate energy. Anaerobic metabolism, however, is less efficient than aerobic metabolism and can be sustained only for a limited time.

In the period during which perfusion is insufficient to meet the myocardial demand, the myocardial cells become ischemic. In order to sustain themselves, myocardial cells with an energy deficiency must uncouple their electrical activation from mechanical contraction and remain in their resting state. Thus, the area of the myocardium that is ischemic cannot participate in the pumping process of the heart.[1,2]

Various areas of the myocardium are more or less susceptible to ischemia. There are several determining factors of this, as follows:

1. Proximity to the Intracavitary Blood Supply.

The internal layers of myocardial cells (endocardium) have a secondary source of nutrients, the intracavitary blood, which provides protection from ischemia.[3,4] The entire myocardium of the right and left atria has so few cell layers that it is essentially all endocardium and subendocardium (Fig. 7.1). In the ventricles, however, only the innermost cell layers are similarly protected. The Purkinje system is located in these layers, and is therefore relatively well protected against ischemia.[5]

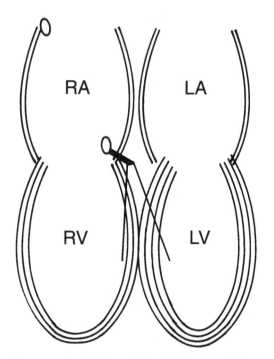

Figure 7.1. Schematic comparison of the relative thicknesses of the myocardium in the four cardiac chambers. The *ovals* indicate the locations of the sinoatrial (SA) and AV nodes; the His bundle (*thick short line*) and right and left bundle branches (*thin longer lines*) descend from the AV node into the interventricular septum. *LA*, left atrium; *LV*, left ventricle; *RA*, right atrium; *RV*, right ventricle. (Modified from Wagner GS, Waugh RA, Ramo BW. Cardiac arrhythmias. New York: Churchill Livingstone, 1983:2.)

2. Distance from the Major Coronary Arteries.

The ventricles consist of multiple myocardial layers that depend on the *coronary arteries* for their blood supply. These arteries arise from the aorta and course along the epicardial surfaces before penetrating the thickness of the myocardium. They then pass sequentially through the epicardial, middle, and subendocardial layers. Since the subendocardial layer is the most distant, innermost layer of the myocardium, it is the most susceptible to ischemia.[6]

3. Workload as Indicated by the Pressure Required to Pump Blood.

The greater the pressure required by a cardiac chamber to pump blood, the greater its workload and the greater its metabolic demand for oxygen. The myocardial workload is smallest in the atria, intermediate in the right ventricle, and greatest in the left ventricle. Therefore, the susceptibility to ischemia is also lowest in the atria, intermediate in the right ventricle, and greatest in the left ventricle.

Ischemia is a relative condition that depends on the balance among the coronary blood supply, the level of oxygenation of the blood, and the myocardial workload. Theoretically, an individual with normal coronary arteries and fully oxygenated blood could develop myocardial ischemia if the workload were increased either by an extremely elevated arterial blood pressure or an extremely high heart rate. Alternatively, an individual with normal coronary arteries and a normal myocardial workload could develop ischemia if the oxygenation of the blood became extremely diminished. Conversely, the myocardium of someone with severe narrowings (stenoses) in all coronary arteries might never become ischemic if the cardiac workload remained low and the blood was well oxygenated.

When ischemia is produced by an increased workload, it is normally reversed by returning to the resting state before the myocardial cells' reserve supply of glycogen is entirely depleted. However, a condition that produces myocardial ischemia by decreasing the coronary blood supply may not be reversed so easily.

Coronary arteries may gradually become partly obstructed by plaques in the chronic process of atherosclerosis. This condition produces ischemia when, even though the myocardial blood supply is sufficient at a resting workload, it becomes insufficient when the workload is increased by either emotional or physical stress. The gradual progression of the atherosclerotic process is accompanied by growth of collateral arteries, which supply blood to the myocardium beyond the level of obstruction. Indeed, these collateral arteries may be sufficient to entirely replace the blood-supplying capacity of the native artery if it becomes completely obstructed by the atherosclerotic plaque.[7]

Partially obstructed atherosclerotic coronary arteries may suddenly become completely obstructed by the acute processes of spasm of their smooth-muscle layer or *thrombosis* within the remaining arterial lumen.[8,9] In either of these condition, ischemia develops immediately unless the resting metabolic demands of the affected myocardial cells can be satisfied by the collateral blood flow. If the spasm is relaxed or the thrombus is resolved (thrombolysis) before the glycogen reserve of the affected cells is severely depleted, the cells promptly resume their contraction. However, if the acute, complete obstruction continues until the myocardial cells' glycogen is severely depleted, they become *stunned*.[10] Even after blood flow is restored, these cells are unable to resume contraction until they have repleted their glycogen reserves. If the complete obstruction further persists until the myocardial cells' glycogen is entirely depleted, the cells are unable to sustain themselves, are irreversibly damaged, and become necrotic. This clinical process is termed a heart attack or *myocardial infarction* (*MI*).

ELECTROCARDIOGRAPHIC CHANGES DURING MYOCARDIAL ISCHEMIA, INJURY, AND INFARCTION

An increase in myocardial demand does not have as profound an effect on myocardial perfusion as that caused by a complete cessation of coronary blood supply, and is therefore manifested on the ECG only by changes in the ST segments and T waves (Table 7.1). The more profound decrease in perfusion that occurs with acute complete coronary occlusion produces a different array of changes in the ST segments and T waves, and may even alter the QRS complex.[11,12] When blood flow does not rapidly return, the more permanent changes typical of infarction occur in the QRS waveforms.

Table 7.1. Insufficient Myocardial Perfusion

Cause	Electrical Process Primarily Affected	ECG Waveforms Altered
Increased demand	Recovery	ST segment, T wave
Decreased supply	Recovery, activation	QRS complex, ST, T wave

The myocardial cell layers most likely to have insufficient perfusion are those located "at the end of the supply line," as discussed earlier and illustrated in Figure 7.2. However, since the cells in the most endocardial layer receive their nutrients directly from the cavitary blood, it is the subendocardial layer that is most susceptible to insufficient perfusion when there is chronic coronary atherosclerosis and either an increase in

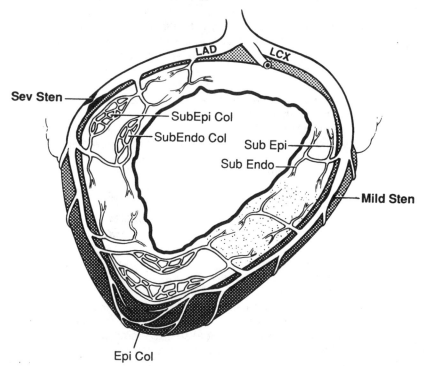

Figure 7.2. A cross-section of the left ventricle from the left anterior oblique view. The epicardial courses of the main branches of the LAD coronary artery and left circumflex (*LCX*) artery and their intramyocardial branches are shown. Subepicardial (*Sub Epi*) and subendocardial (*Sub Endo*) branches are present throughout; epicardial (*Epi Col*), subepicardial (*SubEpi Col*), and subendocardial (*SubEndo Col*) collaterals are present distal to the severe stenosis (*Sev Sten*) in the LAD coronary artery. A mild stenosis (*Mild Sten*) in the LCX coronary artery has not yet produced ischemia, and no collaterals have therefore developed. (From Califf RM, Mark DB, Wagner GS, eds. Acute coronary care, 2nd ed. Chicago: Mosby-Year Book, 1994, with permission.)

myocardial demand or a decrease in blood supply.[3,4] The thicker-walled left ventricle is much more susceptible to insufficient perfusion than is the thinner-walled right ventricle because of both the wall thickness itself and the greater workload of the left ventricle.

In the general presentation given above, the term ischemia is used for the general condition of insufficient myocardial perfusion. However, this condition has two different ECG manifestations: ischemia and *injury*. The ECG changes caused by a potentially reversible increase in myocardial metabolic demand or decrease in coronary blood flow are typically termed "ischemia" when the axis of the T wave is altered in relation to that of the QRS complex (Fig. 7.3B), and "injury" when the level of the ST-segment baseline is deviated from the level of the TP and PR segment baseline (Fig. 7.3C). When the ST segment deviates from the baseline, it attains a spatial direction (axis) as previously described for the P wave, QRS complex, and T wave (Chapter 3, "Interpretation of the Normal Electrocardiogram"). The T-wave changes of ischemia and the ST-segment changes of injury may occur either independently of one another or simultaneously.

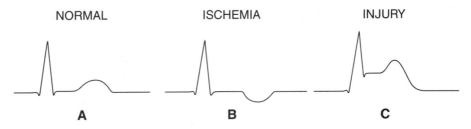

Figure 7.3. Schematic single ventricular cycles from an ECG lead oriented to the cardiac long axis are shown for normal **(A)**, ischemic **(B)**, and injury conditions **(C)**.

When insufficient myocardial perfusion is limited to the subendocardial layer of the left ventricle, the affected cells may lose their ability to maintain the prolonged activation that causes the normal similarity in the spatial directions of the QRS complex and T wave (Chapter 1, "Cardiac Electrical Activity"). The resultant *ischemic T waves* are inverted from positive to negative in many of the ECG leads because the axis of the ischemic T waves is directed away from the involved region of the left ventricle (Fig. 7.4A). When insufficient perfusion extends through all of the myocardial layers (*transmurally*), the resultant epicardial ischemia shifts the T-wave axis toward the involved region of the left ventricle[13] (Fig 7.4B). The resultant *hyperacute T waves* have increased amplitude in many of the ECG leads.

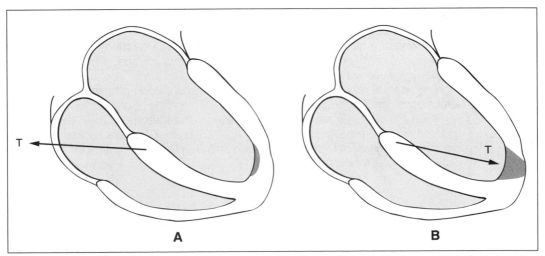

Figure 7.4. The mean direction (*arrow*) of the T wave from baseline in the center of cardiac electrical activity is shown when subendocardial ischemia **(A)** or transmural ischemia **(B)** is present.

Shifting of the ST segment baseline occurs when insufficient perfusion causes the myocardial-cell membranes to become abnormally permeable to the flow of ions. The resulting difference in electrical potential between injured and uninjured myocardium causes a constant flow of *injury current*.[13] When the injury is limited to the subendocardial layer of the left ventricle, the resultant "subendocardial injury" (SEI) shifts the axis of the ST segment generally away from that ventricle, but not specifically away from the involved region (Fig 7.5A). It should be noted that the clinically accepted term represented by the "I" in the abbreviation "SEI" is "ischemia" rather than "injury." When injury extends transmurally, the resultant "epicardial injury" shifts the axis of the ST segment toward the specifically involved region of the left ventricle[14,15] (Fig. 7.5B). "Injury" is the clinically accepted term here, and no abbreviation is used. A nonregional epicardial injury current is caused by pericardial inflammation (termed *pericarditis*), as presented in Chapter 11, "Miscellaneous Conditions."

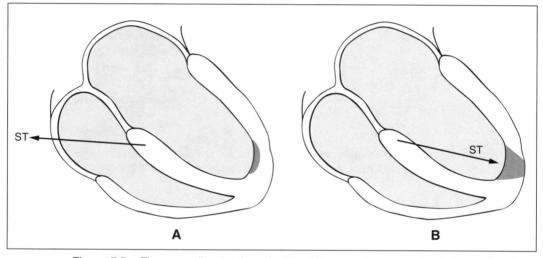

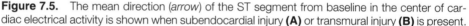

Figure 7.5. The mean direction (*arrow*) of the ST segment from baseline in the center of cardiac electrical activity is shown when subendocardial injury **(A)** or transmural injury **(B)** is present.

Insufficient perfusion of the left ventricle caused by an increase in myocardial metabolic demand is limited to the subendocardial layer of the left ventricle. However, insufficient perfusion caused by a decrease in myocardial blood flow is limited to the subendocardial layer only if the responsible coronary arterial occlusion is incomplete; if the occlusion is complete, the insufficiency of perfusion extends transmurally to the epicardial layer. If a complete occlusion persists, and myocardial reperfusion is not attained while the cells retain their viability, a myocardial infarction occurs (Chapter 10, "Myocardial Infarction"). As the infarction process evolves, the axes of the QRS complex and T wave are directed away from the infarcted area.[16] Unless poor postinfarction myocardial reperfusion occurs, the ST segment soon returns to a position isoelectric with the TP/PR-segment baseline.

The ECG changes associated with each of the three pathologic processes discussed here are presented in the next three chapters: Chapters 8, ("Ischemia Due to Increased Myocardial Demand"), 9 ("Ischemia Due to Insufficient Blood Supply"), and 10 ("Myocardial Infarction").

GLOSSARY

Aerobic metabolism: the intracellular method for converting glucose into energy that requires the presence of oxygen and produces enough energy to nourish the myocardial cell and also to cause it to contract.

Anaerobic metabolism: the intracellular method for converting glucose into energy that does not require oxygen, but produces only enough energy to nourish the cell.

Coronary arteries: either of the two arteries (right or left) that arise from the aorta immediately above the semilunar valves and supply the tissues of the heart itself.

Hyperacute T waves: T waves with an axis that is directed toward the ischemic area of the left-ventricular epicardium. They can be identified in many leads by an increased positive amplitude.

Injury: a term used for the ST-segment deviation that occurs with insufficient perfusion.

Injury current: The current produced because of the difference in electrical potential between ischemic and nonischemic myocardium.

Ischemic T waves: T waves with an axis that is directed away from the ischemic area of the left ventricular subendocardium.

Myocardial infarction: death of myocardial cells as a result of failure of the circulation to provide sufficient oxygen to restore metabolism after the intracellular stores of glycogen have been depleted.

Myocardial ischemia: a reduction in the supply of oxygen to less than the amount required by myocardial cells to maintain aerobic metabolism.

Myocardial perfusion: the flow of oxygen and nutrients into the cells of the heart muscle.

Pericarditis: inflammation of the pericardium.

Stunned myocardium: a region of myocardium consisting of cardiac cells that are using anaerobic metabolism and are therefore ischemic and incapable of contraction, but which are not infarcted.

Thrombosis: the formation or presence of a blood clot within a blood vessel.

Transmural: involving the full thickness of the myocardial wall.

REFERENCES

1. Rushmer RF. Cardiovascular dynamics. Philadelphia: WB Saunders, 1976:367–369.
2. Reimer KA, Jennings RB, Tatum AH. Pathobiology of acute myocardial ischemia: metabolic, functional and intrastructural studies. Am J Cardiol 1983;52:72A–81A.
3. Reimer KA, Lowe JE, Rasmussen MM, et al. The wavefront phenomenon of ischemic cell death: I. Myocardial infarct size vs. duration of coronary occlusion in dogs. Circulation 1977;56:786–794.
4. Reimer KA, Jennings RB. The "wavefront phenomenon" of myocardial ischemic cell death: II. Transmural progression of necrosis within the framework of ischemic bed size (myocardium at risk) and collateral flow. Lab Invest 1979;40:633–644.
5. Hackel DB, Wagner G, Ratliff NB, et al. Anatomic studies of the cardiac conducting system in acute myocardial infarction. Am Heart J 1972;83:77–81.
6. Bauman RP, Rembert JC, Greenfield JC. The role of the collateral circulation in maintaining cellular viability during coronary occlusion. In: Califf RM, Mark DB, Wagner GS, eds. Acute coronary care. 2nd ed. Chicago: Mosby-Year Book, 1994.
7. Cohen M, Reutzop KP. Limitation of myocardial ischemia by collateral circulation during sudden controlled coronary artery occlusion in tumor subjects: a prospective study. Circulation 1906;74:469–476.
8. Davies MJ, Woolf N, Robertson WB. Pathology of acute myocardial infarction with particular reference to occlusive coronary thrombi. Br Heart J 1976;38:659–664.
9. Davies MJ, Fulton WFM, Robertson WB. The relation of coronary thrombosis to ischemic myocardial necrosis. J Pathol 1979;127:99–110.
10. Braunwald E, Kloner RA. The stunned myocardium: prolonged postischemic ventricular dysfunction. Circulation 1982;66:1146–1149.
11. Ekmekci A, Toyoshima HJ, Kwoczynski JK, et al. Angina pectoris: giant R and receding S wave in myocardial ischemia and certain nonischemic conditions. Am J Cardiol 1961;7:521–532.
12. Wagner NB, Sevilla DC, Krucoff MW, et al. Transient alterations of the QRS complex and the ST segment during percutaneous transluminal balloon angioplasty of the left anterior descending artery. Am J Cardiol 1988;62:1038–1042.
13. Beckwith JR. Grant's clinical electrocardiography, 2nd Ed. New York: McGraw-Hill, 1970: 87–111.
14. Arbane M, Goy JJ. Prediction of the site of the total occlusion in the left anterior descending coronary artery using admission electrocardiogram in anterior wall acute myocardial infarction. Am J Cardiol 2000;85:487–491.
15. Menown IB, Mackenzie G, Adgey A. Optimizing the initial 12-lead electrocardiographic diagnosis of acute myocardial infarction. Eur Heart J 2000;21:275–283.
16. Wagner NB, Wagner GS, White RD. The twelve-lead ECG and the extent of myocardium at risk of acute infarction: cardiac anatomy and lead locations, and the phases of serial changes during acute occlusion. In: Califf RM, Mark DB, Wagner GS, eds. Acute coronary care in the thrombolytic era. Chicago: Year Book, 1988: 31–45.

CHAPTER 8

Ischemia and Injury Due to Increased Myocardial Demand

CHANGES IN THE ST SEGMENT

 Normally, the ST segment of the electrocardiogram (ECG) is at the same baseline level as the PR and TP segments (Fig. 1.12). Observation of the stability of the position of the ST segment on the ECG of a patient receiving a graded exercise stress test provides clinical information about the presence or absence of myocardial ischemia.[1] If coronary blood flow is capable of increasing to a degree sufficient to satisfy the metabolic demands even of the cells in the left-ventricular subendocardium, there is minimal alteration in the appearance of the ST segment. A common normal variation in the ECG during exercise stress testing is shown in Figure 8.1.[2] Note the minor depression of the J point with the ST segment upsloping toward the upright T wave.

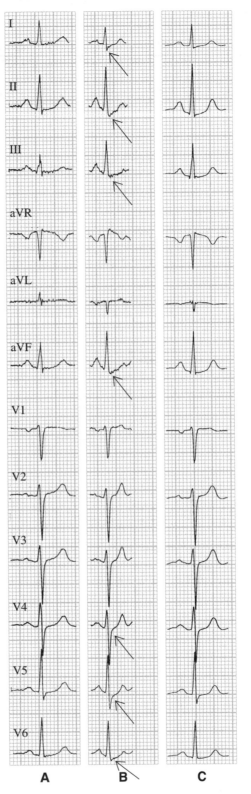

Figure 8.1. Twelve-lead ECGs recorded from a 54-year-old man at rest **(A)**, during and exercise stress test **(B)**, and immediately after the test **(C)**. *Arrows* indicate the depression of the ST-J point in many leads in **B**.

When a partial obstruction within the coronary arteries prevents myocardial blood flow from increasing sufficiently during an exercise stress test, the resulting subendocardial ischemia (SEI) is manifested by horizontal ST-segment depression (Fig. 8.2B).[3] Refer to Chapter 7 ("Myocardial Ischemia and Infarction") for explanation of this process and its terminology. However, the ST-segment depression typically disappears when the demand on the myoicardium is decreased by stopping the exercise (Fig. 8.2C). This suggests that the myocardial cells have been reversibly ischemic (injured) and have not become infarcted.

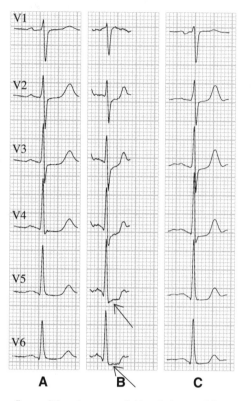

Figure 8.2. Serial recordings of the six precordial leads from a 60-year-old man with a history of exertional chest pain made at rest **(A)**, during exercise at a heart rate of 167/min **(B)**, and 5 minutes after exercise **(C)**. *Arrows* indicate the horizontal ST-segment depression in leads V5 and V6 in **B**.

A combination of two diagnostic criteria (on either a resting or exercise ECG recording) in at least one ECG lead have typically been required for the diagnosis of left ventricular SEI (Fig. 8.3), as follows:

1. A depression of at least 1.0 mm (0.10 mV) at the J point.
2. Either a horizontal or a downward slope toward the end of the ST segment at its junction with the T wave. The T wave may either remain positive (Fig. 8.3*B*) or deviate away from the QRS complex (Fig. 8.3*C*).

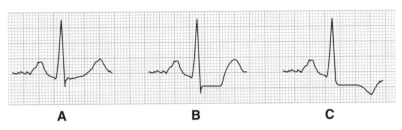

A   **B**   **C**

Figure 8.3. Single schematic cardiac cycles showing the normal condition at rest **(A)** and two variations of the abnormal condition of exercise-induced SEI **(B and C)**.

Lesser deviations of the ST segments, as illustrated in Figure 8.4, could be caused by SEI or could be a variation of normal. Even the ST segment changes "diagnostic" of left-ventricular SEI could be due to an extreme variation of normal. When these ECG changes appear on either resting or exercise recordings, they should be considered in the context of other manifestations of coronary insufficiency, such as precordial pain, decreased blood pressure, or cardiac arrhythmias.[3,4]

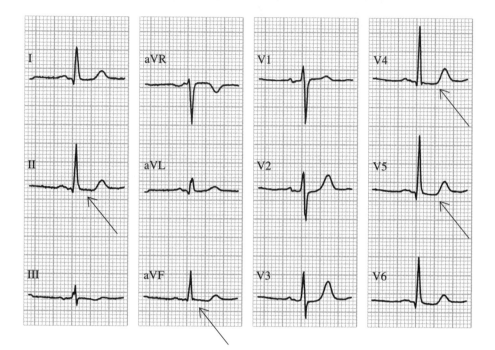

Figure 8.4. Twelve-lead ECG from a 69-year-old woman with severe substernal pain at rest and who was transported by ambulance to the emergency department of a hospital. *Arrows* indicate minimal ST-segment depression in many leads.

Deviation of the junction of the ST segment with the J point, followed by an upsloping ST segment, may also be abnormal.[2] A 0.1- to 0.2-mV depression of the J point, followed by an upsloping ST segment that remains 0.1-mV depressed for 0.08 s,[5] or by a 0.2-mV depression of the J point followed by an upsloping ST segment that remains 0.2-mV depressed for 0.08 second, may also be considered "diagnostic" of SEI[6] (Fig. 8.5).

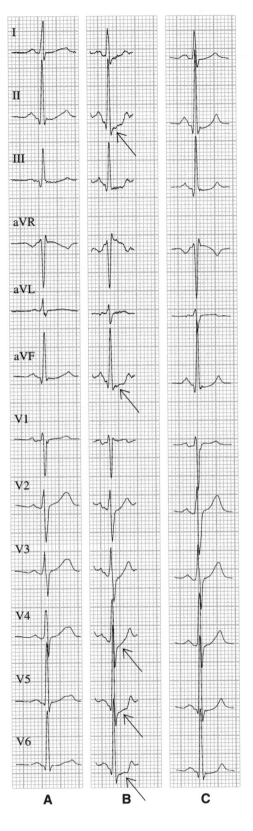

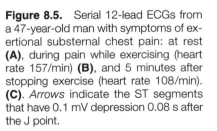

Figure 8.5. Serial 12-lead ECGs from a 47-year-old man with symptoms of exertional substernal chest pain: at rest **(A)**, during pain while exercising (heart rate 157/min) **(B)**, and 5 minutes after stopping exercise (heart rate 108/min). **(C)**. *Arrows* indicate the ST segments that have 0.1 mV depression 0.08 s after the J point.

Another clinical test used in the diagnosis of SEI is continuous ECG monitoring. This method has been termed *Holter monitoring* after its developer, and is discussed in Chapter 2 ("Recording the Electrocardiogram"). Originally, only a single ECG lead was monitored in this method, but current methods provide three leads during ambulatory activity and all 12 standard leads at the bedside. Figure 8.6 illustrates an episode of ST-segment depression during walking, accompanied by nonsustained ventricular tachycardia (Chapter 17, "Reentrant Ventricular Tachyarrhythmias"). An entry to the diary kept to accompany Holter monitoring relates the cardiac event to the precipitating activity (walking) and to the the symptoms perceived (slight breathlessness). Since the episode was not accompanied by any chest pain, it could be considered an example of what has been clinically termed *silent ischemia*.[7-9]

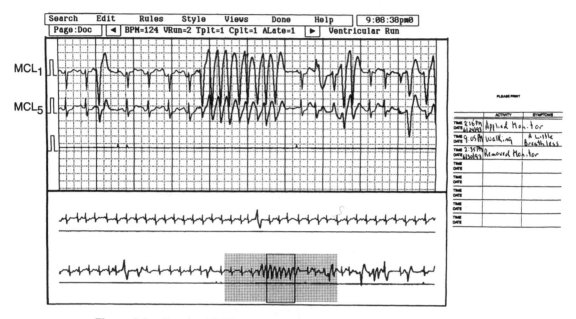

Figure 8.6. Two-lead (*MCL₁* and *MCL₅*), 24-hour ECG recording from a 57-year-old man with symptoms of mild dyspnea.

As indicated in Chapter 2 ("Recording the Electrocardiogram"), the positive poles of most of the standard limb and precordial ECG leads are directed toward the left ventricle. SEI causes the ST axis to point generally away from the left ventricle (Chapter 7, "Myocardial Ischemia and Infarction," Figure 7.5). The changes in the ST segment appear negative or depressed in the leftward (I, aVL, or V4–V6) and inferiorly oriented leads (II, III, and aVF) which have their positive poles directed toward the left ventricle (Fig. 8.7A and B). As previously stated, the location of the ECG leads showing ST-segment depression is not indicative of the involved region of the left ventricular subendocardium. In leads that have their positive poles directed away from the left ventricle (such as limb lead aVR and precordial leads V1 and V2), however, the ST segments may appear elevated, as indicated in Figure 8.7A and B.

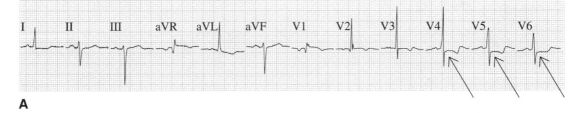

A

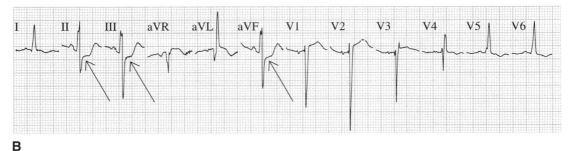

B

Figure 8.7. Twelve-lead ECGs at the times of admission to emergency departments for a 73-year-old woman with 2 hours of nonexertional substernal chest pain **(A)** and a 58-year-old man with a previous infarction and 3 hours of severe chest pain and shortness of breath preceding admission **(B)**. *Arrows* indicate the depressed ST segments in the ECGs in both **A** and **B**.

The change in the ST segments that occurs with left-ventricular SEI is similar to that described in Chapter 4 ("Chamber Enlargement") for left ventricular strain (Fig. 4.8B). However, left-ventricular strain also causes the T waves to be directed away from the left ventricle, and is accompanied by the QRS changes of left-ventricular hypertrophy (LVH). A diagnostic dilemma therefore exists only when SEI is accompanied by both the T-wave changes of subendocardial ischemia and the QRS-complex changes of LVH.

The maximal ST-segment depression during stress tests is almost never seen in leads V1–V3.[10] When these leads do exhibit the maximal ST depression in the ECG, the cause is either right-ventricular strain (Chapter 4, "Chamber Enlargement") or posterior epicardial injury (Chapter 9, "Ischemia Due to Insufficient Blood Supply"). The ST-segment depression of left-ventricular SEI usually resolves in the minutes following removal of the excessive cardiovascular stress. Occasionally, ST-segment depression is observed in the absence of an obvious increase in left-ventricular workload. In this case the possibility of subendocardial infarction should be investigated.[11]

The abnormality of electrical recovery in SEI that is manifested on the ECG by ST-segment deviation occurs for each of the individual subendocardial cells at the time they complete their activation process (Fig. 1.11). Therefore, SEI that manifests itself through depression of the ST segments actually begins during the QRS complex. This results in secondary deviation of the QRS-complex waveforms in the same direction as that of the ST segments shown in Figure 8.8*A* and *B*. This distortion affects the amplitudes but not the durations of the QRS-complex waveforms, and alters their later aspects more than their earlier aspects.[12]

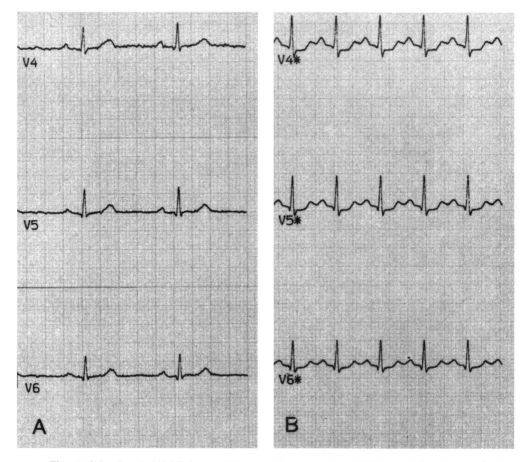

Figure 8.8. Leads V4–V6 from a 67-year-old woman at rest **(A)** and during chest pain at a heart rate of 125/min while performing an exercise stress test **(B)**. The small terminal S waves in all three leads move downward with the ST segments.

CHANGES IN THE T WAVE

Normally, the directions of the QRS complexes and T waves are similar rather than opposite, because of the reversed (epicardial-to-endocardial) direction of ventricular repolarization (Fig. 1.11). Ischemic subendocardial cells cannot maintain prolonged activation, thereby causing the T wave on the ECG to become "inverted" in relation to the QRS complexes (Fig. 8.9). As indicated in Chapter 3 ("Interpretation of the Normal Electrocardiogram"), there is normally an angle of less than 45 degrees between the axes of the QRS complexes and T waves in the frontal plane, and less than 60 degrees between these same axes in the transverse plane.[13] When the angles in the respective planes exceed these limits, in the absence of other abnormal conditions such as ventricular hypertrophy or bundle-branch block (BBB), the presence of ischemic T waves should be considered. Note other leads in Figure 8.9. that show biphasic T waves (leads II, III, and aVF) or both negative QRS complexes and T waves both (leads V1 and V2), which could (if seen in the absence of the changes in leads V3–V6) be variants of normal.

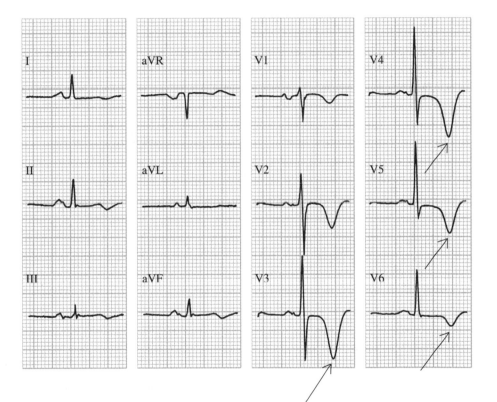

Figure 8.9. Twelve-lead ECGs from a 78-year-old woman presenting to the emergency department with 1 hour of severe substernal chest pain. *Arrows* indicate the T waves in many leads that are directed opposite to the predominant direction of the QRS complex.

As stated in Chapter 7 ("Myocardial Ischemia and Infarction") (Fig. 7.4), the axis of the T wave deviates away from the ischemic region in the left-ventricular subendocardium. Therefore, it is possible to identify this region as the site of ischemia by noting those ECG leads that show inverted T waves. Figure 8.10 illustrates the typical lead groups that localize ischemia in the distributions of the three major coronary arteries: the left anterior descending (LAD) coronary artery (Fig 8.10*A*), the right coronary artery (Fig 8.10*B*), and the left circumflex (LCX) artery (Fig 8.10*C*). In Figure 8.10*B*, the inverted T waves in inferiorly oriented leads are accompanied by abnormally tall positive T waves in anteriorly oriented leads, indicating that the ischemia also involves the posterior free wall of the left ventricle.

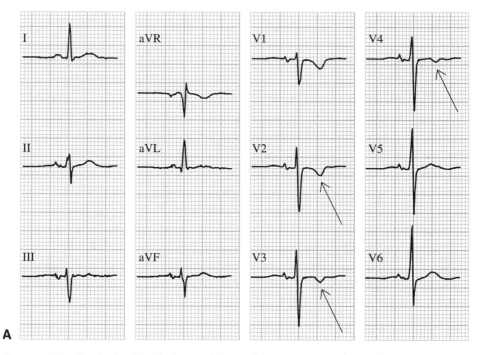

A

Figure 8.10. Twelve-lead ECGs from a 63-year-old woman presenting to the emergency department with 2 hours of substernal chest pain **(A)**, a 78-year-old man with an occluded RCA vein graft 3 days after coronary bypass surgery **(B)**, and an 83-year-old man with a previous anterior infarct and recurrent resting chest pain following abdominal surgery **(C)**. Coronary angiography revealed high-grade stenosis of the proximal LCX artery. *Arrows* in **A**, **B**, and **C** indicate abnormally directed T waves.

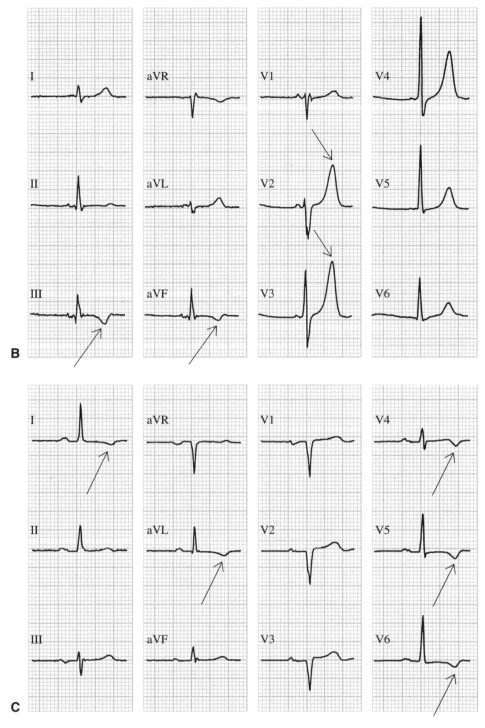

Figure 8.10. *(continued)*

T-wave changes are both less specific and less sensitive than ST-segment changes for diagnosing insufficient myocardial perfusion caused by increased demand. Inversion of T waves occurs in the absence of ischemia (low specificity), either as a normal variant or with other cardiac or noncardiac conditions.[14] Also, inversion of T waves sometimes fails to occur in the presence of ischemia (low sensitivity), as during an abnormal exercise stress test. Figure 8.11A and B, shows examples of stress tests positive for the existence of SEI as documented by the typical ST-segment changes of SEI in both the presence and absence of T-wave inversion.

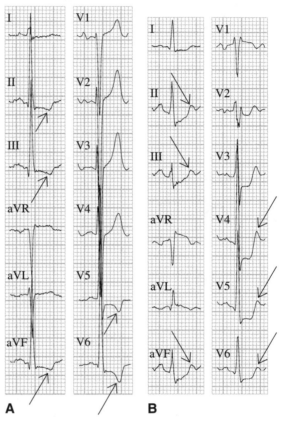

Figure 8.11. Resting and exercise 12-lead ECGs from a 47-year-old man **(A)** and a 72-year-old man with sustained chest pain during exercise stress testing **(B)**. *Arrows* indicate negative T waves in **A** and positive T waves in **B** following the diagnostically depressed ST segments.

Like ST-segment depression, T-wave inversion usually resolves when the increased left ventricular workload that causes it is removed. Unlike ST-segment depression, however, T-wave inversion is typically present for a prolonged period after the acute phase of myocardial infarction. This chronic T-wave inversion should not be considered evidence for persistent ischemia. It represents an alteration in electrical recovery caused by the infarction-induced changes in electrical activation of the myocardium.

(Fig. 8.12*A* and *B*). In Figure 8.12*B*, the "T-wave inversion" appears as increased positivity when the infarct is located in the posterior free wall of the left ventricle (note the prominent R wave in lead V2, discussed in Chapter 10, "Myocardial Infarction.")

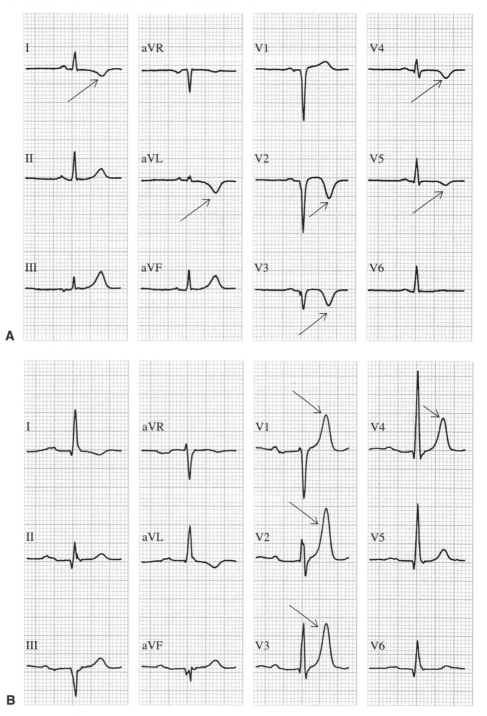

Figure 8.12. Twelve-lead ECGs from two patients at 6 weeks after hospital discharge for acute myocardial infarction: **A.** ECG of a 62-year-old man who developed Q waves in leads V1 to V3. **B.** ECG of a 75-year-old man with a remote inferior infarction who at the time of this ECG had developed increased R waves in leads V2–V4 after a documented thrombotic occlusion of the LCX artery. *Arrows* indicate the inverted negative T waves in **A** and the inverted positive T waves in **B**.

GLOSSARY

Holter monitoring: continuous ECG recording of one or more leads, either for the detection of abnormalities of morphology suggestive of ischemia or abnormalities of rhythm.

Silent ischemia: evidence of myocardial ischemia appearing on an ECG recording in the absence of any awareness of symptoms of ischemia.

Subendocardial ischemia (SEI): a condition marked by deviation of the ST segments of an ECG away from the ventricle (always the left ventricle),

and in which only the inner part of the myocardium is ischemic. The "I" in the abbreviation should more accurately represent injury, since the ST segment is shifted away from the TP-PR baseline by a current of injury.

TP segment: the period from the end of the T wave to the onset of the P wave in the ECG.

Ventricular strain: deviation of the ST segments and T waves of an ECG away from the ventricle in which there is either a severe systolic overload or marked hypertrophy.

REFERENCES

1. Sheffield LT, Holt JH, Reeves TJ. Exercise graded by heart rate in electrocardiographic testing for angina pectoris. Circulation 1965;32:622–629.
2. Stuart RJ, Ellestad MH. Upsloping ST segments in exercise stress testing. Am J Cardiol 1976;37:19–22.
3. Ellestad MH, Cooke BM, Greenberg PS. Stress testing; clinical application and predictive capacity. Prog Cardiovasc Dis 1979;21:431–460.
4. Ellestad MH, Savitz S, Bergdall D, et al. The false-positive stress test: multivariate analysis of 215 subjects with hemodynamic, angiographic and clinical data. Am J Cardiol 1977;40:681–685.
5. Rijneki RD, Ascoop CA, Talmon JL. Clinical significance of upsloping ST segments in exercise electrocardiography. Circulation 1980;61:671–678.
6. Kurita A, Chaitman BR, Bourassa MG. Significance of exercise-induced junctional ST depression in evaluation of coronary artery disease. Am J Cardiol 1977;40:492–497.
7. Wolf F, Tzivoni D, Stern S. Comparison of exercise tests and 24-hour ambulatory electrocardiographic monitoring in detection of ST-T changes. Br Heart J 1974;36:90–95.
8. Selwyn A, Fox K, Eves M, et al. Myocardial ischemia in patients with frequent angina pectoris. Br Med J 1978;2:1594–1596.
9. Krucoff MW, Pope JE, Bottner RK, et al. Dedicated ST-segment monitoring in the CCU after successful coronary angioplasty: incidence and prognosis of silent and symptomatic ischemia. In: van Armin T, Maseri A, eds. Silent ischemia: current concepts and management. Darmstadt: Steinkopff Verlag, 1987:140–146.
10. Shah A, Wagner GS, Green CL, et al. Electrocardiographic differentiation of the ST-segment depression of acute myocardial injury due to left circumflex artery occlusion from that of myocardial ischemia of nonocclusive etiologies. Am J Cardiol 1997;80:512–513.
11. Hurst JW, Logue RB. The heart: arteries and veins. New York: McGraw-Hill, 1966:147.
12. Glazier JJ, Chierchia S, Margonato A, et al. Increase in S-wave amplitude during ischemic ST-segment depression in stable angina pectoris. Am J Cardiol 1987;59:1295–1299.
13. Beckwith JR. Grant's clinical electrocardiography, 2nd ed. New York: McGraw-Hill, 1970:60.
14. Taggart P, Carruthers M, Joseph S, et al. Electrocardiographic changes resembling myocardial ischaemia in asymptomatic men with normal coronary arteriograms. Br Heart J 1979;41:214–225.

CHAPTER 9

Ischemia and Injury Due to Insufficient Blood Supply

CHANGES IN THE ST SEGMENT

 Just as changes in the ST segment of the electrocardiogram (ECG) are reliable indicators of myocardial injury (although it is commonly termed "ischemia") caused by increased myocardial demand, they are also reliable indicators of injury from insufficient coronary blood flow. Observation of the position of the ST segments (relative to the PR and TP segments) in a patient experiencing acute precordial pain provides clinical evidence of the presence or absence of severe myocardial injury or developing myocardial infarction. However, many normal individuals show marked ST-segment elevation on routine standard ECGs (Fig. 9.1).[1-3]

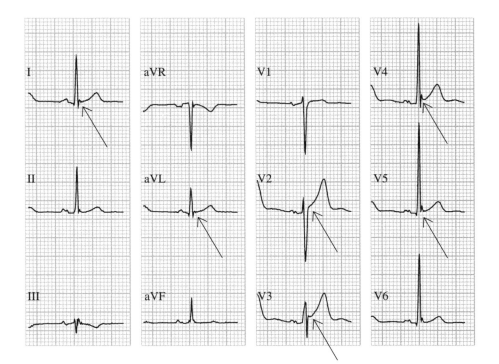

Figure 9.1. Twelve-lead ECG from a 34-year-old man with a strong family history of heart disease presenting for the fourth time within a year to an emergency department with severe chest pain. *Arrows* indicate ST-segment elevation in many leads.

When a sudden, complete occlusion of a coronary artery prevents any blood flow from reaching an area of myocardium, the resulting epicardial injury[4-6] is manifested by deviation of the ST segment toward the involved region. However, as shown in the ECG of a patient receiving brief therapeutic balloon occlusion during percutaneous transluminal coronary angioplasty (PTCA) (Fig. 9.2A to C), the ST-segment changes typically disappear abruptly when coronary blood flow is restored by deflating the angioplasty balloon after a brief period. This indicates that the myocardial cells have been reversibly "injured" and have not actually become infarcted.

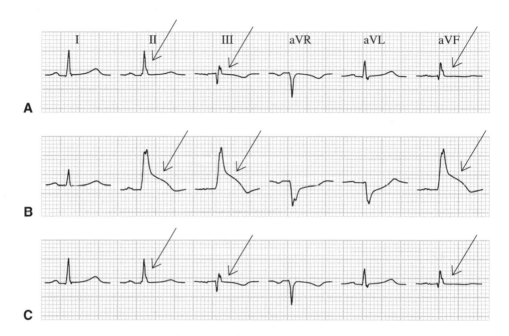

Figure 9.2. The six limb leads of the ECG recorded serially from a 58-year-old man with chest pain on exertion caused by a 90% obstruction of the RCA. **A:** Before the PTCA procedure. **B:** After 2 minutes of angioplasty balloon occlusion of the RCA. **C:** After 2 minutes of reperfusion following balloon deflation. *Arrows* indicate the ST segments in leads II, III, and aVF that move toward the involved myocardial region during balloon occlusion.

It may be difficult to differentiate the abnormal changes in the ST segment produced by epicardial injury from variations of normal when the deviation of the ST segment is minimal. Presence of one of the following criteria is typically required for diagnosis of epicardial injury:

1. Elevation of the origin of the ST segment at its junction (J point) with the QRS complex of: (a) ≥0.10 mV in two or more limb leads or precordial leads V4 to V6 or (b) ≥0.20 mV in two or more precordial leads V1 to V3.
2. Depression of the origin of the ST segment at the J point of (0.10 mV in two or more of precordial leads V1 to V3.

The greater threshold is required for ST-segment elevation in leads V1 to V3 because a normal slight, elevation of the ST segment is often present. When the amplitude and duration of the terminal S wave is further increased in these leads as a result of left-ventricular hypertrophy or left bundle-branch block (LBBB), an even greater normal elevation of the ST segment is present. A recent study has shown that elevation of the ST segment to ≥0.5 mV is required in leads V1 to V3 to diagnose acute anterior epicardial injury in the presence of LBBB.[7] However, the 0.1 mV threshold remains applicable for diagnosis of acute epicardial injury when the deviation of the ST segment is in the same direction (concordant with) as that of the terminal QRS waveform.

The deviated ST segment may be horizontal (Fig. 9.3A), downsloping (Fig. 9.3B), or upsloping (Fig. 9.3C). The sloping produces different amounts of deviation of the ST segment as it moves from the J point toward the T wave. Various positions along the ST segment are sometimes selected for measurement of ST-segment deviation either for establishing the diagnosis of epicardial injury or for estimating its extent. "J" and "J + 0.08 s" have been used in some clinical situations, and are illustrated in Figure 9.3. Note that the J point is more elevated than the J + 0.08-s point in Figure 9.3A, equally elevated in Figure 9.3B, and less elevated in Figure 9.3C. The ECG criteria for epicardial injury may be accompanied by other manifestations of insufficient myocardial perfusion, such as typical or atypical precordial pain, decreased blood pressure, or cardiac arrhythmias.

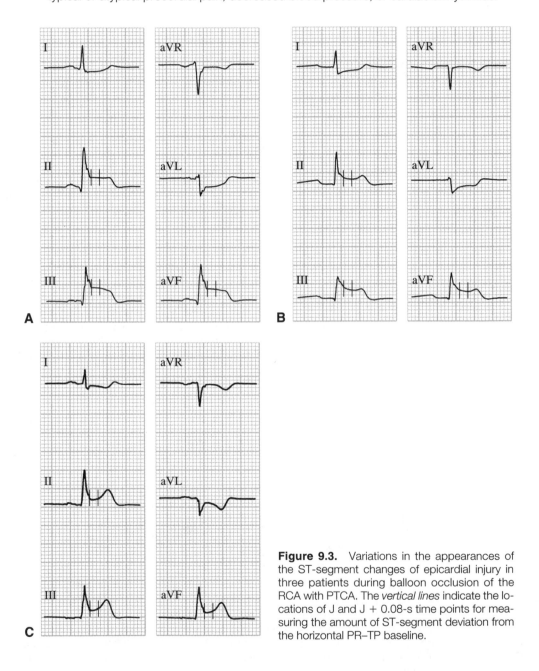

Figure 9.3. Variations in the appearances of the ST-segment changes of epicardial injury in three patients during balloon occlusion of the RCA with PTCA. The *vertical lines* indicate the locations of J and J + 0.08-s time points for measuring the amount of ST-segment deviation from the horizontal PR–TP baseline.

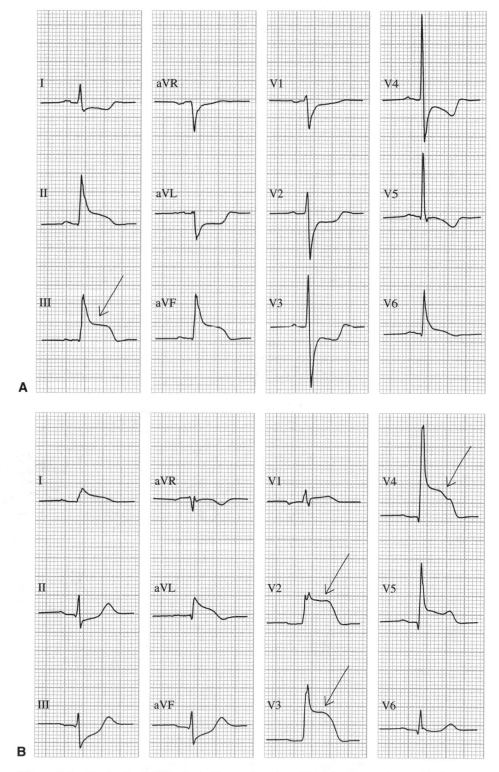

Figure 9.4. Twelve-lead ECGs illustrating acute epicardial injury after 1 minute of balloon occlusion in the mid-RCA of a 47-year-old man with symptoms of unstable angina **(A)** and the proximal LAD of a 73-year-old woman with a recent acute anterior infarction **(B)**. *Arrows* indicate the maximal ST-segment deviation directed toward the involved regions.

Since the ST-segment axis in epicardial injury deviates toward the involved area of myocardium, these changes described above appear positive or elevated in leads with their positive poles pointing toward injured inferior (Fig. 9.4A) or anterior (Fig. 9.4B) aspects of the left ventricle. Often, both ST-segment elevation and depression appear in different leads of a standard 12-lead ECG. Usually, as in Figure 9.3, the direction of the greater deviation should be considered primary and the direction of the lesser deviation should be considered secondary or *reciprocal*. When epicardial injury involves both inferior and posterior aspects of the left ventricle, the ST-segment depression of posterior involvement in leads V1 to V3 may equal or exceed the elevation produced by inferior involvement in leads II, III, and aVF.

When inferior epicardial injury is accompanied by left-ventricular subendocardial injury (SEI), the ST-segment depression in leads V4 to V6 may equal or exceed the ST-segment elevation in leads II, III and aVF. The SEI results from increased metabolic demand in myocardium supplied by subtotally occluded arteries that is remote from the site of acute occlusion. This is equivalent to a positive stress test induced by the hemodynamic abnormality resulting from acute transmural ischemia (Chapter 8, "Ischemia and Injury Due to Increased Myocardial Demand").

Epicardial injury most commonly occurs in the distal aspect of the area of the left-ventricular myocardium supplied by one of the three major coronary arteries, as indi-

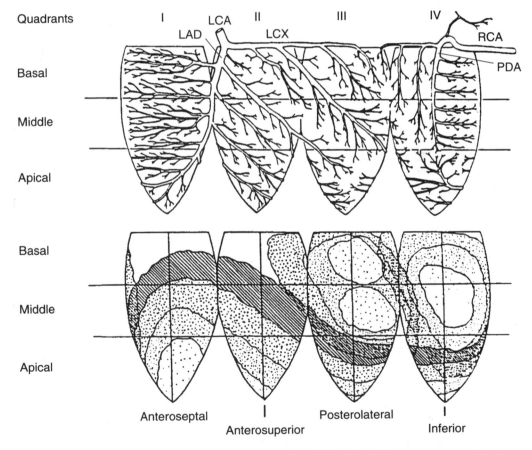

Figure 9.5. The 12 sectors of the LV myocardium defined by the four quadrants and the three levels. The distributions of the coronary arteries [*LCA, LAD, LCX, RCA*, and posterior descending (*PDA*)] **(top)** are related to the distributions of insufficient blood supply resulting from occlusions of the respective arteries **(bottom)**. The four grades of *shading* from light to dark indicate the size of the involved region as small, medium, large, and very large, respectively. (From Califf RM, Mark DB, Wagner GS. Acute coronary care in the thrombolytic era. 1st ed. Chicago: Year Book, 1988:20–21.)

cated in Figure 9.5.[8] Note that two areas are indicated in the posterolateral quadrant because occlusion may be in the main left circumflex artery (LCX) (top area of the quadrant) or a large (marginal) branch of the artery (bottom area of the quadrant). The relationships among the coronary artery, left-ventricular quadrant, sectors of that quadrant, and diagnostic ECG leads are indicated in Table 9.1.

Table 9.1.   Injury Terminology Relationships

Coronary Artery	LV Quadrant	Sectors	Diagnostic Leads	Common Terms
Left anterior descending	Anteroseptal	All	V1–V3 (elevation)	Anterior
	Anterosuperior	All	I, aVL (elevation)	Lateral
	Inferior	Apical	V4-V6 (elevation)	Lateral
	Posterolateral	Apical	V4-V6 (elevation)	Lateral
Posterior descending	Inferior	Basal, middle	II, III, aVF (elevation)	Inferior
Left circumflex	Posterolateral	Basal, middle	V1-V3 (depression)	Posterior

In about 90% of individuals, the posterior descending coronary artery (PDA) originates from the right coronary artery (RCA) and the LCX supplies only part of a single left-ventricular quadrant. This has been termed *right coronary dominance*. In the other 10% of individuals, with left coronary dominance, the PDA originates from the LCX, and the RCA supplies only the right ventricle.

The basal and middle sectors of the posterior–lateral quadrant of the left ventricle typically supplied by the LCX and its branches are located distant from the positive poles of all 12 of the standard ECG leads. Therefore, posterior–lateral epicardial injury is typically indicated by depression rather than elevation of the ST segment in these leads (Fig. 9.6). Note that no ST-segment elevation is present in any standard lead. Additional leads on the posterior–lateral thorax would be required to record ST-segment elevation due to epicardial injury in this area.[9]

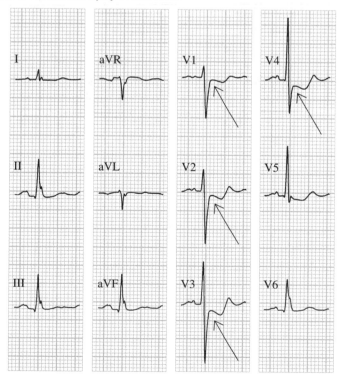

Figure 9.6.   A 12-lead ECG recorded after 1 minute of balloon occlusion in the mid-LCX of a 54-year-old man with symptoms of acute unstable angina. *Arrows* indicate the posterior epicardial injury appearing as ST-segment depression in leads V1 to V4.

Epicardial injury may also involve the thinner-walled right-ventricular myocardium when its blood supply via the RCA becomes insufficient. Right-ventricular epicardial injury is represented on the standard ECG as ST-segment elevation in lead V1 (Fig. 9.7). There may also be ST elevation in lead V2, but the elevation in lead V1 is greater than that in lead V2. There would be even greater elevation in the more rightward additional leads V3R and V4R than in lead V1, which could also be considered lead V2R.

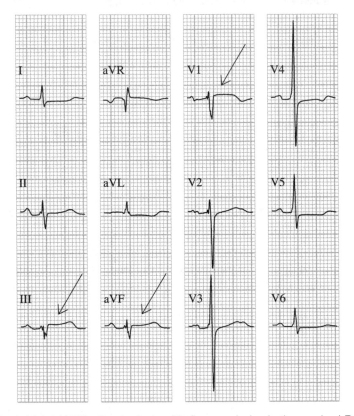

Figure 9.7. A 12-lead ECG after 1 minute of balloon occlusion in the proximal RCA in a 65-year-old woman presenting with acute precordial pain of sudden onset. *Arrows* indicate the inferior epicardial injury appearing as ST-segment elevation in leads III and aVF, and right-ventricular epicardial injury appearing as ST-segment elevation in lead V1.

As illustrated in Figure 9.2, the entire ST-segment elevation caused by PTCA disappears abruptly when epicardial injury persists for only the 1 to 2 minutes required for PTCA. However, epicardial injury produced by coronary thrombosis typically persists throughout the minutes to hours required for clinical administration of some form of reperfusion therapy, and then only resolves gradually after the restoration of blood flow. Figure 9.8A illustrates the resolution of ST-segment elevation in the anterior precordial leads (V2 and V4) following angiographically documented thrombolysis in the left anterior descending coronary artery (LAD) at 2 h after the onset of acute precordial pain. The disappearance of epicardial injury may reveal the already developed QRS-complex changes of infarction that were previously obscured by the injury current. In some patients, multiple episodes of ST-segment elevation and resolution (e.g., in precordial leads V2 and V4

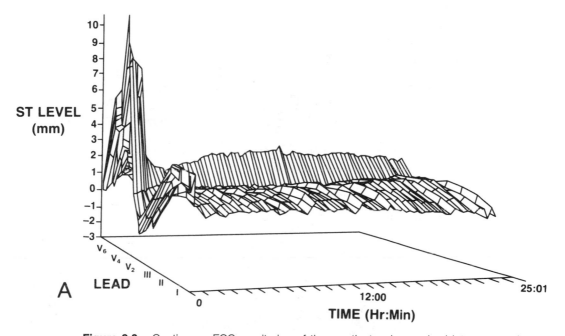

Figure 9.8. Continuous ECG monitoring of three patients who received intravenous thrombolytic therapy after presenting with ECG evidence of acute epicardial injury. The magnitude of ST-segment deviation (in millimeters) is indicated on the y axis, in each of the six representative ECG leads indicated on the x axis, over the periods of time following initiation of the therapy, as indicated on the z axis. (**A** from Krucoff MW, Wagner NB, Pope JE, et al. The portable programmable microprocessor-driven real-time 12-lead electrocardiographic monitor: a preliminary report of a new device for the noninvasive detection of successful reperfusion or silent coronary reocclusion. Am J Cardiol 1990;65:143–148, with permission. **B** and **C** from Krucoff MW, Croll MA, Pope JE, et al. Continuous 12-lead ST-segment recovery analysis in the TAMI 7 study. Circulation 1993;88;437–446, with permission. Copyright 1993 American Heart Association.)

in Figure 9.8*B*) have been documented by continuous monitoring after the initiation of intravenous thrombolytic therapy (Fig. 9.8*B*). In the absence of successful thrombolytic therapy, there is eventual gradual resolution of the ST-segment elevation (e.g., in limb leads II and III in Figure 9.8*C*) as the area with epicardial injury becomes infarcted.[10,11]

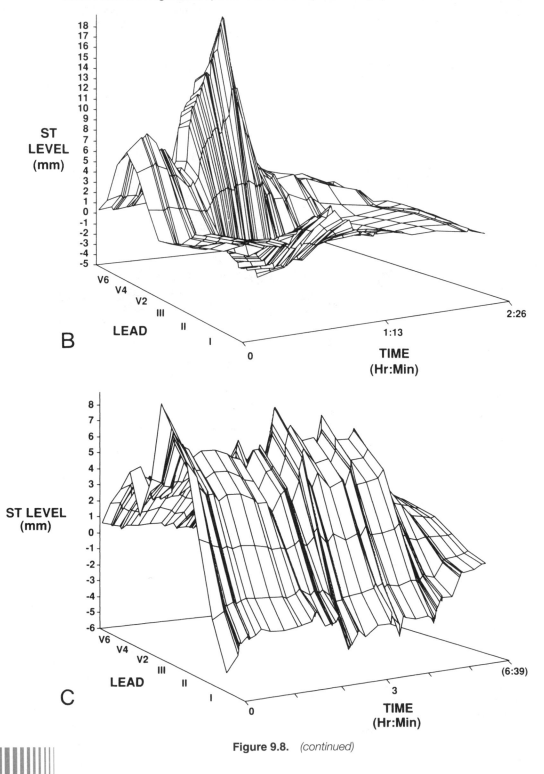

Figure 9.8. *(continued)*

CHANGES IN THE T WAVE

Just as changes in the T wave are unreliable indicators of ischemia caused by increased myocardial demand, they are also unreliable indicators of ischemia from insufficient coronary blood supply. Figure 9.9 presents the changes in ST segments and T waves immediately after acute balloon inflation in the LAD of two patients. In both examples the ECG waveform axes of the ST segments and T waves deviate toward the involved anterior aspect of the left ventricle. In some patients, the degree of deviation of the T-wave axis is similar to that of the ST segment (Fig. 9.9A), and should therefore be considered secondary. In other patients there is the markedly greater deviation of the T-wave axis that is characteristic of hyperacute T waves, as in Figure 9.9B. These primary T-wave elevations typically persist for only a brief period after acute coronary thrombosis.[12] Hyperacute T waves may therefore be useful in timing the duration of epicardial injury when a patient presents with acute precordial pain.

Sclarovsky and colleagues have introduced an ECG method for grading the severity of acute ischemia caused by decreased blood supply, as follows: Grade I = hyperacute T waves only; Grade II = elevation of the ST segment with or without hyperacute T waves but with preserved appearance of the QRS complex; and Grade III = distortion of the terminal portion of the QRS complex by disappearance of the S wave, as in Figure 9.9B. This grading scale indicates the amount of protection against ischemia provided by either collateral flow or metabolic "preconditioning" developed in response to prior ischemia (Grade I = most protected and Grade III = least protected). The greater the protection, the longer the time that can elapse before infarction occurs.[13]

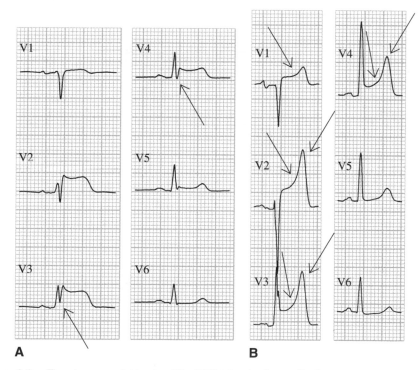

Figure 9.9. The six precordial leads of the ECG after 1 minute of balloon occlusion of the LAD in **A:** a 74-year-old woman with a 5-year history of exertional angina; and **B:** a 51-year-old man with an initial episode of precordial pain. *Arrows* indicate ST-segment elevation and hyperacute T waves in **A** and disappearance of the S wave from below the TP-PR segment baseline in **B**.

Definition of the amplitude of the T wave required to identify the hyperacute changes that occur alone in ischemia of Grade I severity or that accompany epicardial injury in ischemia of Grade II severity requires reference to the upper limits of T-wave amplitudes in the various ECG leads of normal subjects. Table 9.2 presents the upper limits of T-wave amplitudes (in millivolts) in each of the 12 standard ECG leads for females and males in the over-40-year-old age group in the normal data base from Glasgow, Scotland.[14] A rough estimate of the normal upper limits of T-wave amplitude would be at least 0.50 mV in the limb leads and at least 1.00 mV in the precordial leads. Amplitudes exceeding these limits are required to identify the hyperacute T waves that may appear during the earliest phase of acute transmural ischemia.

Table 9.2.[a, b]   T Wave Amplitude Limits

Lead	Males 40–49	Females 40–49	Males 50+	Females 50+
aVL	0.30	0.30	0.30	0.30
I	0.55	0.45	0.45	0.45
-aVR	0.55	0.45	0.45	0.45
II	0.65	0.55	0.55	0.45
aVF	0.50	0.40	0.45	0.35
III	0.35	0.30	0.35	0.30
V1	0.65	0.20	0.50	0.35
V2	1.45	0.85	1.40	0.70
V3	1.35	0.85	1.35	0.85
V4	1.15	0.85	1.10	0.75
V5	0.90	0.70	0.95	0.70
V6	0.65	0.55	0.65	0.50

[a] Modified from Macfarlane PW, Lawrie TDV. In: *Comprehensive electrocardiology.* vol. 3. New York: Pergamon Press, 1989:1446–1457.
[b] Presentation of upper-limit T-wave amplitudes (in millivolts rounded to the nearest 0.05) in each lead by gender and age for normal subjects from Glasgow, Scotland. The leads are arranged in the panoramic sequence.

CHANGES IN THE QRS COMPLEX

 The ECG manifestation of epicardial injury, like that of the SEI described previously, begins during the QRS complex. This may result in secondary deviation of the waveforms of the QRS complex in the same direction as that of the waveforms of the ST segments, as illustrated in balloon inflation 2 of Figure 9.10. The deviation affects the amplitudes of the later QRS waveforms to a greater extent than those of the earlier QRS waveforms.[15] During inflation 1, the distortion of the QRS complex is much greater than could be produced by the current of the injury. A primary alteration in the mid- and late QRS waveforms is apparent.[15]

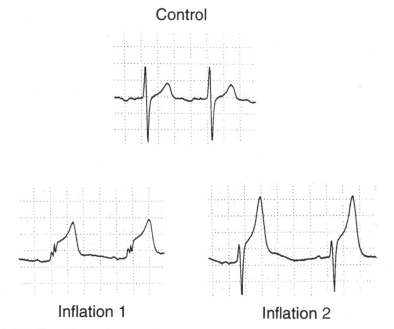

Figure 9.10. Recordings of two cardiac cycles in lead V2 from baseline (control) and after 2 minutes each of two different periods of balloon occlusion of the LAD (From Wagner NB, Sevilla DC, Krucoff MW, et al. Transient alterations of the QRS complex and the ST segment during percutaneous transluminal balloon angioplasty of the left anterior descending coronary artery. Am J Cardiol 1988;62:1038–1042, with permission.)

The primary changes in the QRS complexes in acute ischemia of Grade III severity may occur after the onset of epicardial injury, as seen in inflation 1 of Figures 9.10 and 9.11. The deviation of the axis of the QRS complex toward the area of epicardial injury is considered primary because the change in amplitude of the QRS-complex waveforms is greater than that of the ST-segment waveforms (lead V2 of Fig. 9.11B). The duration of the QRS complex may also be prolonged as in the patient whose ECG is shown in the figure. Typically, acute ischemia of a higher grade of severity (Sclarovsky Grade III) occurs during initial balloon occlusion when either collateral arteries or preconditioning provide the least protection. The most likely cause of the primary deviation of the QRS complex is an ischemia-induced delay in myocardial electrical activation. The epicardial layer of the area with epicardial injury is activated late, thereby producing an unopposed positive QRS-complex waveform. With epicardial injury in the posterior–lateral left ventricle, the QRS complex would deviate in the negative direction in leads V1–V3.[16]

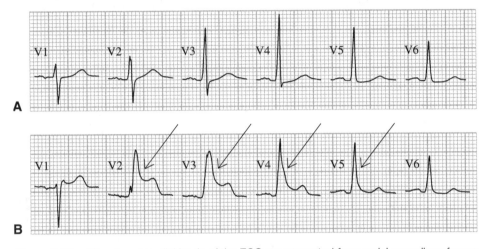

Figure 9.11. The six precordial leads of the ECG are presented from serial recordings from a 64-year-old man with acute unstable angina. **A:** Baseline recording prior to angiography after pain had resolved. **B:** After 2 minutes of the initial balloon occlusion of the LAD. *Arrows* indicate the increased duration of the QRS complex in **B** that is is apparent in leads V2 to V5.

The deviation of the ST segments in epicardial injury confounds measurement of the amplitudes of the QRS-complex waveforms of the ECG because there are no longer isoelectric PR-ST-TP segments. As illustrated in Figure 9.12, the baseline of the PR segment remains as the reference for the initial waveform of the QRS complex, but with secondary deviation of the QRS complex, the terminal waveform maintains its relationship with the ST-segment baseline. The amplitude of the S wave measured from the ST-segment baseline is the same in Figure 9.12*A* and *B*. With primary distortion of the QRS complex, even this relationship is absent. Methods such as that of Sclarovsky and colleagues, which require waveform quantitation of the QRS complex, use the TP-PR level for reference.

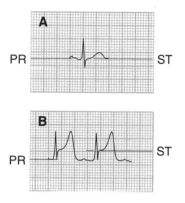

Figure 9.12. **A:** An ECG recording made before balloon inflation, in which the PR and ST baselines are at the same level and a 0.03-mV S wave is present. **B:** During balloon occlusion, the ST segment is elevated by 0.03 mV by the epicardial injury current, and the S wave also deviates upward so that it just reaches the PR-segment baseline.

GLOSSARY

Epicardial injury: transmural ischemia or pericardial irritation causing deviation of the ST segments of the ECG.

Left coronary dominance: an unusual coronary artery anatomy in which the PDA is a branch of the LCX.

Reciprocal: a term referring to deviation of the ST segments in the opposite direction from that of their maximal deviation.

Right coronary dominance: the usual coronary artery anatomy in which the PDA is a branch of the right coronary artery.

REFERENCES

1. Prinzmetal M, Goldman A, Massumi RA, et al. Clinical implications of errors in electrocardiographic interpretations: heart disease of electrocardiographic origin. JAMA 1956;161:138.
2. Levine HD. Non-specificity of the electrocardiogram associated with coronary artery disease. Am J Med 1953;15:344.
3. Marriott HJL. Coronary mimicry: normal variants, and physiologic, pharmacologic and pathologic influences that simulate coronary patterns in the electrocardiogram. Ann Intern Med 1960;52:411.
4. Vincent GM, Abildskov JA, Burgess MJ. Mechanisms of ischemic ST-segment displacement: evaluation by direct current recordings. Circulation 1977; 56:559–566.
5. Kleber AG, Janse MF, van Capelle FJL, Durrer D. Mechanism and time course of S–T and T–Q segment changes during acute regional myocardial ischemia in the pig heart determined by extracellular and intracellular recordings. Circ Res 1978;48:603–613.
6. Janse MJ, Cinca J, Morena H, et al. The "border zone" in myocardial ischemia: an electrophysiological, metabolic and histochemical correlation in the pig heart. Circ Res 1979;44:576–588.
7. Sgarbossa EB, Pinski SL, Barbagelata A, et al. Electrocardiographic diagnosis of evolving acute myocardial infarction in the presence of left bundle-branch block. N Engl J Med 1996; 334:481–487.
8. Wagner GS, Wagner NB. The 12-lead ECG and the extent of myocardium at risk of acute infarction: anatomic relationships among coronary, Purkinje, and myocardial anatomy. In: Califf RM, Mark DB, Wagner GS, eds. Acute coronary care in the thrombolytic era. Chicago: Year Book, 1988:20–21.
9. Seatre HA, Startt-Selvester RH, Solomon JC, et al. 16-lead ECG changes with coronary angioplasty: location of ST-T changes with balloon occlusion of five arterial perfusion beds. J Electrocardiol 1991;24 [Suppl]:153–162.
10. Krucoff MW, Croll MA, Pope JE, et al. Continuously updated 12-lead ST-segment recovery analysis for myocardial infarct artery patency assessment and its correlation with multiple simultaneous early angiographic observations. Am J Cardiol 1993;71:145–151.
11. Kondo M, Tamura K, Tanio H, et al. Is ST segment re-elevation associated with reperfusion an indicator of marked myocardial damage after thrombolysis? J Am Coll Cardiol 1993;21:62–67.
12. Dressler W, Roesler H. High T waves in the earliest stage of myocardial infarction. Am Heart J 1947; 34:627–645.
13. Sclarovsky S, ed. Electrocardiography of acute myocardial ischemic syndromes. London: Martin Dunitz, 1999.
14. Macfarlane PW, Lawrie TDV, eds. Comprehensive electrocardiography. New York: Pergamon Press, 1989: 1446–1457.
15. Wagner NB, Sevilla DC, Krucoff MW, et al. Transient alterations of the QRS complex and ST segment during percutaneous transluminal balloon angioplasty of the left anterior descending artery. Am J Cardiol 1988;62: 1038–1042.
16. Selvester RH, Wagner NB, Wagner GS. Ventricular excitation during percutaneous transluminal angioplasty of the left anterior descending coronary artery. Am J Cardiol 1988;62:1116–1121.

CHAPTER 10

Myocardial Infarction

CHANGES IN THE QRS COMPLEX

When insufficient coronary blood supply persists after myocardial energy reserves have been depleted, the myocardial cells become irreversibly ischemic and the process of necrosis termed "myocardial infarction" occurs.[1,2] The QRS complex is the most useful aspect of the electrocardiogram (ECG) for evaluating the presence, location, and extent of myocardial infarction. As indicated in Chapter 9 ("Ischemia and Injury Due to Insufficient Blood Supply"), almost immediately after a complete coronary artery occlusion, the QRS axis deviates toward the involved myocardial region; secondarily as a result of the epicardial current of injury and primarily because of a delay in myocardial activation. Because the process of infarction begins in the most poorly perfused subendocardial layer of the myocardium, the initial deviation of the QRS complex toward the involved region is replaced by deviation of the initial QRS waveforms away from the infarcted region.[3] Absence of any electrical activation of the infarcted myocardium has replaced the delayed activation of the severely ischemic myocardium, as illustrated in Figure 10.1A and B. Note that the infarction has shifted the arrow that indicates the summated QRS forces at 0.02 to 0.03 s (20 to 30 ms) away from the anterior myocardium and overlying precordium.

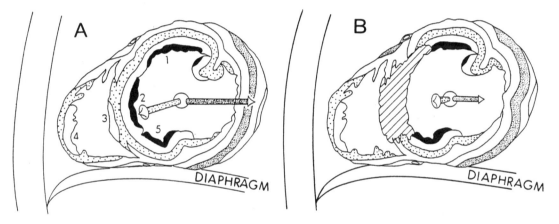

Figure 10.1. Schematic cross-sections of the right and left ventricles with isochronic lines at 10-ms intervals, viewed from an apical perspective. The anterior precordium is at the left in both **A** and **B**. The normal sequence of activation **(A)** is contrasted with the abnormal sequence resulting from an anterior infarction (*hatched area* in **B**). The numbers in **A** indicate the sites of the endocardial insertions of the anterior (*1*), and posterior fascicles (*2*), and the septal fibers (*5*) of the left bundle branch, and the septal (*3*) and right-ventricular (*4*) fibers of the right bundle branch. The 0- to 10-ms isochrones are in *black*, the 20- to 30-ms isochrones are in light *stippling*, and the 50- to 60-ms isochrones are in *dark stippling*. The *arrows* indicate the summated directions of the 20- to 30-ms isochrones before and after anterior infarction. (From Selvester RH, Wagner NB, Wagner GS. Ventricular excitation during percutaneous transluminal angioplasty of the left anterior descending coronary artery. Am J Cardiol 1988;62:1117–1120, with permission.)

The evolving appearance of the abnormalities of the QRS complex produced by an *anterior infarction* during continuous monitoring for ischemia are illustrated in Figure 10.2. Secondary changes in the morphology of the QRS complex during epicardial injury have shifted the axis of the complex toward the anterior left-ventricular wall. Myocardial reperfusion is accompanied by rapid resolution of the epicardial injury and a shift of the axis of the QRS complex away from the anterior left-ventricular wall. Although it may appear that the reperfusion itself has caused the infarction, it is much more likely that the infarction had already occurred before initiation of the therapy that led to reperfusion, but that its detection on the ECG was obscured by the secondary changes of the QRS complex caused by the epicardial injury.

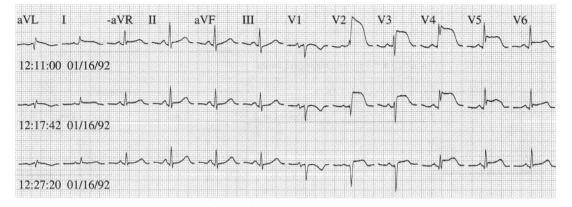

Figure 10.2. Continuous ECG monitoring during the first 27 minutes of intravenous thrombolytic therapy (begun at 12:00:00) in a 69-year-old man with acute thrombotic occlusion of the LAD. The 12 standard leads of the ECG are presented in the panoramic format after 11, 17, and 27 minutes of therapy.

Epicardial injury involving the thin right-ventricular free wall may be manifested on the ECG by deviation of the ST segment (Chapter 9, "Ischemia and Injury Due to Insufficient Blood Supply"), but right-ventricular infarction is not manifested by significant alteration of the QRS complex. This is because activation of the right-ventricular free wall is insignificant in comparison with activation of the thicker interventricular septum and left-ventricular free wall. Myocardial infarction evolves from epicardial injury in the distal aspects of the left-ventricular myocardium supplied by one of the three major coronary arteries, as previously illustrated in Table 9.1 and Figure 9.5.[4]

QRS COMPLEX CRITERIA FOR DIAGNOSING INFARCTION

 ## Abnormal Q Waves

The initial portion of the axis of the QRS complex deviates most prominently away from the area of infarction and is represented on the ECG by a prolonged Q-wave duration. As presented in Figure 3.4, the initial QRS waveform may normally be negative in all leads except V1 to V3. The presence of any Q wave is considered abnormal only in these three of the 12 standard ECG leads. Table 10.1 indicates the upper limits of normal of the Q wave duration in the various ECG leads.[5] The duration of the Q wave should be the primary measurement used in the definition of abnormality, because the amplitudes of the individual QRS waveforms vary with the overall amplitude of the QRS complex. As discussed in the next section, Q-wave amplitude should be considered abnormal only in relation to the amplitude of the following R wave.

Table 10.1.[a] **Wave Duration Limits**

Limb Leads		Precordial Leads	
Lead	Upper Limit	Lead	Upper Limit
I	<0.03 s	V1	Any Q
II	<0.03 s	V2	Any Q
III	None	V3	Any Q
aVR	None	V4	<0.02 s
aVL	<0.03 s	V5	<0.03 s
aVF	<0.03 s	V6	<0.03 s

[a] Modified from Wagner GS, Freye CJ, Palmeri ST, Roark SF, Stack NC, Ideker RE, Harrell FE Jr, Selvester RH. Evaluation of a QRS scoring system for estimating myocardial infarct size. I. Specificity and observer agreement. Circulation 1982;65:345.

Many cardiac conditions other than myocardial infarction are capable of producing abnormal initial QRS waveforms. As indicated in Chapters 4 to 6 ("Abnormal Wave Morphology," "Intraventricular Conduction Abnormalities," and "Ventricular Preexcitation"), ventricular hypertrophy, intraventricular conduction abnormalities, and ventricular preexcitation commonly prolong the duration of the Q wave. The term "Q wave" as used here also refers to the Q-wave equivalent of abnormal R waves in leads such as V2 and V3. Therefore, the following steps should be considered in the evaluation of Q waves for the presence of myocardial infarction:

1. Are abnormal Q waves present in any lead?
2. Are criteria present for other cardiac conditions that can produce abnormal Q waves?
3. Does the extent of Q-wave abnormality exceed that which could have been produced by some other cardiac condition?

Abnormal R Waves

The deviation of the QRS axis away from the area of a myocardial infarction may, in the absence of abnormal Q waves, be represented by diminished R waves. Table 10.2 indicates the leads in which R waves of less than a certain amplitude or duration may be indicative of myocardial infarction.[6]

Table 10.2.   R Wave Lower Limits

Limb Leads		Precordial Leads	
Lead	Criteria for Abnormal	Lead	Criteria for Abnormal
I	R amp ≤ 0.20 mV[a]	V1	None
II	None	V2	R dur ≤ 0.01 s or amp ≤ 0.10 mV
III	None	V3	R dur ≤ 0.02 s or amp ≤ 0.20 mV
aVR	None	V4	R amp ≤ 0.70 mV or ≤ Q amp
aVL	R amp ≤ Q amp	V5	R amp ≤ 0.70 mV or ≤ 2 × Q amp
aVF	R amp ≤ 2 × Q amp	V6	R amp ≤ 0.60 mV or ≤ 3 × Q amp

[a] amp, amplitude; dur, duration.

Infarction in the posterior–lateral region of the left ventricle is represented by a positive rather than a negative deviation of the QRS complex. This results in an increased rather than a decreased R-wave duration and amplitude in precordial leads V1 and V2[7] (Table 10.3)

Table 10.3.   R Wave Upper Limits

Lead	Criteria for Abnormal
V1	R dur ≥ 0.04 s, R amp ≥ 0.60 mV, R amp ≥ S amp
V2	R dur ≥ 0.05 s, R amp ≥ 1.50 mV, R amp ≥ 1.5 × S amp

QRS COMPLEX CRITERIA FOR LOCALIZING INFARCTION

Table 10.4 indicates the relationships among the coronary arteries, left-ventricular quadrants, and ECG leads that provide a basis for localizing myocardial infarctions.[4] It may also be helpful to continually refer back to figure 9.5 as this learning unit is read.

Table 10.4. Infarction Terminology Relationships

Coronary Artery	LV Quadrant	Sectors	Diagnostic Leads	Common Terms
Left arterior descending	Anteroseptal	All	V1-V3 (away (from)	Arterior
	Anterosuperior	All	I, aVL (away from)	Lateral
	Inferior	Apical	V4-V6 (away from)	Lateral
	Posterolateral	Apical	V4-V6 (away from)	Lateral
Posterior descending	Inferior	Basal, middle	II, III, aVF (away from)	Inferior
Left circumflex	Posterolateral	Basal, middle	V1-V3 (toward)	Posterior

An infarct produced by insufficient blood flow via the left anterior descending coronary artery (LAD) and limited to the anterior–septal quadrant (Fig. 10.3A) is termed an "anterior infarct." When the infarct extends into the anterior–superior quadrant (Fig. 10.3B) and/or into the apical sectors of other quadrants (Fig. 10.3C) it is commonly referred to as an "anterior–*lateral*" infarct. Although these two additional myocardial regions that may be infarcted by occlusion of the LAD are anatomically separate from one another, they commonly share the same "lateral" designation.

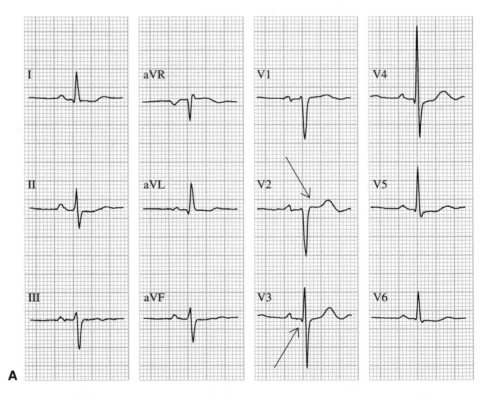

A

Figure 10.3. Twelve-lead ECGs from a 75-year-old man with a previous anterior infarct **(A)**, a 61-year-old man with a previous anterior infarct involving the anterosuperior quadrant **(B)**, and a 55-year-old man with a previous anterior infarct involving multiple apical sectors **(C)**. *Arrows* indicate the abnormal initial QRS forces (Q waves or diminished R waves).

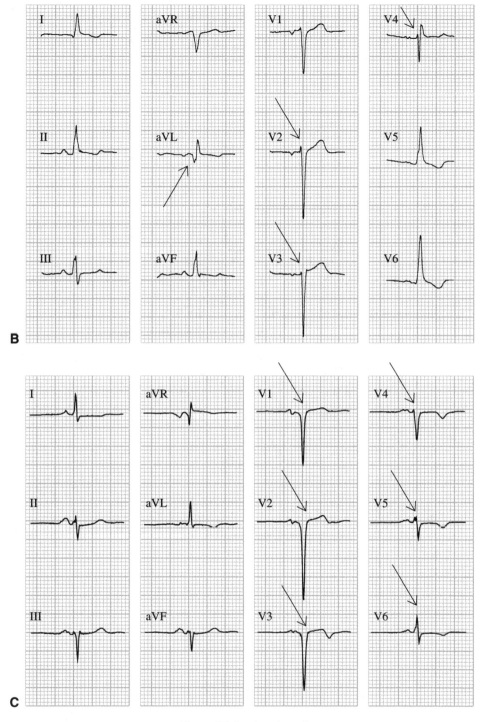

Figure 10.3. *(continued)*

In most individuals, the right coronary artery (RCA) is "dominant" (supplying the posterior descending artery), and its sudden complete obstruction typically produces an "*inferior*" infarction involving the basal and middle sectors of the inferior quadrant (Fig. 10.4). Abnormal Q waves appear only in the three limb leads with inferiorly oriented positive poles (leads II, III, and aVF).

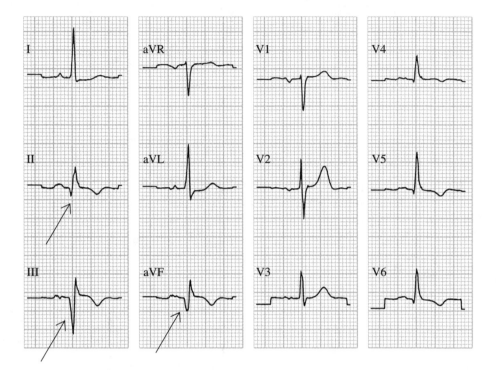

Figure 10.4. A 12-lead ECG from a 72-year-old woman 3 days after an acute inferior myocardial infarction. *Arrows* indicate abnormal Q waves.

Also, when the RCA is dominant, the typical distribution of the left circumflex artery (LCX) supplies only the left-ventricular free wall between the distributions of the anterior and posterior descending arteries. The basal and middle sectors of this posterior–lateral quadrant are located away from the positive poles of all 12 of the standard ECG leads. Therefore, "*posterior*" infarction is indicated by a positive rather than a negative deviation of the QRS complex (Fig. 10.5). Additional leads on the posterior thorax would be required to record the elevation of the ST segment caused by epicardial injury and the negative deviation of the QRS complex caused by myocardial infarction in this region.[7]

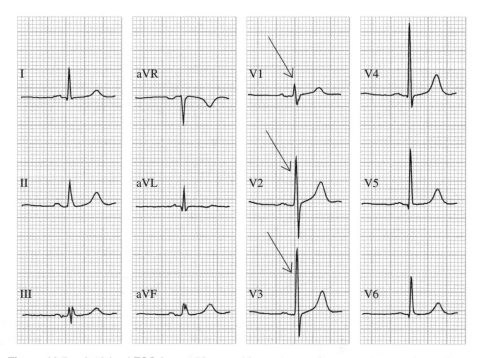

Figure 10.5. A 12-lead ECG from a 70-year-old man 1 year after an acute posterior-wall myocardial infarction. Coronary angiography showed complete occlusion of a non-dominant LCX (the RCA supplied the posterior descending artery). *Arrows* indicate the increased R waves in leads V1 to V3.

Figure 10.6 presents an example of the almost complete QRS-axis deviation away from the left-ventricular free wall that would be expected from more extensive posterior infarction. Note the almost completely positive QRS forces in leads V1 to V3 and the abnormal Q wave in lead V6.

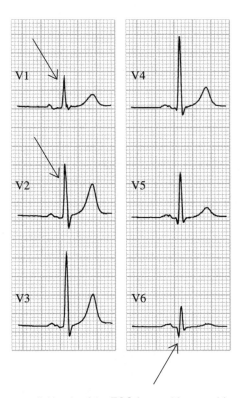

Figure 10.6. The six precordial leads of the ECG from a 63-year-old man 1 week after an acute posterior infarction. *Arrows* indicate the abnormal R waves in leads V1–V2 and the abnormal Q wave in lead V6.

When the left coronary artery (LCA) is dominant (supplying the posterior descending artery), a sudden complete obstruction of the RCA can produce infarction only in the right ventricle, which is not likely to produce changes in the QRS complex. The LCX supplies the middle and basal sectors of both the posterior–lateral and inferior quadrants, and its obstruction can produce an inferior–posterior infarction (Fig. 10.7). This same combination of left-ventricular locations can be involved when there is dominance of the RCA and one of its branches extends into the typical distribution of the LCX. The ECG in this instance indicates the region infarcted, but not whether the RCA or the LCX is the "culprit artery."

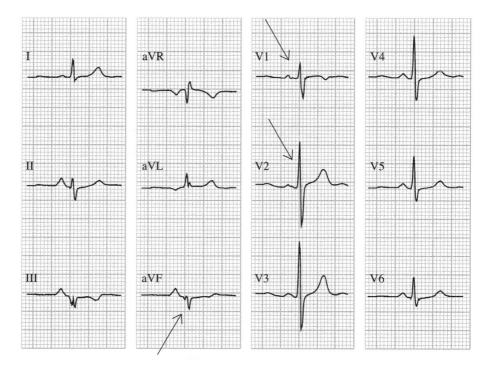

Figure 10.7. A 12-lead ECG from a 70-year-old woman with a healed inferior–posterior infarction. *Arrows* indicate the abnormal Q wave in lead aVF and abnormally prominent R waves in leads V1–V2.

The posterior region of the apex of the heart may be involved when either a dominant RCA or LCX is acutely obstructed, and inferior, posterior, and apical locations of infarctions are apparent on the ECG, as illustrated in Figure 10.8. A baseline ECG is shown in Figure 10.8A without abnormal QRS forces. The ECG at the time of hospital admission (Fig. 10.8B) already shows abnormal Q waves, and the recording at hospital discharge (Fig. 10.8C) shows that an abnormally prominent R wave has appeared in leads V1 and V2.

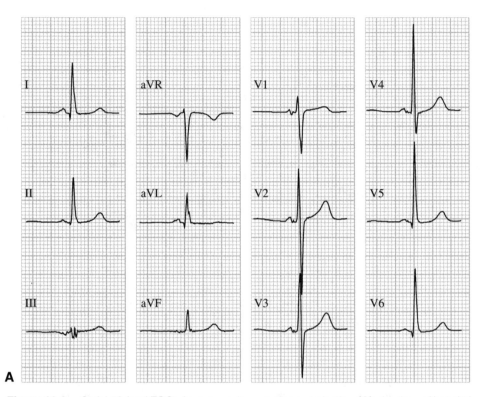

A

Figure 10.8.   Serial 12-lead ECGs from a previous routine examination **(A)**, the time of hospital admission **(B)**, and the time of hospital discharge of an 81-year-old man **(C)**. *Arrows* indicate abnormal initial QRS forces in **B** and **C**.

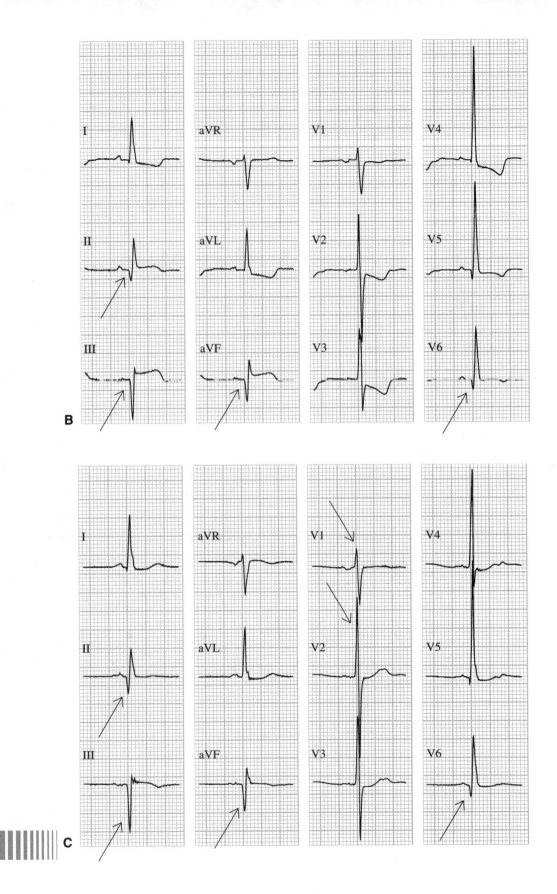

QRS COMPLEX CRITERIA FOR ESTIMATING INFARCT SIZE

An individual patient may have single or multiple infarcts in the regions of any of the three major coronary arteries. Selvester and coworkers developed a method for estimating the total percentage of the left ventricle that is infarcted by using a weighted scoring system.[8] Computerized simulation of the sequence of electrical activation of the normal human left ventricle provided the basis for their 31-point scoring system, with each point accounting for 3% of the left ventricle.[8,9] The Selvester QRS scoring system includes 50 criteria from 10 of the 12 standard ECG leads, with weights ranging from one to three points per criterion (Fig. 10.9). There are criteria in precordial leads V1 and V2 for both anterior and posterior infarct locations. In addition to the Q-wave and decreased R-wave criteria typically used for diagnosis and localization of infarcts, this system for estimating infarct size also contains criteria relating to the S wave.[6]

Complete 50-Criteria, 31-Point QRS Scoring System*

Lead	Maximum Lead Points	Criteria	Points
I	(2)	Q≥30 ms	(1)
		{ R/Q ≤1	(1)
		{ R≤0.2 mV	(1)
II	(2)	{ Q≥40 ms	(2)
		{ Q≥30 ms	(1)
aVL	(2)	Q≥30 ms	(1)
		R/Q ≤1	(1)
aVF	(5)	{ Q≥50 ms	(3)
		{ Q≥40 ms	(2)
		{ Q≥30 ms	(1)
		{ R/Q ≤1	(2)
		{ R/Q ≤2	(1)

V1
- Anterior (1): Any Q (1)
- Posterior (4): R/S ≥1 (1)
  - { R≥50 ms (2)
  - { R≥1.0 mV (2)
  - { R≥40 ms (1)
  - { R≥0.6 mV (1)
- Q and S≤0.3 mV (1)

V2
- Anterior (1):
  - { Any Q (1)
  - { R≤10 ms (1)
  - { R≤0.1 mV (1)
  - { R≤R V, mV (1)
- Posterior (4): R/S ≥1.5 (1)
  - { R≥60 ms (2)
  - { R≥2.0 mV (2)
  - { R≥50 ms (1)
  - { R≥1.5 mV (1)
- Q and S≤0.4 mV (1)

V3 (1)
- Any Q (1)
- R≤20 ms (1)
- R≤0.2 mV (1)

V4 (3)
- Q≥20 ms (1)
- { R/S ≤0.5 (2)
- { R/Q ≤0.5 (2)
- { R/S ≤1 (1)
- { R/Q ≤1 (1)
- { R≤0.7 mV (1)

V5 (3)
- Q≥30 ms (1)
- { R/S ≤1 (2)
- { R/Q ≤1 (2)
- { R/S ≤2 (1)
- { R/Q ≤2 (1)
- { R≤0.7 mV (1)

V6 (3)
- Q≥30 ms (1)
- { R/S ≤1 (2)
- { R/Q ≤1 (2)
- { R/S ≤3 (1)
- { R/Q ≤3 (1)
- { R≤0.6 mV (1)

Figure 10.9. The maximal number of points that can be awarded for each lead is shown in parentheses following each lead name (or left-ventricular region within a lead for leads V1 and V2), and the number of points awarded for each criterion is indicated in parentheses after each criterion name. The QRS criteria from 10 of the 12 standard ECG leads are indicated. Only one criterion can be selected from each group of criteria within a bracket. All criteria involving R/Q or R/S ratios consider the relative amplitudes of these waves. (Modified from Selvester RH, Wagner GS, Hindman NB. The Selvester QRS scoring system for estimating myocardial infarct size. The development and application of the system. Arch Intern Med 1985;145:1877–1881. Copyright 1985 American Medical Association.)

In the Selvester scoring system, Q-wave duration is heavily considered. This measurement is easy when the QRS complex has discrete Q and R waves, as illustrated in Figure 10.10A, B, C, E, and G.[6] The other panels in the figure (Fig. 10.10D and F) present small upward deflections in a generally negative QRS complex that cannot be termed R waves because they never reach the positive side of the baseline. This QRS-complex variation should be termed "QS." The true Q-wave duration should be measured along the ECG baseline from the onset of the initial negative deflection to the point directly at or above the peak of the notch in the negative deflection.

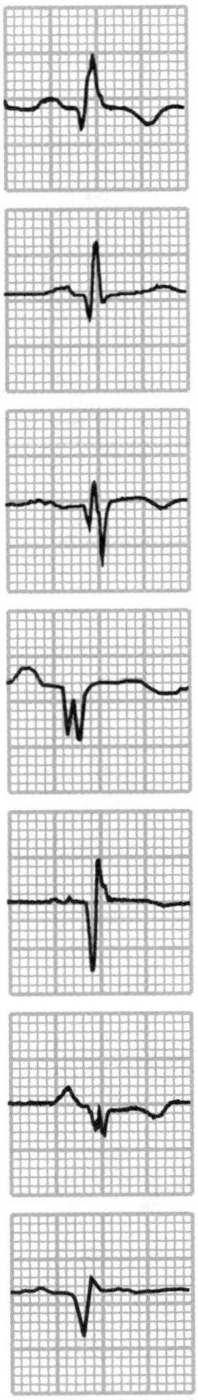

	LEAD aVF	Q DURATION	R/Q RATIO	TOTAL POINTS
A		.03 sec (1)		1
B		.03 sec (1)	≤2:1 (1)	2
C		.03 sec (1)	≤1:1 (2)	3
D		.03 sec (1)	≤1:1 (2)	3
E		.04 sec (2)	≤1:1 (2)	4
F		.04 sec (2)	≤1:1 (2)	4
G		≥.05 sec (3)	≤1:1 (2)	5

Figure 10.10. **A–G.** Variations in the appearance of the QRS complex in lead aVF representing the changes of inferior infarction. The numbers of QRS points awarded for the Q-wave duration and the R/Q amplitude ratio criteria met in the various ECGs given as examples are indicated in parentheses. The total number of QRS points awarded for lead aVF is indicated for each example in the final column. (Modified from Wagner GS, Freye CJ, Palmeri ST, et al. Evaluation of a QRS scoring system for estimating myocardial infarct size. I. Specificity and observer agreement. Circulation 1982;65:342–347.)

Satisfaction of only a single Selvester scoring criterion may represent either a normal variant or an extremely small infarct. Two infarcts located in opposite sectors of the left ventricle, however, may confound the application of this system. The opposing effects on the summation of the ventricular electrical forces may cancel each other, producing falsely negative ECG changes. Figure 10.11*A* and *B* illustrates the coexistence of both anterior and posterior infarcts and the potential for underestimation of the total percentage of the left ventricle that is infarcted. The 0.04 R wave in lead V1 indicates the posterior involvement, and the small Q wave preceding the R wave in leads V2 and V3 indicates the anterior involvement.

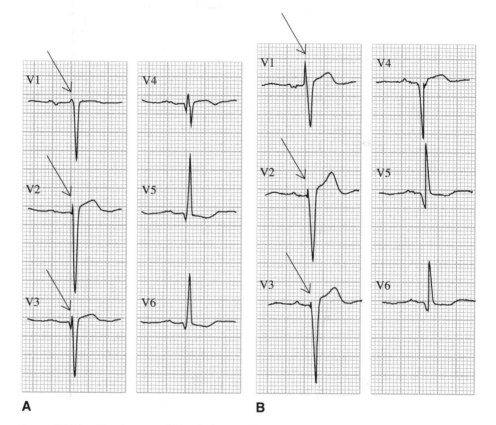

A　　　　　　　　　**B**

Figure 10.11. The 6 precordial leads from a 66-year-old man **(A)** and a 58-year-old man **(B)** with previous anterior and posterior infarcts. The arrows indicate the abnormal initial positive QRS waveform in lead V1 and the abnormal initial negative QRS waveforms in V2 and V3. Note there are also abnormal initial negative QRS waveforms in V4–V6 in both **A** and **B**.

A method has been developed for predicting final myocardial infarct size by quantitating initial changes in the ST segment. Aldrich and colleagues developed formulas for both anterior and inferior MI locations as follows:[10]

% anterior LV infarcted = 3[1.5 (number of leads with ST elevation − 0.4)]
% inferior LV infarcted = 3[0.6 (Σ ST elevation in leads II, III, aVF) + 2.0]

Abnormal Q waves already present on the initial ECG recorded from a patient with suspected acute infarction typically indicate that some of the involved myocardium has already been irreversibly damaged. Anderson and colleagues have developed an ECG acuteness score to augment the timing of acute symptom onset in guiding the clinician about the potential for myocardial salvage.[11] This is a two-step process, as follows:

1. The phase of the infarction process (from I A to II B) is determined in all leads with either ST-segment elevation or abnormally tall T waves (Tables 9.2):

   I = no abnormal Q waves; A = tall T waves; B = positive but not tall T waves.
   II = abnormal Q waves; A = tall T waves; B = positive but not tall T waves.

2. The overall acuteness score (from 4.0 to 1.0) is determined for the entire 12-lead ECG:

$$\frac{4(\text{\# leads I A}) + 3(\text{\# leads I B}) + 2(\text{\# leads II A}) + (\text{\# leads II B})}{\text{Total \# leads I A, I B, II A, or II B.}}$$

CHANGES IN THE ST SEGMENT

The changes in the ST segment that are prominent during epicardial injury typically disappear when the jeopardized myocardium either infarcts or regains sufficient perfusion. The time course of resolution of injury is shortened by reperfusion via the culprit artery, as discussed in Chapter 9 ("Ischemia and Injury Due to Insufficient Blood Supply"). When reelevation of the ST segments is observed, further epicardial injury is suggested and is typically limited to a particular region of the left ventricle. When the ST-segment elevation occurs in leads representing multiple left-ventricular regions, acute bleeding into the pericardium should be considered (Fig. 10.12).[12] This may be the first indication that an infarct has caused a myocardial rupture with leakage of blood into the pericardial sac. If this process remains undetected, cardiac arrest may result from *pericardial tamponade*, in which myocardial relaxation is restricted by the blood in the enclosed pericardial space. The ECG changes in such a case are similar to those of acute pericarditis, discussed in Chapter 11 ("Miscellaneous Conditions").

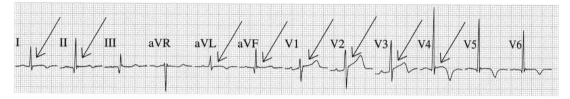

Figure 10.12. A 12-lead ECG from a 68-year-old man 4 days after thrombolytic therapy for an acute inferior infarction. Acute chest pain has returned. *Arrows* indicate ST-segment elevation in multiple leads.

In some patients, the ST-segment elevation does not completely resolve during the acute phase of a myocardial infarction (Fig. 10.13). This condition more commonly occurs with anterior infarcts than with those in the other locations in the left ventricle.[12] The lack of ST-segment resolution has been associated acutely with failure to reperfuse, and chronically with thinning of the left-ventricular wall caused by infarct expansion.[13,14] The extreme manifestation of infarct expansion (ventricular aneurysm) may be prevented by successful reperfusion therapy.

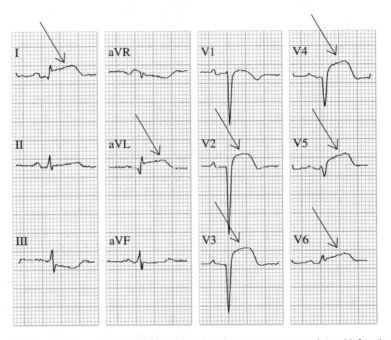

Figure 10.13. A 12-lead ECG obtained 2 weeks after an acute anterolateral infarction. *Arrows* indicate persistent ST-segment elevation without evolution of T-wave inversion.

CHANGES IN THE T WAVE

 The movement of the T-wave axis toward an area of epicardial injury, like that of the ST segment, resolves as the jeopardized myocardium either recovers or infarcts. Unlike the ST segment, however, the T waves do not typically return to their normal positions as the process of infarction evolves. The T waves move past the isoelectric baseline until they are directed away from the area of infarction.[15] They assume an appearance identical to that described in Chapter 7 ("Myocardial Ischemia, Injury, and Infarction") as "ischemic T waves," even though there is no ongoing myocardial ischemia. This evolution of the T-wave axis, from being directed toward the jeopardized region to being directed away from the infarcted region, is illustrated in Figure 10.14*A* and *B*. Typically, the terminal portion of the T wave is the first to become inverted, followed by the middle and initial portions.

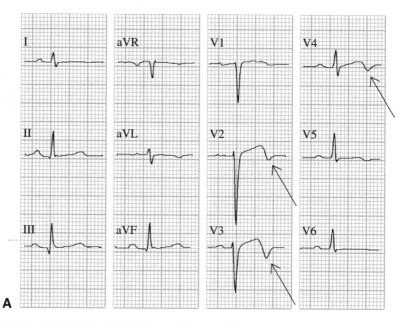

Figure 10.14. Serial 12-lead ECGs from a 64-year-old woman at 3 days **(A)** and 7 days **(B)** after an uncomplicated acute anterior infarction. *Arrows* indicate the terminal T-wave negativity by 3 days and total T-wave negativity by 7 days.

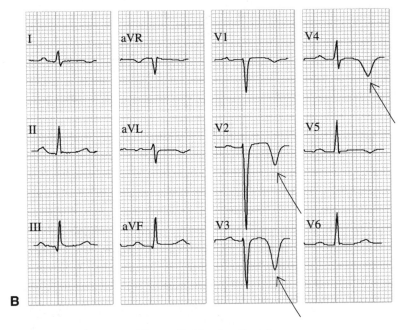

Figure 10.14. *(continued)*

Similarly, when the posterior–lateral quadrant of the left ventricle is involved, the T waves eventually become markedly positive. Figure 10.15 illustrates the prominent positive T waves in leads V1 and V2 that accompany the negative T waves in other leads during the healing phase of an inferior–posterior–lateral infarction.

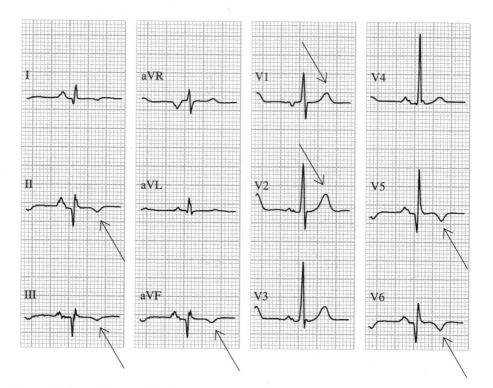

Figure 10.15. A 12-lead ECG from a 53-year-old man 5 days after an inferior–posterior–lateral infarction. *Arrows* indicate negative T waves in leads with abnormal Q waves but positive T waves in leads with abnormal R waves.

GLOSSARY

Anterior infarction: an infarction in the distribution of the LAD, involving primarily the middle and apical sectors of the anterior–septal quadrant of the left ventricle.

Apical infarction: an infarction in the distribution of any of the major coronary arteries, involving primarily the apical sectors of the posterior–lateral and inferior quadrants of the left ventricle.

Collateral blood supply: the perfusion of an area of myocardium via arteries that have developed to compensate for an obstruction of one of the principal coronary arteries.

Infarct expansion: partial disruption of the myocardial wall in the area of a recent infarction that results in thinning of wall and dilation of the involved chamber.

Inferior infarction: an infarction in the distribution of the posterior descending coronary artery, involving primarily the basal and middle sectors of the inferior quadrant of the left ventricle, but often extending into the posterior aspect of the right ventricle.

Lateral infarction: an infarction in the distribution of a "diagonal" or "marginal" coronary artery, involving primarily the basal and middle sectors of the anterior–superior quadrant of the left ventricle.

Myocardial rupture: complete disruption of the myocardial wall in the area of a recent infarction, resulting in leakage of blood out of the involved chamber.

Necrosis: death of a living tissue; termed an infarction when it is caused by insufficient supply of oxygen via the circulation.

Pericardial tamponade: filling of the pericardial sac with fluid, which restricts the relaxation of the cardiac chambers.

Posterior infarction: infarction in the distribution of the LCX, involving primarily the basal and middle sectors of the posterior–lateral quadrant of the left ventricle.

Ventricular aneurysm: the extreme of infarct expansion, in which the ventricular wall becomes so thin that it bulges outward (dyskinesia) during systole.

REFERENCES

1. Reimer KA, Lowe JE, Rasmussen MM, et al. The wavefront phenomenon of ischemic cell death: I. Myocardial infarct size vs. duration of coronary occlusion in dogs. Circulation 1977;56:786–794.
2. Reimer KA, Jennings RB. The "wavefront phenomenon" of myocardial ischemic cell death: II. Transmural progression of necrosis within the framework of ischemic bed size (myocardium at risk) and collateral flow. Lab Invest 1979;40:633–644.
3. Wagner NB, White RD, Wagner GS. The 12 lead ECG and the extent of myocardium at risk of acute infarction: cardiac anatomy and lead locations, and the phases of serial changes during acute occlusion. In: Califf RM, Mark DB, Wagner GS, eds. Acute coronary care in the thrombolytic era. Chicago: Year Book, 1988:36–41.
4. Wagner GS, Wagner NB. The 12-lead ECG and the extent of myocardium at risk of acute infarction: anatomic relationships among coronary, Purkinje, and myocardial anatomy. In: Califf RM, Mark DB, Wagner GS, eds. Acute coronary care in the thrombolytic era. Chicago: Year Book, 1988:16–30.
5. Wagner GS, Freye CJ, Palmeri ST, et al. Evaluation of a QRS scoring system for estimating myocardial infarct size. I. Specificity and observer agreement. Circulation 1982;65:342–347.
6. Hindman NB, Schocken DD, Widmann M, et al. Evaluation of a QRS scoring system for estimating myocardial infarct size. V. Specificity and method of application of the complete system. Am J Cardiol 1985;55:1485–1490.
7. Flowers NC, Horan LG, Sohi GS, et al. New evidence for inferior–posterior myocardial infarction on surface potential maps. Am J Cardiol 1976;38:576–581.
8. Selvester RH, Wagner JO, Rubin HB. Quantitation of myocardial infarct size and location by electrocardiogram and vectorcardiogram. In: Boerhave course in quantitation in cardiology. Leyden, The Netherlands: Leyden University Press, 1972:31.
9. Selvester RH, Soloman J, Sapoznikov D. Computer simulation of the electrocardiogram. In: Computer techniques in cardiology. New York: Marcel Dekker, 1979:417.
10. Aldrich HR, Wagner NB, Boswick J, et al: Use of initial ST segment deviation for prediction of final electrocardiographic size of acute myocardial infarcts. Am J Cardiol 1988;61:749–753.
11. Corey KE, Maynard C, Pahlm O, et al. Combined historical and electrocardiographic timing of acute anterior and inferior myocardial infarcts for prediction of reperfusion achievable size limitation. Am J Cardiol 1999;83:826–831.
12. Arvan S, Varat MA. Persistent ST-segment elevation and left ventricular wall abnormalities: 2-dimensional echocardiographic study. Am J Cardiol 1984;53:1542–1546.
13. Lindsay J Jr, Dewey RC, Talesnick BS, et al. Relation of ST segment elevation after healing of acute myocardial infarction to the presence of left ventricular aneurysm. Am J Cardiol 1984;54:84–86.
14. Oliva PB, Hammill SC, Edwards WD. Electrocardiographic diagnosis of post infarction regional pericarditis: ancillary observations regarding the effect of reperfusion on the rapidity and amplitude of T wave inversion after acute myocardial infarction. Circulation 1993;88:896–904.
15. Mandel WJ, Burgess MJ, Neville J Jr, et al. Analysis of T wave abnormalities associated with myocardial infarction using a theoretic model. Circulation 1968;38:178–188.

CHAPTER 11

Miscellaneous Conditions

The previous chapters in Section II of this book have presented the electrocardiographic waveform changes that represent abnormal conditions within the heart itself. The present chapter concludes the section on abnormal wave morphology by presenting seven miscellaneous conditions that can be diagnosed by interpretation of the electrocardiogram (ECG). This chapter begins with the general abnormalities of the myocardium (cardiomyopathies) and includes both the late effects of volume and pressure overloads (Chapter 4, "Chamber Enlargement") and insufficient blood supply (Chapters 7 to10, "Myocardial Ischemia and Infarction," "Ischemia and Injury Due to Increased Myocardial Demand," "Ischemia and Injury Due to Insufficient Blood Supply," and "Myocardial Infarction"). The following Learning Units consider the ECG waveform changes representing abnormalities of the pericardial linings of the heart and the other major intrathoracic organ, the lungs. Conditions affecting more remote parts of the body, including the brain and endocrine glands, and abnormal amounts of either internally produced or ingested substances in the circulating blood that may also be suspected or even diagnosed by ECG waveform changes, are considered in the final section of this chapter.

CARDIOMYOPATHIES

Cardiomyopathy is a general term applied to all conditions in which the myocardium does not function normally. The primary diagnostic classifications of cardiomyopathy are "ischemic" and "nonischemic." Ischemic cardiomyopathy may either be potentially reversible (*hibernating*) or irreversible (infarction), resulting in the ECG changes of ischemia, injury, and infarction discussed in Chapters 7 to10. *Hypertrophic cardiomyopathy* is a common nonischemic cardiomyopathy that occurs when a hypertrophied ventricle either fails to maintain or interferes with normal function. The hypertrophy may either be secondary to pressure overload (Chapter 4, "Chamber Enlargement") or may be a primary cardiac condition. Primary hypertrophic cardiomyopathy may involve both ventricles, one entire ventricle, or only a portion of one ventricle. A common localized variety of this condition is hypertrophic obstructive cardiomyopathy (HOCM), in which the hypertrophied interventricular septum obstructs the aortic outflow tract during systole, resulting in *subaortic stenosis*. HOCM is associated with many different ECG manifestations, none of which is typical.

A spectrum of ECG changes may occur in hypertrophic cardiomyopathy regardless of whether or not the problem is localized to the septum[1,2]:

1. Typical left-ventricular hypertrophy (LVH) (see Chapter 4, "Chamber Enlargement").
2. Marked LAD (see Chapter 3, "Interpretation of the Normal Electrocardiogram").
3. Deep, narrow Q waves in the leftward-oriented leads.
4. Atrial enlargement (see Chapter 4, "Chamber Enlargement").

The changes that may occur in HOCM are illustrated in Figure 11.1.

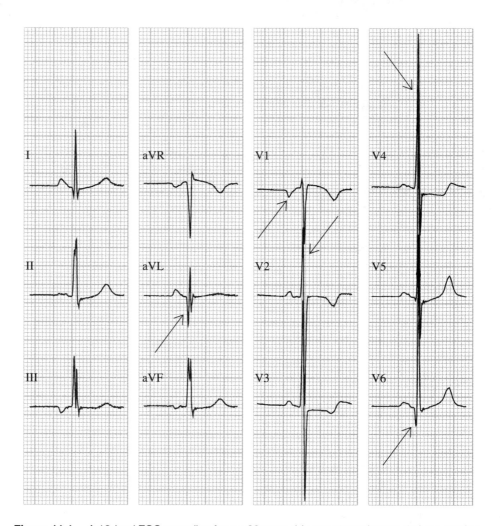

Figure 11.1. A 12-lead ECG recording from a 29-year-old asymptomatic man during a routine health evaluation. *Arrows* indicate the waveforms most characteristic of hypertrophic obstructive cardiomyopathy, including the prominent Q waves in leads aVL and V6, tall precordial R waves in leads V2 to V5, and increased terminal P-wave negativity in lead V1.

Amyloidosis

An abnormal protein called amyloid is deposited in the heart during various disease processes. Its accumulation causes cardiac amyloidosis, which eventually produces heart failure. Amyloidosis may be suspected when the following combination of ECG changes appears[3]:

1. Low voltage of all waveforms in the limb leads.
2. Marked left-axis deviation typical of left anterior fascicular block (LAFB).
3. QS or minimal R waves in leads V1 to V4.
4. A prolonged atrioventricular (AV) conduction time.

Characteristics 1 and 3 are apparent in the example presented in Figure 11.2.

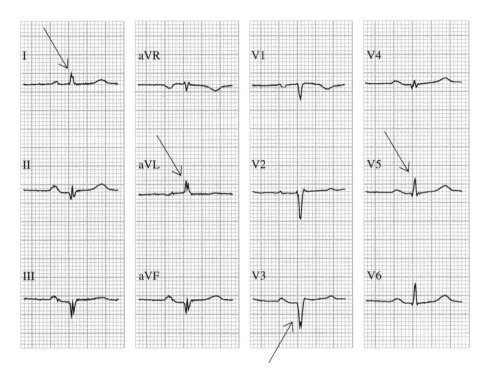

Figure 11.2. A 12-lead ECG recording from an 87-year-old man with severe heart failure but no history of ischemic heart disease. *Arrows* indicate the extremely low voltage in both limb and precordial leads. (From Marriott HJL. Correlations of electrocardiographic and pathologic changes. In: Pathology of the heart and blood vessels. Springfield, IL: Charles C Thomas, 1968.)

PERICARDIAL ABNORMALITIES

A small, fluid-filled space called the *pericardial sac* separates the heart from the other structures in the thorax. The sac is lined by two layers of connective tissue referred to as the *pericardium*. The innermost of these two layers (visceral pericardium) adheres to the myocardium, while the outer layer (parietal pericardium) encloses the pericardial fluid. These two layers of tissue can become inflamed for many reasons (*pericarditis*). The inflammation usually resolves after an acute phase, but may progress to a chronic phase. The acute phase may be complicated by the collection of excess pericardial fluid, a condition termed *pericardial effusion*. Chronic persistence of the inflammatory process may result in thickening of the pericardial tissues and is called *constrictive pericarditis*.

Acute Pericarditis

Typically, acute pericarditis persists for 3 or 4 weeks, and the ECG changes it produces evolve through two stages. The characteristic ECG abnormality during the earliest stage of acute pericarditis is elevation of the ST segments in many leads, accompanied by upright T waves (Fig. 11.3A).[4] Depression of the PR segment was also present in 28 of a series of 44 consecutive patients with acute pericarditis.[5] When the ST segments return to the isoelectric level, the ECG may appear normal (Fig. 11.3B).

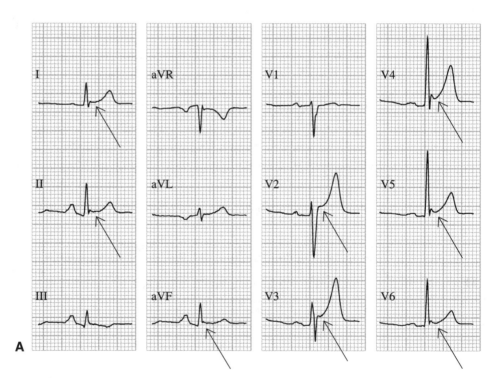

Figure 11.3. A 12-lead ECG recording from a 60-year-old man upon presenting to an emergency facility with acute chest pain **(A)** and 1 month after complete resolution of all symptoms **(B)**. *Arrows* indicate widespread ST-segment elevation in **A** and resolution to baseline level with T-wave inversion in **B**.

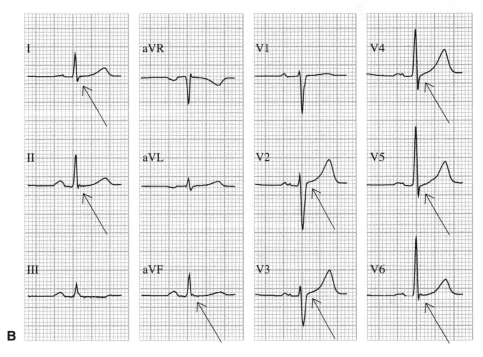

Figure 11.3. *(continued)*

More typically, when the ST-segment elevation resolves, there is progression to the second stage[6] of acute pericarditis, with widespread T-wave inversion, as in Figure 11.4.

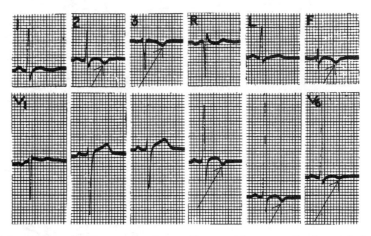

Figure 11.4. A 12-lead ECG recording from a 19-year-old woman after 1 week in the hospital with acute pericarditis. *Arrows* indicate T wave inversion in many leads.

The ST-segment elevation in the first stage of acute pericarditis occurs because the inflammation also involves the immediately adjacent epicardial layer of myocardium, producing the epicardial injury discussed in Chapter 9 ("Ischemia and Injury Due to Insufficient Blood Supply"). When the epicardial injury is caused by insufficient myocardial perfusion, the ST-segment elevation is restricted to the ECG leads that overlie the myocardial region supplied by the obstructed coronary artery. Pericarditis usually involves the entire epicardium, which results in ST-segment elevation in all of the standard leads except aVR. However, differentiation between acute pericarditis and acute epicardial injury becomes difficult when the pericarditis is localized, creating ST-segment elevation in only a few leads (Fig. 11.5). In both of these conditions, the patient may present with precordial pain, making an additional clinical evaluation necessary to reach the correct diagnosis.

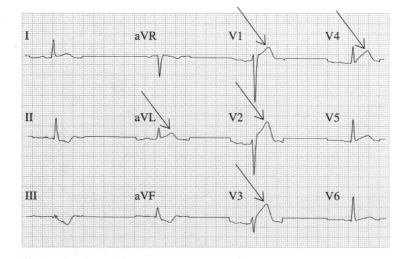

Figure 11.5. A 12-lead ECG recording from a 57-year-old woman with carcinoma of the breast and acute chest pain. *Arrows* indicate leads with ST-segment elevation.

Acute pericarditis must also be differentiated from early repolarization as a normal variant, discussed in Chapter 3 ("Interpretation of the Normal Electrocardiogram"). As Spodick[4] has suggested, pericarditis is more likely to present with:

1. ST-segment elevation in both the limb and precordial leads.
2. A frontal plane ST-segment axis to the left of the T-wave axis.
3. ST-segment depression in lead V1.

Figure 11.6 presents a typical example that could represent either a normal variant or the first stage of acute pericarditis.

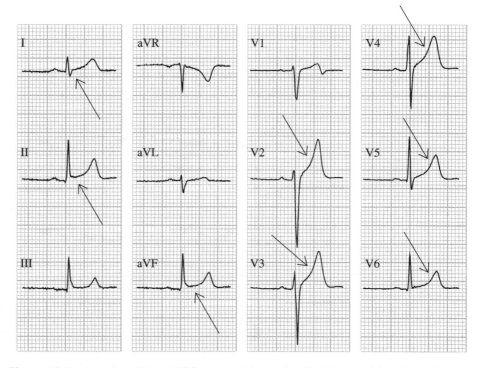

Figure 11.6. A routine 12-lead ECG recorded from a healthy 25-year-old male medical student. *Arrows* indicate the multiple leads with ST-segment elevation.

Pericardial Effusion and Chronic Constriction

Small and even moderate amounts of pericardial effusion or constriction may have little or no effect on the ECG. However, a generalized decrease in all of the ECG waveform amplitudes (low voltage) occurs if significant pericardial effusion or thickening develops. This probably occurs because the cardiac impulses are dampened by the pericardial fluid or fibrotic thickening. Since both of these pathologic conditions have similar effects on the cardiac electrical activity and its transmission to the body surface, they are considered together. A triad of ECG changes that is virtually diagnostic of pericardial effusion or constriction is presented below (Fig. 11.7):

1. Low voltage.
2. Widespread ST-segment elevation.
3. *Total electrical alternans*.

Total electrical alternans refers to the alternating high and low voltages of all ECG waveforms between cardiac cycles within a given lead.[7,8]

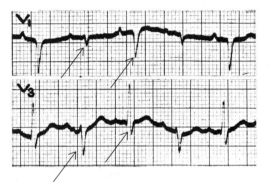

Figure 11.7. ECG leads V1 and V3 recorded from a 64-year-old man with carcinoma of the lung and malignant pericardial effusion. *Arrows* indicate the markedly different P wave and QRS-complex waveforms alternating on consecutive cardiac cycles.

Besides the foregoing ECG effects, chronic constrictive pericarditis may be accompanied by the T-wave inversion that defines the second stage of acute pericarditis.[9] The depth of inversion of the T waves has been reported to correlate with the degree of pericardial adherence to the myocardium.[10] This may be clinically important because surgical "stripping" of the thickened pericardium is more difficult when it is adhered tightly to the myocardium.

PULMONARY ABNORMALITIES

When a pulmonary abnormality creates an increased resistance to blood flow from the right side of the heart, a condition of systolic or pressure overload develops (Chapter 4, "Chamber Enlargement"). This condition has been termed *cor pulmonale*, and can occur either acutely or chronically. The most common cause of acute cor pulmonale is *pulmonary embolism*. Chronic cor pulmonale may be produced by the pulmonary congestion that occurs with left-ventricular failure or by the pulmonary hypertension that develops either as a primary disease or as a secondary disease to chronic obstructive pulmonary disease. Right-atrial enlargement commonly occurs with acute and chronic cor pulmonale. In the acute condition, there is right-ventricular dilation, whereas in the chronic condition there is right ventricular hypertrophy (RVH). Since chronic RVH is discussed in detail in Chapter 4 ("Chamber Enlargement"), only acute cor pulmonale is included here.

Chronic obstructive pulmonary disease is often characterized by emphysema, in which the lungs become overinflated. This produces anatomic changes that affect the ECG in unique ways, as presented in Table 11.1.

Table 11.1. Emphysema and the ECG

Anatomic Changes	ECG Changes
Compression of the heart into a more vertical position	Vertical P wave
Lowering of the diaphragm	Rightward QRS axis in the frontal plane
Increased volume of the thorax	Decreased amplitudes of ECG waveforms (low voltage)

The ECG changes of pulmonary emphysema may occur alone or in combination with the changes of RVH, since emphysema may or may not produce chronic cor pulmonale.

Acute Cor Pulmonale

In typical acute cor pulmonale, changes appear in the frontal-plane leads that mimic those in acute inferior myocardial infarction (Chapter 10, "Myocardial Infarction"). Lead III is mainly involved, with:

1. An increase in the size of the normal Q wave.
2. Slight ST-segment elevation.
3. Shallow inversion of the T wave.

In contrast to the case with inferior infarction, there are minimal if any changes in leads II and aVF. The size of the S wave is increased in lead I, indicating a rightward shift of the QRS axis, as seen in Figure 11.8.[11]

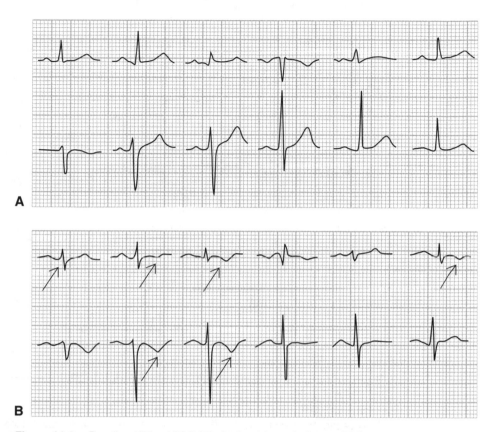

Figure 11.8. Baseline 12-lead ECG **(A)** obtained 1 year before an ECG recorded at the time of a documented pulmonary embolism **(B)**. The *arrow* in lead I indicates an increased S wave due to the rightward shift of the frontal-plane axis, and the *arrows* in leads II, III, aVF, and V2 to V3 indicate T-wave inversion. The limb leads above and precordial leads below are presented in their typical sequences in both **A** and **B**.

In the precordial leads, elevated ST segments and inverted T waves are sometimes seen over the right ventricle, while S waves may become more prominent over the left ventricle. The typical changes of right bundle-branch block (RBBB) may be apparent in lead V1, as illustrated in Figure 11.9.

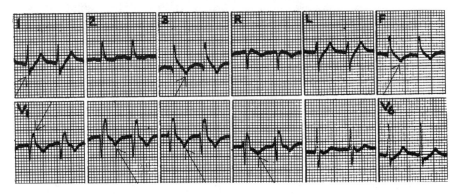

Figure 11.9. A 12-lead ECG (showing two cardiac cycles in each lead) from a 63-year-old woman with a massive pulmonary embolism. The *arrows* indicates the rightward axis shift in lead I; the inverted T waves in leads III, aVF, and V2 to V4; and the prominent R' wave of RBBB in lead V1.

Pulmonary Emphysema

The five most typical findings in emphysema have been grouped together as follows[12]:

1. Prominent P waves in leads II, III, and aVF.
2. Exaggerated atrial repolarization (TP) waves producing ≥0.10 mV ST segment depression in leads II, III, and aVF.
3. Rightward shift of the axis of the QRS complex in the frontal plane.
4. Decreased progression of the R-wave amplitudes in the precordial leads.
5. Low voltage of the QRS complexes, especially in the left precordial leads.

Figure 11.10 presents a typical example of pulmonary emphysema with rightward shifts of both the P waves and QRS complexes, and a low voltage in the left (V4–V6) precordial leads.

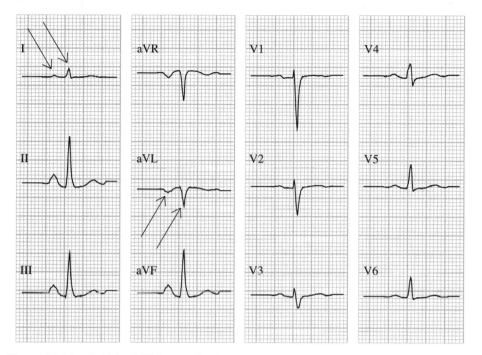

Figure 11.10. A 12-lead ECG recording from a 68-year-old man with severe dyspnea and a chest radiograph diagnostic of advanced pulmonary emphysema. *Arrows* indicate the rightward shift of the P waves and QRS complexes (negative in lead aVL and only slightly positive in lead I).

The QRS axis in the frontal plane is occasionally indeterminate, as in Figure 11.10.[13] This occurs because pulmonary emphysema directs the QRS complex posteriorly, so that minimal upward or downward deviation will swing the frontal-plane axis of the complex from +90 degrees to −90 degrees. Figure 11.11 also illustrates criteria 1, 2, 3, and 4 in the list given above.

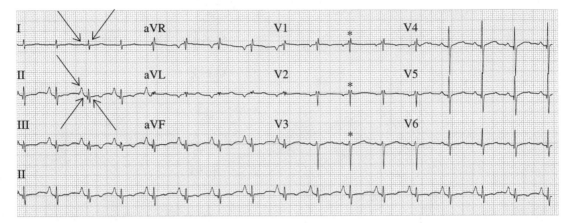

Figure 11.11. A 12-lead ECG recording from a 72-year-old woman with pulmonary emphysema. The *arrows* in lead I indicate the isoelectric P wave and low-voltage QRS complex, and the *arrows* in lead II indicate the prominent P wave and PR and ST segments depressed below the TP-segment baseline. *Asterisks* indicate the absence of decreased R wave progression from leads V1 to V3.

Selvester and Rubin have developed quantitative ECG criteria for both definite and possible emphysema,[14] as presented in Table 11.2.

Table 11.2. ECG Criteria for Emphysema[a]

Definite Emphysema	Possible Emphysema

A. P axis > +60 degrees in limb leads
   and either
	P axis > +60 degrees in limb leads
	   and either

B. 1. R and S amp ≤ 0.70 mV in limb leads
   and
	1. R and S amp ≤ 0.70 mV in limb leads
	   or

2. R amp ≤ 0.70 mV in V6 or	2. R amp ≤ 0.70 mV in V6
C. SV4 ≥ RV4	

[a] From Rubin LJ, ed. Pulmonary heart disease. Boston: Martinus Nijhoff, 1984:122.

These criteria achieve approximately 65% sensitivity for the diagnosis of emphysema and 95% specificity for the exclusion of emphysema in normal control subjects and in patients with congenital heart disease or myocardial infarction.[13] This good performance relative to that of other systems is most likely the result of combining quantitative criteria for the frontal-plane P-wave axis with criteria for both the frontal- and transverse-plane amplitudes of the QRS complex.

INTRACRANIAL HEMORRHAGE

Hemorrhage into either the intracerebral or subarachnoid spaces can produce dramatic changes in the ECG, presumably because of increased intracranial pressure.[15–18] Less severe ECG changes occur with nonhemorrhagic cerebrovascular accidents.[19] The three most common ECG changes in intracranial hemorrhage are:

1. Widening and inversion of T waves in the precordial leads.
2. Prolongation of the QTc interval.
3. Bradyarrhythmias.

Figure 11.12 presents a typical example of criterion 1.

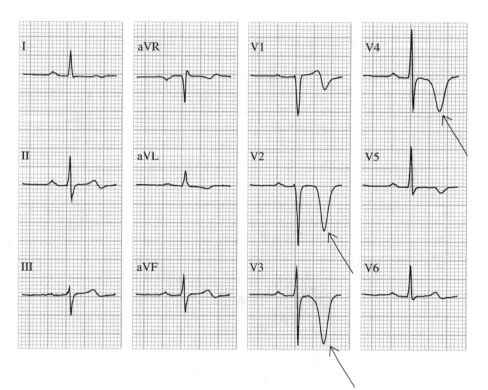

Figure 11.12. A 12-lead ECG recording from a 78-year-old woman with severe headache of sudden onset followed by loss of consciousness. The clinical diagnosis was an intracerebral hemorrhage. *Arrows* indicate the unusually prominent inverted T waves.

ENDOCRINE AND METABOLIC ABNORMALITIES

Thyroid Abnormalities

The hypothyroid condition is termed *myxedema* and the hyperthyroid condition is termed *thyrotoxicosis*. Both are often accompanied by typical changes in ECG waveform morphology. Since the thyroid hormone thyroxin mediates sympathetic nervous activity, a hypothyroid state is accompanied by a slowing of the sinus rate (sinus bradycardia). Conversely, a hyperthyroid state is accompanied by an acceleration of the sinus rate (sinus tachycardia).[20] Similarly, AV conduction may be impaired in hypothyroidism and accelerated in hyperthyroidism.[21]

Myxedema

The diagnosis of myxedema should be suspected when the following combination of ECG changes is present (Fig. 11.13):

1. Low voltage of all waveforms.
2. Inverted T waves without ST-segment deviation in many or all leads.
3. Sinus bradycardia.

These changes may be related to cardiac deposits of the gelatinous connective tissue typical of myxedema, to diminished sympathetic nervous activity, and/or the effect on the myocardium of reduced levels of the thyroid hormone thyroxin.[22]

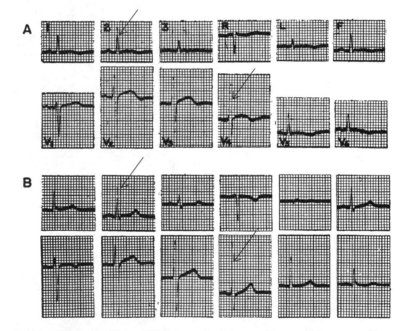

Figure 11.13. Two serial 12-lead ECG recordings from a 43-year-old woman with myxedema, the first made at the time of initial presentation with typical symptoms of hypothyroidism **(A)** and the second after 10 weeks of treatment with thyroid extract **(B)**. *Arrows* indicate contrasting R-wave amplitudes in leads 2(II) and V4 before and after treatment.

Thyrotoxicosis

The diagnosis of thyrotoxicosis should be suspected when the amplitudes of all of the ECG waveforms are increased.[23] This simulates right-atrial and left-ventricular enlargement as discussed in Chapter 4 ("Abnormal Wave Morphology"). The heart rate is rapid because of the increased levels of thyroxin. The cardiac rhythm may reflect an acceleration of normal sinus impulse formation (*sinus tachycardia*), or the abnormal atrial tachyarrhythmia known as *atrial fibrillation* (Chapter 15, "The Atrial Flutter/Fibrillation Spectrum"). Although the QT interval decreases as the heart rate increases, the corrected QT interval (QTc) may be prolonged.[24]

Obesity

Obesity has the potential for affecting the ECG through several effects, as follows:

1. Displacement of the heart by elevating the diaphragm.
2. Increasing the cardiac workload.
3. Increasing the distance between the heart and the recording electrodes.

In a study of more than 1,000 obese individuals, the heart rate, PR interval, QRS interval, QRS voltage, and QTc interval all showed an increase with increasing obesity.[25] The QRS axis also tended to shift leftward. Interestingly, only 4% of this population had low QRS voltage. One study has reported an increased incidence of false-positive criteria for inferior myocardial infarction in both obese individuals and in women in the final trimester of pregnancy (presumably because of diaphragmatic elevation).[26]

Hypothermia

Hypothermia has been defined as a rectal temperature below 36°C or 97°F. At these lower temperatures, characteristic ECG changes develop, as illustrated in Figure 11.14. All intervals of the ECG (including the RR, PR, QRS, and QT intervals) may lengthen. Characteristic *Osborn waves* appear as deflections at the J point in the same direction as that of the QRS complex.[27] The height of the Osborn waves is roughly proportional to the degree of hypothermia.

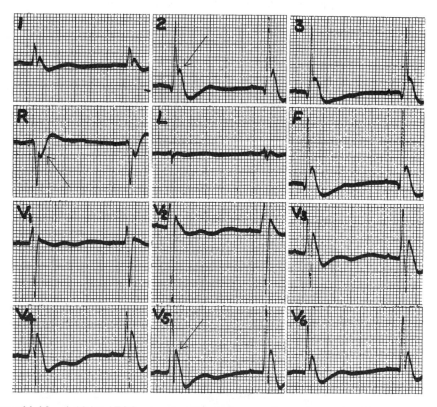

Figure 11.14. A 12-lead ECG recording showing two cardiac cycles per lead from an 82-year-old man exposed to the cold for 48 hours and who presented with a body temperature of 91°F. *Arrows* indicate the Osborn waves in several leads where they are most prominent.

ELECTROLYTE ABNORMALITIES

 Either abnormally low (hypo-) or high (hyper-) serum levels of the electrolytes potassium or calcium may produce marked abnormalities of the ECG waveforms. Indeed, typical ECG changes may provide the first clinical evidence of the presence of these conditions.

Potassium

The terms *hypo-* and *hyperkalemia* are commonly used for alterations in serum levels of potassium. Since abnormalities in either of these conditions may be life threatening, an understanding of the ECG changes they produce is important.

Hypokalemia

Hypokalemia may have many causes,[28] and often occurs with other electrolyte disturbances (e.g., reduced serum magnesium levels) and the presence of digitalis. The typical ECG signs of hypokalemia may appear when the serum potassium concentration is within normal limits, and conversely, the ECG may be normal when serum levels of potassium are elevated. The ECG changes in hypokalemia, as illustrated in Figures 11.15 and 11.16, are[29]:

1. Flattening or inversion of the T wave.
2. Increased prominence of the U wave.
3. Slight depression of the ST segment.
4. Increased amplitude and width of the P wave.
5. Prolongation of the PR interval.
6. Premature beats and sustained tachyarrhythmias.
7. Prolongation of the QTc interval.

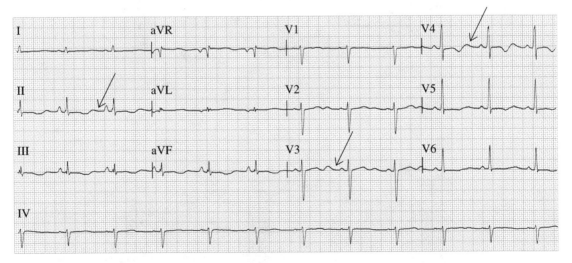

Figure 11.15. A multilead ECG recording from a 53-year-old man receiving diuretic therapy for chronic heart failure. The patient's serum potassium level was 1.7 mEq/L; the normal range is from 4.0 to 5.0 mEq/L. *Arrows* indicate the markedly prolonged QT interval (0.710 s). Three cycles are included for each lead, to indicate the heart rate of 65 beats/min and therefore a QTc of 0.719 s [0.710 + (0.00175 × 5)].

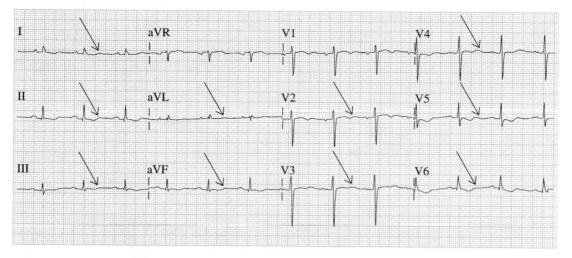

Figure 11.16. A 12-lead ECG recording from a 75-year-old man on long-term diuretic therapy for congestive heart failure. The patient's serum potassium level was 3.2 mEq/L. *Arrows* indicate generally "flattened" T waves, with slightly depressed ST segments in some leads.

The characteristic reversal in the relative amplitudes of the T and U waves is the most characteristic change in waveform morphology in hypokalemia. The U-wave prominence is caused by prolongation of the recovery phase of the cardiac action potential. This can lead to the life-threatening *torsades de pointes* type of ventricular tachyarrhythmia, as discussed in Chapter 17 ("Ventricular Tachyarrhythmias").[30] Hypokalemia also potentiates the tachyarrhythmias produced by digitalis toxicity, discussed in Chapter 22 ("Dr. Marriott's Systematic Approach to the Diagnosis of Arrhythmias").

Hyperkalemia

As in hypokalemia, there may be a poor correlation between serum potassium levels and the typical ECG changes of hyperkalemia.[31] The earliest ECG evidence of hyperkalemia usually appears in the T waves, as illustrated in Figure 11.17. The variety of changes include:

1. Increased amplitude and peaking of the T wave.
2. Prolongation of the PR interval.
3. Prolongation of the QRS interval.
4. Flattening of the P wave.

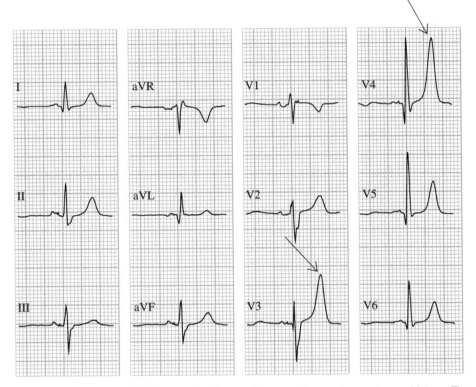

Figure 11.17. A 12-lead ECG recording from a 42-year-old man with acute renal failure. The patient's serum potassium level was 7.1 mEq/L. *Arrows* indicate the unusually prominent and peaked positive T waves.

The AV conduction in hyperkalemia may become so delayed that advanced AV block appears, as discussed in Chapter 22 ("Dr. Marriott's Systematic Approach to the Diagnosis of Arrhythmias").[32] Prolongation of the QRS complex and flattening of the P waves occur because the high potassium levels in hyperkalemia delay the spread of the cardiac activating impulse through the myocardium. This abnormally slow conduction can lead to cardiac arrest from ventricular fibrillation, as discussed in Chapter 19 ("Decreased Automaticity").[33]

The P waves may totally disappear from the ECG, as illustrated in Figure 11.18A. The T waves and the QRS complexes return to their normal duration and the P waves reappear when the serum potassium concentration returns to normal (Fig. 11.18B). Hyperkalemia may also reduce the myocardial response to artificial pacemaker stimulation.[34]

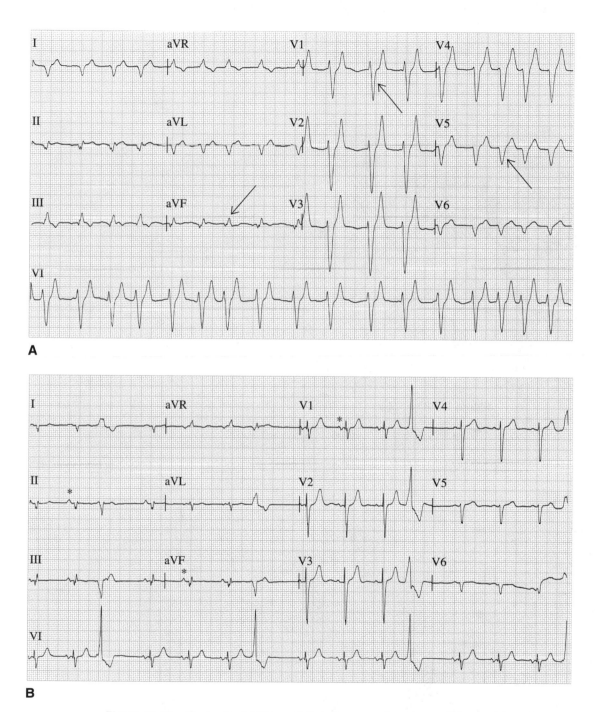

Figure 11.18. Twelve-lead ECG and V1 rhythm recordings from a 72-year-old woman with end-stage renal disease. The patient's serum potassium level was initially 7.8 mEq/L **(A)** and was then corrected to 4.5 mEq/L **(B)** after dialysis. *Arrows* indicate the markedly prolonged QRS complexes in **A**, and *asterisks* indicate the reappearing P waves in **B**.

Calcium

The ventricular recovery time, as represented on the ECG by the QTc interval (Chapter 3, "Interpretation of the Normal Electrocardiogram"), is altered by the extremes of serum calcium levels:

Deficiency = Hypocalcemia → Prolonged QTc interval
Excess = Hypercalcemia → Shortened QTc interval

The change in the QTc interval is produced by an increase or decrease in duration of the ST segment while the T wave remains relatively normal (Fig. 11.19).[35]

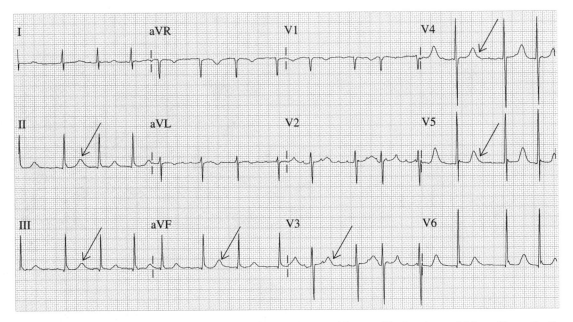

Figure 11.19. A 12-lead ECG from a 49-year-old man with chronic renal failure. The patient's serum calcium level was 7.2 mg/100 m; the normal range is from 9.0 to 11.0 mg/100 ml. *Arrows* indicate the prolonged QT interval of 0.434 s, and since the ventricular rate is 88 beats/min, the QTc interval is 0.483 s [0.434 + (0.00175 × 28)] (using the Hodges formula).

In *hypocalcemia*, the prolonged QT interval may be accompanied by terminal T-wave inversion in some leads (Fig. 11.20).

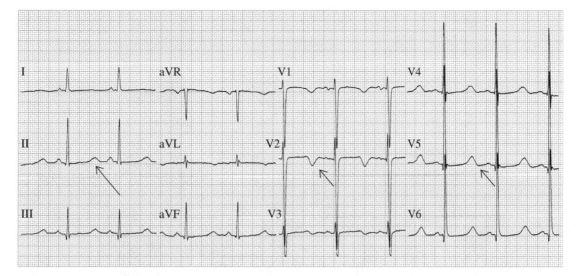

Figure 11.20. A 12-lead ECG from a 24-year-old woman with chronic renal failure. The patient's serum calcium level was 4.7 meq/L. *Arrows* indicate the markedly prolonged QT interval (0.500 s). The ventricular rate is 100 beats/min, and therefore the QTc = 0.570 s [0.500 + (0.00175 × 40)] (using the Hodges formula).

In *hypercalcemia*, the proximal limb of the T wave abruptly slopes to its peak, and the ST segment may not be apparent, as illustrated in Figure 11.21.[36] In extreme hypercalcemia, an increase in amplitude of the QRS complex, diphasic T waves, and Osborn waves has been described.[37,38]

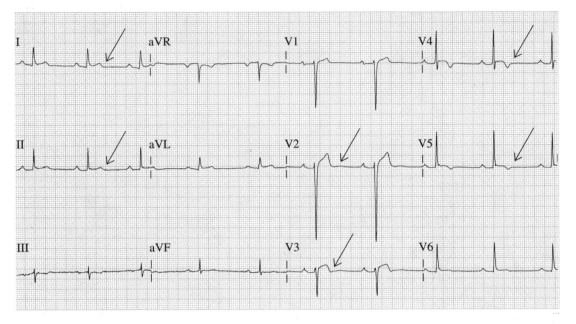

Figure 11.21. A 12-lead ECG recording from a 33-year-old man with hyperparathyroidism (a serum calcium level of 15 mg/100 ml). *Arrows* indicate the QT interval of 0.307 s, and since the heart rate is 56 beats/min, the QTc is 0.300 s [0.307 + (0.00175 × −4)].

DRUG EFFECTS

Either therapeutic or toxic cardiac effects of various medications can sometimes be detected on the ECG. The term "drug effect" refers to the therapeutic cardiac manifestations of a drug on the ECG, while the term "drug toxicity" refers to the cardiac *arrhythmias* caused by various medications (Chapter 22, "Dr. Marriott's Systematic Approach to the Diagnosis of Arrhythmias"). The level of a drug in blood and tissue at which toxicity occurs can vary widely, depending on the underlying pathology for which the drug is being used, the patient's premedication ECG status, the variations in electrolytes such as potassium, and the presence of other drugs.

Digitalis

Digitalis is a drug commonly used to treat cardiac failure and to slow the ventricular rate in atrial tachyarrhythmias. It causes characteristic ECG changes termed "digitalis effect" because the recovery or repolarization of the myocardial cells occurs earlier than it normally does, as illustrated in Figure 11.22. This is manifested on the ECG by:

1. "Coved" ST-segment depression.
2. A flattened T wave.
3. A decreased QTc interval.

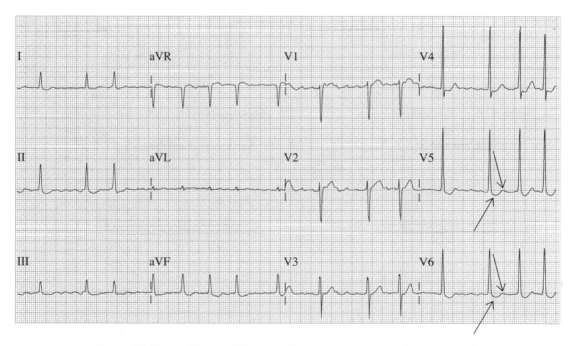

Figure 11.22. A 12-lead ECG from a 71-year-old woman on long-term digitalis management for atrial fibrillation. *Arrows* indicate the coved ST segments and flattened T waves.

Occasionally, the ST-J point is depressed, mimicking myocardial injury (Fig. 11.23). This extreme example of digitalis effect usually occurs only in those leads with tall R waves. Another manifestation of digitalis effect is the vagally mediated slowing of AV-nodal conduction (Chapter 22, "Dr. Marriott's Systematic Approach to the Diagnosis of Arrhythmias"). In sinus rhythm, there is a slight increase in the PR interval, and in atrial fibrillation there is a decrease in the ventricular rate (Chapter 15, "The Atrial Flutter/Fibrillation Spectrum").

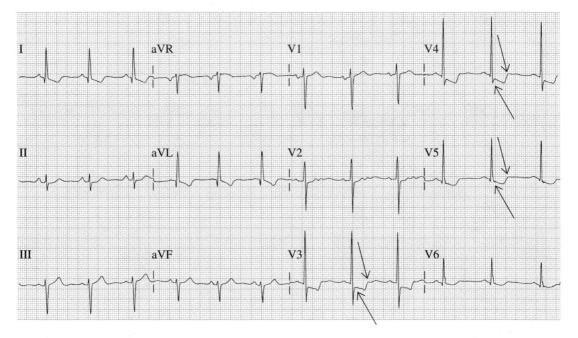

Figure 11.23. A 12-lead ECG recording from a 77-year-old woman with congestive heart failure. The ECG changes, including ST-segment depression, developed at the time of administration of the digitalis loading dosages. *Arrows* indicate the marked ST-segment depression with decreased T-wave amplitude.

Antiarrhythmic Drugs

The effect of an antiarrhythmic drug may be modified by the underlying cardiac disorder for which it is being used, by coexisting electrolyte imbalance, and by interaction of the drug with other drugs. An example of the last of these would be a marked increase in blood levels of Drug A (e.g., digitalis) that occurs with the introduction of Drug B (e.g., quinidine and amiodarone). The commonly used antiarrhythmic drugs are classified as follows according to Vaughan Williams and associates.[39,40]

Class 1 Drugs

Drugs in Class 1 of the Vaughn Williams classification have direct action on the myocardial cell membrane, and have been subdivided according to their effect on the different phases of the action potential. These drugs and their effects on the action potential are as follows:

Quinidine (Including Procainamide and Diisopyramide).   In contrast to digitalis, the effect of quinidine is produced by a delay in the recovery or repolarization of myocardial cells. This results in prolongation of the QTc interval,[41] a decreased T-wave amplitude, and an increased U-wave amplitude, as illustrated in Figure 11.24. In this example, the QT interval is 0.39 s, and since the ventricular rate is 100 beats/min, the QTc interval is prolonged to 0.49 s. Minimal prolongation of the QRS complex occurs rarely with quinidine effect; an increase in duration of the QRS complex of 25% to 50% is evidence of quinidine toxicity (Chapter 22, "Dr. Marriott's Systematic Approach to the Diagnosis of Arrhythmias"). Also, quinidine effect is exaggerated by the presence of digitalis. The phenothiazine group of drugs, which are commonly used in treating psychiatric disorders, produce ECG changes similar to quinidine effect.

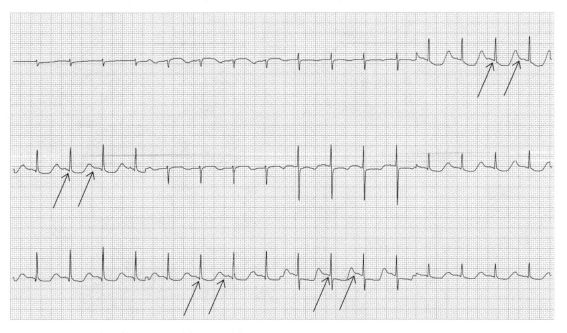

Figure 11.24.   A 12-lead ECG recording from a 68-year-old woman with recent acute anterior infarction complicated by ventricular tachycardia. The arrhythmia has been controlled by quinidine, and a quinidine effect appears on the ECG. *Arrows* indicate the markedly prolonged QT interval, extending from the onset of the QRS complex to the end of the T wave.

Lidocaine and Mexilitine.   Usually the surface ECG is unaltered by lidocaine and mexiletene.

Flecainide.   Flecainide produces broadening of the QRS complex, with the interval between the J point and the end of the T wave remaining unaltered, thus slightly prolonging the QT interval.

Class 2 Drugs

The drugs in Class 2 of the Vaughn Williams classification system are the β-adrenergic blocking agents. By decreasing sympathetic effect on the heart, there is a slowing of rate due to the decreased sinoatrial (SA) node impulse formation. Conduction through the AV node is also delayed, prolonging the PR interval of the ECG. If there is underlying SA- or AV-nodal dysfunction, these changes may be increased.

Class 3 Drugs

The drugs in Class 3 of the Vaughn Williams system prolong myocardial repolarization, and may therefore markedly prolong the QTc interval on the ECG. Among the Class 3 drugs are:

Sotalol.   Sotalol has both Class 2 and Class 3 drug effects, and may therefore produce SA- and AV-nodal suppression and also prolongation of the QTc interval.

Amiodarone.   Amiodarone has Class 1, Class 2, and Class 3 effects.

Class 4

Drugs in Class 4 of the Vaughn Williams classification system block calcium channels, and as a result slow both SA- and AV-nodal functions. Their effects are therefore similar to those of drugs in Class 2.

GLOSSARY

Arrhythmia: any cardiac rhythm other than regular sinus rhythm.

Atrial Fibrillation: the tachyarrhythmia at the rapid end of the flutter/fibrillation spectrum, produced by macroreentry within multiple circuits in the atria and characterized by irregular multiform f waves.

Constrictive pericarditis: thickening of the pericardium caused by chronic inflammation and resulting in interference with myocardial function.

Cor pulmonale: an acute or chronic pressure overload of the right side of the heart, caused by increased resistance to blood flow through the lungs.

Digitalis: a drug that occurs naturally in the foxglove plant and is used both to increase contraction of the cardiac muscle and decrease conduction through the AV node.

Emphysema: a pulmonary disease in which the alveoli are destroyed and the lungs become overinflated.

Hypercalcemia: an abnormally increased level of serum calcium (Ca^{++}), with a serum Ca^{++} concentration above 11.0 mg/100 ml.

Hyperkalemia: an abnormally increased level of serum potassium (K^+), with a serum K^+ concentration above 5.0 mEq/L.

Hypertrophic cardiomyopathy: a condition in which cardiac performance is decreased because of decreased contraction capability of the thickened myocardium.

Hypocalcemia: an abnormally decreased level of serum calcium (Ca^{++}), with a serum Ca^{++} concentration below 9.0 mg/100 ml.

Hypokalemia: an abnormally decreased level of serum potassium (K^+) with a serum K^+ concentration below 4.0 mEq/L.

Hypothermia: subnormal temperature of the body defined as temperature under 36°C or 97°F.

Low voltage: a total amplitude of the QRS complex that is less than 0.70 mV in all limb leads and less than 1.0 mV in all precordial leads.

Myxedema: severe hypothyroidism characterized by a decreased metabolic state and firm, inelastic edema, dry skin and hair, and loss of mental and physical vigor.

Osborn waves: abnormal ECG waveforms caused by hypothermia.

Pericardial effusion: an increase in the amount of fluid in the pericardial sac.

Pericardial sac: the fluid-filled space between the two layers of the pericardium.

Pericarditis: acute or chronic inflammation of the pericardium.

Pericardium: the two-layered membrane that encloses the heart and the roots of the great blood vessels.

Procainamide: a compound related to the local anesthetic procaine that is used in the treatment of reentrant tachyarrhythmias.

Pulmonary embolism: the sudden obstruction of a pulmonary artery by a dislodged clot or fat originating from the legs or the pelvic region.

Quinidine: a drug that occurs naturally in the bark of the cinchona tree and which prolongs myocardial recovery time and protects against some tachyarrhythmias. However, quinidine and other related drugs may also produce tachyarrhythmias by overprolongation of recovery time.

Sinus tachycardia: an acceleration of the normal sinus rhythm beyond the upper limit of 100 beats/min.

Subaortic stenosis: narrowing of the outflow passage from the left ventricle proximal to the aortic valve to a degree sufficient to obstruct the flow of blood.

Thyrotoxicosis: severe hyperthyroidism characterized by an increased metabolic condition, sweating, and protruding eyes.

Torsades de pointes: a variety of ventricular tachycardia resulting from prolongation of the ventricular recovery time. The term is French for "turning of the points" or turning of the directions of the QRS complex alternately between positive and negative.

Total electrical alternans: alternation in the amplitudes of all of the ECG waveforms in the presence of a regular cardiac cycle lengths.

REFERENCES

1. Bahl OP, Massie E. Electrocardiographic and vectorcardiographic patterns in cardiomyopathy. Cardiovasc Clin 1972;4:95–112.
2. Spodick DH. Hypertrophic obstructive cardiomyopathy of the left ventricle (idiopathic hypertrophic subaortic stenosis). Cardiovasc Clin 1972;4:133–165.
3. Farrokh A, Walsh TJ, Massie E. Amyloid heart disease. Am J Cardiol 1964;13:750.
4. Spodick DH. Differential characteristics of the electrocardiogram in early repolarization and acute pericarditis. N Engl J Med 1976;295:523–526.
5. Bruce MA, Spodick DH. Atypical electrocardiogram in acute pericarditis; characteristics and prevalence. J Electrocardiol 1980;13:61–66.
6. Spodick DH. Pathogenesis and clinical correlations of the electrocardiographic abnormalities of pericardial disease. Cardiovasc Clin 1977;8:201–213.
7. Bashour FA, Cochran PA. The association of electrical alternans with pericardial effusion. Dis Chest 1963;44: 146.
8. Nizet PM, Marriott HJL. The electrocardiogram and pericardial effusion. JAMA 1966;198:169.

9. Dalton JC, Pearson RJ, White PD. Constrictive pericarditis: a review and long term follow-up of 78 cases. Ann Intern Med 1956;45:445.
10. Evans W, Jackson F. Constrictive pericarditis. Br Heart J 1952;14:53.
11. Sreeram N, Cheriex EC, Smeets JLRM, et al. Value of the 12-lead electrocardiogram at hospital admission in the diagnosis of pulmonary embolism. Am J Cardiol 1994;73:298–303.
12. Wasserburger RH, Kelly JR, Rasmussen HK, et al. The electrocardiographic pentalogy of pulmonary emphysema: a correlation of roentgenographic findings and pulmonary function studies. Circulation 1959;20: 831–841.
13. Grant RP. Left axis deviation. An electrocardiographic–pathologic correlation study. Circulation 1956; 14:233.
14. Selvester RH, Rubin HB. New criteria for the electrocardiographic diagnosis of emphysema and cor pulmonale. Am Heart J 1965;69:437–447.
15. Burch GE, Meyers R, Abildskov JA. A new electrocardiographic pattern observed in cerebrovascular accidents. Circulation 1954;9:719.
16. Hersch C. Electrocardiographic changes in subarachnoid haemorrhage, meningitis, and intracranial space-occupying lesion. Br Heart J 1964;26:785.
17. Surawicz B. Electrocardiographic pattern of cerebrovascular accident. JAMA 1966;197:913.
18. Shuster S. The electrocardiogram in subarachnoid haemorrhage. Br Heart J 1960;22:316–320.
19. Fentz V, Gormsen J. Electrocardiographic patterns in patients with cerebrovascular accidents. Circulation 1962;25:22–28.
20. Williams GH, Braunwald E. Endocrine and nutritional disorders and heart disease. In: Heart disease. Philadelphia: WB Saunders, 1980:1825–1853.
21. Vanhaelst L, Neve P, Chailly P, et al. Coronary disease in hypothyroidism: observations in clinical myxoedema. Lancet 1967;2:800–802.
22. Surawicz B, Mangiardi ML. Electrocardiogram in endocrine and metabolic disorders. Cardiovasc Clin 1977; 8:243–266.
23. Surawicz B, Mangiardi ML. Electrocardiogram in endocrine and metabolic disorders. In: Electrocardiographic correlations. Philadelphia: FA Davis, 1977:243–266.
24. Harumi K, Ouichi T. Q-T prolongation syndrome (in Japanese). In: Naika mook. Tokyo: Kinbara, 1981:210.
25. Frank S, Colliver JA, Frank A. The electrocardiogram in obesity: statistical analysis of 1,029 patients. J Am Coll Cardiol 1986;7:295–299.
26. Starr JW, Wagner GW, Behar VS, et al. Vectorcardiographic criteria for the diagnosis of inferior myocardial infarction. Circulation 1974;49:829–836.
27. Okada M, Nishimura F, Yoshino H, et al. The J wave in accidental hypothermia. J Electrocardiol 1983;16:23–28.
28. Salerno DM, Asinger RW, Elsperger J, et al. Frequency of hypokalemia after successfully resuscitated out-of-hospital cardiac arrest compared with that in transmural acute myocardial infarction. Am J Cardiol 1987;59: 84–88.
29. Surawicz B. The interrelationship of electrolyte abnormalities and arrhythmias. In: Cardiac arrhythmias: their mechanisms, diagnosis, and management. Philadelphia: JB Lippincott, 1980:83.
30. Krikler DM, Curry PVL. Torsade de pointes, an atypical ventricular tachycardia. Br Heart J 1976;38:117–120.
31. Surawicz B. Relationship between electrocardiogram and electrolytes. Am Heart J 1967;73:814–834.
32. Ettinger PO, Regan TJ, Oldewurtel HA. Hyperkalemia, cardiac conduction, and the electrocardiogram. A review. Am Heart J 1974;88:360–371.
33. Sekiya S, Ichikawa S, Tsutsumi T, et al. Nonuniform action potential durations at different sites in canine left ventricle. Jpn Heart J 1983;24:935–945.
34. Bashour TT. Spectrum of ventricular pacemaker exit block owing to hyperkalemia. Am J Cardiol 1986;57: 337–338.
35. Bronsky D, Dubin A, Waldstein SS, et al. Calcium and the electrocardiogram. II. The electrocardiographic manifestations of hyperparathyroidism and of marked hypercalcemia from various other etiologies. Am J Cardiol 1961;7:833–839.
36. Nirenburg DW, Ransil BJ. Q-aTc interval as a clinical indicator of hypercalcemia. Am J Cardiol 1979;44: 243–248.
37. Douglas PS, Carmichael KA, Palevsky PM. Extreme hypercalcemia and electrocardiographic changes. Am J Cardiol 1984;54:674–679.
38. Sridharan MR, Horan LG. Electrocardiographic J wave in hypercalcemia. Am J Cardiol 1984;54:672–673.
39. Vaughan Williams EM. Classification of antiarrhythmic drugs. In: Sandoe E, Flensted-Jensen E, Olsen KH, eds. Cardiac arrhythmias. Sodertalje, Sweden: Astra. 1970: 449–472.
40. Singh BN, Vaughan Williams EM. A fourth class of antidysrhythmic action? Effect of verapramil on ouabain toxicity, on artial and ventricular intracellular potentials, and on other features of cardiac function. Cardiovascular Res 1972;6:109–119.
41. Watanabe Y, Dreifus LS. Interactions of quinidine and potassium on atrioventricular transmission. Circ Res 1967;20:434–446.

III

ABNORMAL RHYTHMS

CHAPTER 12

Introduction to Arrhythmias

APPROACH TO ARRHYTHMIA DIAGNOSIS

The nine features that should be examined in every analysis of the electrocardiogram (ECG) are presented in Chapter 3 ("Interpretation of the Normal Electrocardiogram"). The two of these features that are of primary importance in the evaluation of cardiac rhythm are:

1. Rate and regularity.
9. Identification of the rhythm.

The method for determining the rates of both regular and irregular rhythms should be reviewed before proceeding with this chapter. Normal sinus rhythm, with its rate limit of 60 to100 beats/min, and its slight irregularity due to respiratory variation, is also presented in Chapter 3 ("Interpretation of the Normal Electrocardiogram"). Of the original nine features presented in Chapter 3, the additional ECG features that are important aspects of many of the abnormalities of cardiac rhythm include:

2. P-wave morphology.
3. PR interval.
4. QRS-complex morphology.
8. QTc interval.

The term "arrhythmia" is very general, referring to all rhythms other than regular sinus rhythm. Even the slight variation in sinus rate caused by altered autonomic balance during the respiratory cycle is termed "sinus arrhythmia." The term *dysrhythmia* has been proposed by some as an alternative, but "arrhythmia," meaning "imperfection in a regularly recurring motion," is the commonly accepted term for rhythms other than regular sinus rhythm. The presence of an arrhythmia does not necessarily reflect cardiac disease, as indicated by the broad array of abnormal rhythms that commonly occur in healthy individuals of all ages. Arrhythmias are primarily classified according to their rate, and usually the atria and ventricles have the same rates. However, there are many different atrial/ventricular relationships among the cardiac arrhythmias, as listed below:

1. The atrial and ventricular rhythms are associated and have the same rate, but (a) the rhythm originates in the atria; or (b) the rhythm originates in the ventricles.
2. The atrial and ventricular rhythms are associated, but the atrial rate is faster than the ventricular rate (the rhythm must originate in the atria).
3. The atrial and ventricular rhythms are associated, but the ventricular rate is faster than the atrial rate (the rhythm must originate in the ventricles).
4. The atrial and ventricular rhythms are independent (atrioventricular [AV] dissociation) and: (a) the atrial and ventricular rates are the same (isorhythmic dissociation); or (b) the atrial rate is faster than the ventricular rate; or (b) the ventricular rate is faster than the atrial rate.

When the atrial and ventricular rhythms are associated but have differing rates, the rhythm is named according to the rate of the chamber (atrial or ventricular) from which it originates (e.g., when a rapid atrial rhythm is associated with a slower ventricular rate, the name "atrial tachyarrhythmia" is used). When the atrial and ventricular rhythms are dissociated, names should be given to both of the rhythms (e.g., atrial tachyarrhythmia with ventricular tachyarrhythmia).

The term *bradyarrhythmia* is used to identify any rhythm with a rate <60 beats/min, and "tachyarrhythmia" is used to identify any rhythm with a rate >100 beats/min. There are also many arrhythmias that do not alter the rate beyond these normal limits. In contrast to the general terms brady- and tachyarrhythmia, the terms brady- and tachycardia refer to specific arrhythmias such as sinus bradycardia and sinus tachycardia.

The two important aspects of arrhythmias that are basic to their understanding are:

1. Their mechanism.
2. Their site of origin.

The mechanisms that produce arrhythmias are either:

1. Problems of impulse formation (*automaticity*).
2. Problems of impulse conduction (block or reentry).

PROBLEMS OF AUTOMATICITY

Arrhythmias caused by problems of automaticity can originate in any cell in the pacemaking and conduction systems that is capable of spontaneous depolarization. Such cells, termed *pacemaker cells*, are present in the:

1. Sinus node.
2. Purkinje cells scattered through the atria.
3. Common (His) bundle.
4. Right and left bundle branches.
5. Purkinje system in the fascicles and peripheral network.

Normally, the automaticity of the sinoatrial (SA) node exceeds that of all other parts of the pacemaking and conduction systems, allowing it to control the cardiac rate and rhythm. This is important because of both the location of the SA node and its relationship to the parasympathetic and sympathetic components of the autonomic nervous system (Chapter 3, "Interpretation of the Normal Electrocardiogram"). A site below the SA node can initiate the cardiac rhythm either because it usurps control from the SA node by accelerating its own automaticity, or because the SA node abdicates its role by decreasing its automaticity. The term "ectopic" is often applied to rhythms that originate from any site other than the SA node. Cardiac cells function as pacemakers by forming electrical impulses called action potentials via the process of *spontaneous depolarization* (Fig. 12.1). When the automaticity of cardiac cells is severely impaired, the therapeutic use of an artificial pacemaker may be required (Chapter 21, "Artificial Cardiac Pacemakers"). The acceleration of automaticity is limited by the maximal rate of impulse formation in pacemaker cells, and therefore rarely causes a clinically important tachyarrhythmia.

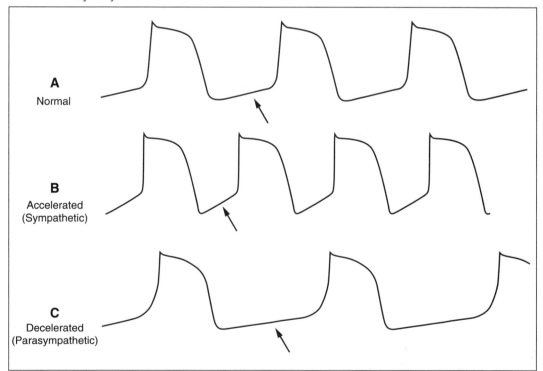

Figure 12.1. Schematic action potentials of a pacemaking cell. Sinus rhythm is shown in **A.** Excess sympathetic activity increases the slope of the slow spontaneous depolarization, creating an accelerated rhythm in **B.** Excess parasympathetic activity decreases the slope of the slow spontaneous depolarization, creating a decelerated rhythm in **C.** *Arrows* indicate the slow spontaneous depolarization in all three conditions.

The mechanism by which a tachyarrhythmia is perpetuated determines the treatment required for its management. Accelerated automaticity can best be treated by eliminating the cause of the acceleration rather than by treating the acceleration itself. When the accelerated automaticity originates from the sinus node, the cause is increased sympathetic nervous activity resulting from systemic conditions such as exertion, anxiety, fever, decreased cardiac output, or thyrotoxicosis. When the accelerated automaticity originates from another location, the most common causes are ischemia and digitalis toxicity. Therefore, accelerated sinus automaticity is treated by removing the responsible systemic condition, and accelerated nonsinus automaticity is treated by removing the responsible cardiac condition.

PROBLEMS OF IMPULSE CONDUCTION: BLOCK

The term *block* is used to refer to the situation in which conduction is slowed or fails to occur at all [e.g., AV block (Chapter 20, "Atrioventricular Block") or bundle-branch block (Chapter 5, "Intraventricular Conduction Abnormalities")]. Cardiac impulses can be either partly blocked, causing conduction delay (e.g., a prolonged PR interval), or totally blocked, causing conduction failure (e.g., complete AV block). With a partial block of impulses, there is no change in cardiac rate, but with a total block of impulses a bradyarrhythmia is produced. Either partial or total block can occur at any site within the pacemaking and conduction system.

PROBLEMS OF IMPULSE CONDUCTION: REENTRY

Although conduction abnormalities sufficient to produce block can occur only within the pacemaking and conduction systems, uneven or *inhomogeneous conduction* can occur in any part of the heart. This inhomogeneous spread of electrical impulses can result in reentry of an impulse into an area that has just previously been depolarized and repolarized.[1] Reentry produces a circular movement of the impulse, which continues as long as the impulse encounters receptive cells, resulting in a single *premature beat*, multiple premature beats, a nonsustained tachyarrhythmia, or even a sustained tachyarrhythmia.

There are three prerequisites to the development of reentry:

1. An available circuit.
2. A difference in the refractory periods of the two pathways (limbs) in the circuit.
3. Conduction that is sufficiently slow somewhere in the circuit to allow the remainder of the circuit to recover its responsiveness by the time the impulse returns.

In Figure 12.2, the diagrams represent three different situations regarding the homogeneity of pathway receptiveness to impulse conduction: (a) Both limbs of the pathway are receptive (Fig. 12.2*A*). The left and right limbs have completed the recovery process and are receptive to the entering impulse. (b) Both limbs of the pathway are refractory (Fig. 12.2*B*). The left and right limbs are still refractory (because of the persisting depolarized state) to being reactivated by the entering impulse. (c) One limb of the pathway is receptive and the other is refractory (Fig. 12.2*C1*). The left limb of the pathway is refractory and the right limb is receptive. By the time the impulse reaches the distal end of the left limb (by traveling down the right limb), it is able to reenter because repolarization has been completed (Fig. 12.2*C2*). The impulse will continue to cycle within the reentry circuit as long as it encounters receptive cells, thus producing a reentrant tachyarrhythmia.

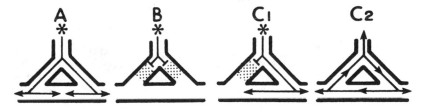

Figure 12.2. *Asterisks* indicate sites of impulse formation, *arrows* indicate the directions of impulse conduction, *perpendicular lines* indicate block of impulse conduction, and *shaded areas* indicate areas that have not completed the repolarization process.

An example of the development of a *reentry circuit* in the presence of an accessory AV conduction pathway is presented in Figure 12.3. During sinus rhythm (Fig. 12.3A), both the AV node and the Bundle of Kent have had time to recover from their previous activation. The premature atrial beat in Figure 12.3B encounters persisting refractoriness in the nearby Bundle of Kent, but encounters receptiveness in the more distant AV node, a situation analogous to that shown in Figure 12.2C1. This leads to the development of a reentry circuit (Fig. 12.3C) analogous to that in Figure 12.2C2. Reentry circuits vary in size from a local area of myocardial fibers (Fig. 12.2C2) to two cardiac chambers (Fig. 12.3C).

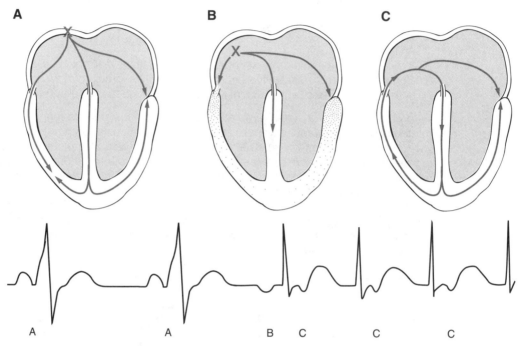

Figure 12.3. **Top:** The presence of a Kent bundle is indicated by the open space between the right atrium and ventricle, and the AV node by the open space at the summit of the interventricular septum. *X* indicates the site of the pacemaker: in the sinus node **(A)** and in the right atrium **(B)**. No pacemaking is required in **C.** The *arrows* indicate the directions of impulse conduction. **Bottom:** the corresponding ECG, indicating sinus rhythm with a normal P wave immediately followed by the QRS complex, indicating ventricular preexcitation **(A)**, an inverted P preceding the QRS complex, indicating an atrial premature beat without preexcitation **(B)**, and an inverted P wave following the QRS complex, indicating a reentrant junctional tachycardia **(C)**. (Modified from Wagner GS, Waugh RA, Ramo BW. Cardiac arrhythmias. New York: Churchill Livingstone, 1983:13.)

The term *microreentry* describes the mechanism that occurs when a reentry circuit is too small for its activation to be represented by a waveform on the surface ECG. The impulses formed within the reentry circuit spread through the surrounding myocardium just as they would spread from an automatic or pacemaking site. The P waves and QRS complexes on the ECG are produced by this passive spread of activation through the atria and ventricles. Microreentry commonly occurs in the AV node (Chapter 16, "Reentrant Junctional Tachycardias") and in the ventricles (Chapter 17, "Reentrant Ventricular Tachyarrhythmias").

The term *macroreentry* describes the mechanism that occurs when a reentry circuit is large enough for its own activation to be represented on the surface ECG (Fig. 12.3). Cycling of the activating impulse through the right atrium (Fig. 12.3C) is represented by a portion of the P wave, with the remainder of the P wave produced by spread of the impulse through the uninvolved left atrium. Cycling of the impulse through the right ventricle (Fig. 112.3C) is represented by a portion of the QRS complex, with the remainder of the QRS complex produced by spread of the impulse through the uninvolved left ventricle.

There are also forms of macroreentry in which the reentry circuit is entirely within either the atrial or ventricular myocardium. When this occurs, sawtoothlike or undulating ECG waveforms replace discrete P waves (Chapter 15, "Atrial Flutter/Fibrillation Spectrum") or QRS complexes (Chapter 17, "Reentrant Ventricular Tachyarrhythmias").

In attempting to treat reentry, it is important to understand its mechanism. For any reentry circuit to perpetuate itself, the advancing head of the recycling impulse must not catch up with the refractory tail (Fig. 12.4A). Thus, there must always be a gap of nonrefractory cells between the head and the tail of the recycling impulse. A sustained reentrant tachyarrhythmia can be terminated by:

1. Administering drugs that accelerate conduction of the impulse in the reentry circuit so that it encounters an area that has not yet recovered (Fig. 12.4B). Termination would also result if a drug prolonged the recovery time.
2. Introducing an impulse from an artificial pacemaker that depolarizes (captures) part of the reentry circuit, thereby rendering it nonreceptive to the returning impulse (Fig. 12.4C).
3. Introducing a precordial electrical shock, termed *cardioversion*, that captures all receptive parts of the heart, including those in the reentry circuit, rendering the circuit nonreceptive to the returning impulse (Fig. 12.4D).
4. Performing surgical or catheter ablation of one limb of the tissue required for the reentry circuit. For example, ablation of the accessory AV pathway in a patient with ventricular preexcitation (Fig. 12.4F).

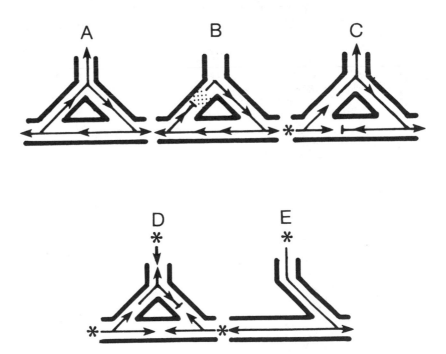

Figure 12.4. The diagram in Figure 12.2 is used to illustrate reentry **(A)** and the four mechanisms of termination **(B** to **E)**. *Asterisks, arrows, perpendiculars,* and *shaded areas* have the same meanings as in Figure 12.3. The *asterisk* in **C** indicates an ectopic site of impulse formation, the *three asterisks* in **D** indicate impulse reception from all sides from the shock, and the *asterisk* in **E** indicates SA-node impulse formation.

CLINICAL METHODS FOR DETECTING ARRHYTHMIA

The introduction of coronary care units (CCUs) in the early 1960s stimulated rapid advances in the diagnosis and treatment of cardiac arrhythmias. In the CCU, patients who have either arrhythmias or a high risk of developing them because of conditions such as acute myocardial infarction are continuously monitored via a single ECG lead (Chapter 2, "Recording the Electrocardiogram"). A modified lead V1 (MCL$_1$) is commonly used for this because it provides both a good view of atrial activity and of differentiation between right- and left-ventricular activity (Fig. 12.5).[2]

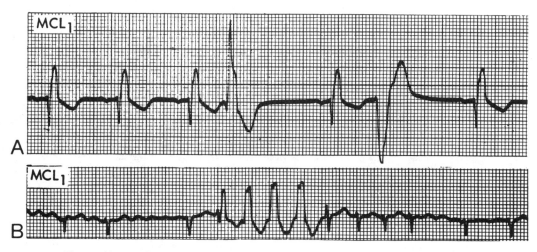

Figure 12.5. In **A**, there is right bundle-branch block during sinus rhythm, and both lead V1-positive (fourth beat) and lead V1-negative (sixth beat) VPBs (Chapter 17, "Reentrant Ventricular Tachyarrhythmias"). In **B**, the basic rhythm is atrial fibrillation, with most beats conducted normally, but beats four through seven are conducted abnormally through the right bundle. Note the typical triphasic appearance of the initial wide QRS complex.

DYNAMIC (HOLTER) MONITORING

A method for continuous ECG monitoring of ambulatory patients in their own environment was developed in the 1960s by Holter, and has since been further developed.[3] In this method, the patient is attached via chest electrodes to a portable tape recorder that records one or two ECG leads for 24 hours. The patient keeps a diary of activities so that symptoms, activity, and cardiac rhythm can be correlated. Thus, the patient is monitored during situations that actually occur in real life situations. Holter monitoring is used to identify any correlation between an arrhythmia and symptoms such as palpitations, dizziness, syncope, or chest pain (Fig. 12.6).

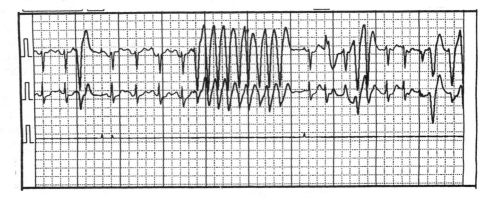

Figure 12.6. Holter recording (as in Figure 8.6) of leads MCL_1 and MCL_5, revealing VPBs and ventricular tachycardia in a 57-year-old man with dyspnea and palpitations following hospital discharge for an acute myocardial infarction.

In a study of 371 patients who underwent a 24-hour period of Holter monitoring for detection of cardiac arrhythmias, 174 (47%) had symptoms during this period. However, symptoms coincided with a disturbance of cardiac rhythm in only 48 (27%) of the patients; the remaining 126 patients (73%) experienced their symptoms when their rhythm was entirely normal. Thus, of the original 371 patients who underwent monitoring, the Holter method revealed whether symptoms were or were not due to the arrhythmia in approximately half. However, the 48 patients in whom arrhythmia was the cause of the symptoms represented only about one of eight of the original 371 patients.[4]

Holter monitoring is also of value in specific cardiac diseases, or in conditions in which information about the heart's rhythm is important for prognosis and management. These conditions are ischemic heart disease, mitral valve prolapse, cardiomyopathy, conduction disturbances, evaluation of pacemaker function, or Wolff–Parkinson–White syndrome. Holter monitoring may also be helpful in the asymptomatic patient in whom an arrhythmia has been detected on routine examination. In addition, Holter monitoring may be of value in assessing the therapeutic effect of antiarrhythmic drugs and adjusting drug dosages. In this context, however, it is important to realize that the frequency of an arrhythmia may show day-to-day spontaneous variation of up to 90%,[5] and that a marked and consistent reduction in the incidence of the arrhythmia must occur before its successful treatment can be assumed. The limited span of (usually) 24 hours of Holter monitoring makes it unsuitable for detecting infrequent disturbances in cardiac rhythm.

TRANSTELEPHONIC MONITORING

The problem of detecting infrequent arrhythmias by Holter monitoring has been largely overcome by *transtelephonic monitoring*.[6,7] When using this method, the patient carries a pocket-sized transmitter and transmits his or her cardiac rhythm via telephone when symptoms occur. This permits more efficient and economical monitoring than with Holter monitoring, and for periods of days or even weeks if necessary (Fig. 12.7).

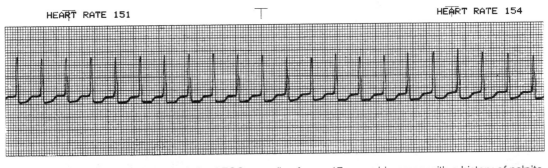

Figure 12.7. A single-lead ECG recording from a 17-year-old woman with a history of palpitations, who transmits this rhythm strip by telephone Immediately after the recurrence of her symptoms.

MEMORY-LOOP MONITORING

 It is often clinically important to observe the initiation of an intermittently occuring symptomatic cardiac arrhythmia. This requires a "memory loop" that continually stores the patient's cardiac rhythm for a set period of time.[8] The patient manually activates the permanent recording function of the arrhythmia monitor as soon as symptoms begin. The prior period of rhythm, that has been stored on the memory loop, is captured to reveal the onset of an arrhythmia accompanying the patient's symptoms. This system may reveal the transition from normal rhythm to abnormal brady- or tachyarrhythmias (Fig. 12.8).

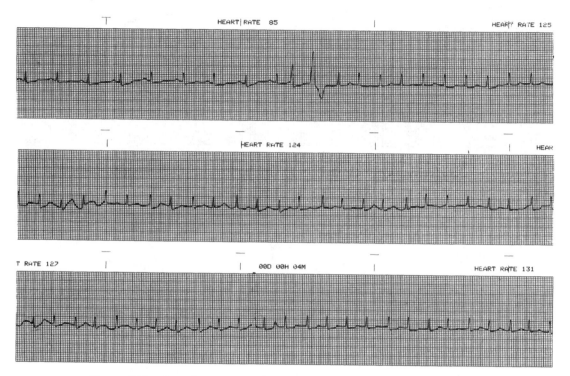

Figure 12.8. A continuous recording of the 30 seconds of rhythm stored by the memory-loop monitor preceding manual activation (indicated by the *mark in the middle of the bottom strip*). This 72-year-old man had a history of recurrent shortness of breath, and activated his recorder as soon as his symptoms began, 20 seconds after the onset of his supraventricular tachycardia.

INVASIVE METHODS OF RECORDING THE ELECTROCARDIOGRAM

Monitoring systems that record via electrodes on the body surface provide access only to electrical activity from the atrial and ventricular myocardia. Furthermore, the atrial activity may be obscured during a tachyarrhythmia because of superimposed QRS complexes and T waves. When the use of alternate body-surface sites for electrodes fails to reveal atrial activity, either transesophageal or intraatrial recording may be necessary. Figure 12.9 illustrates the ability of intraatrial recording to reveal diagnostic atrial activity when none is clearly visible on the body surface.

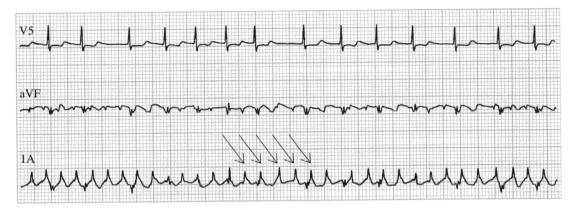

Figure 12.9. Simultaneous recording from surface leads V5 **(top)** and aVF **(middle)**, and from an intraatrial electrode (IA) **(bottom)** from an 81-year-old woman with congestive heart failure. Only an irregularly irregular ventricular rhythm is apparent in lead V5, and intermittent atrial activity can be detected in lead aVF. The diagnosis of the rapid atrial rhythm (flutter–fibrillation) with variable AV block is confirmed by the intraatrial recording, with *arrows* indicating the atrial rate of 330 beats/min.

Positioning of a multipolar catheter across the tricuspid valve provides direct access to recording from the common or His bundle,[9-11] and even from the right bundle branch. With a more proximal electrode in the right atrium, simultaneous recording from multiple intracardiac locations is possible, as illustrated in Figure 12.10.

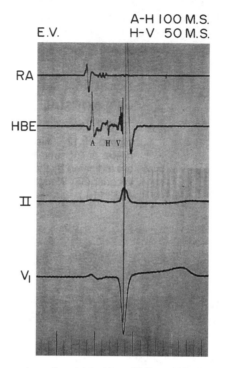

Figure 12.10. Electrograms from the right atrium (*RA*) and His bundle (*HBE*) are presented, along with recordings from standard leads II and V1. The atrium-to-His (*A–H*) and His-to-ventricle (*H–V*) intervals combine to form the PR interval. (From Wagner GS, Waugh RA, Ramo BW. Cardiac arrhythmias. New York: Churchill Livingstone, 1983:117, with permission.)

Recording from the His bundle provides partitioning of the PR interval into two components: from the atria through the AV node to the His bundle (atrium-to-His [AH] interval), and from the His bundle to the ventricles (His-to-ventricle [HV] interval). This method provides direct identification of the site of an AV block (Fig. 12.11).[12] His-bundle recordings have provided proof for many originally assumed electrocardiographic principles that will be discussed in later chapters.

A. PROXIMAL BLOCK–A-V NODE

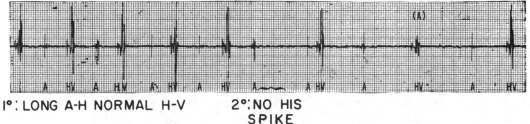

I°: LONG A-H NORMAL H-V   2°: NO HIS
                                    SPIKE

B. DISTAL BLOCK–BUNDLE BRANCHES

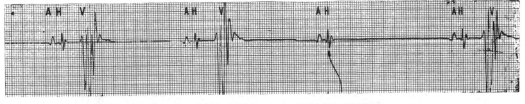

I°: NORMAL A-H LONG H-V   2°: HIS SPIKE
                                    PRESENT

Figure 12.11. His-bundle electrograms from two patients with delay (1°) and even complete (2°) failure of AV conduction. Conduction delays proximal **(A)** and distal **(B)** to the His bundle are indicated by the relationships among atrial (*A*), His (*H*), and ventricular (*V*) spikes. In **A**, during the initial slowly conducted beats (1–4), the A-H time is long but the H-V time is normal; however, in **B**, during the initial slowly conducted beats (1–2), the A-H time is normal and the H-V time is long. When A-V conduction fails to occur in **A** (during the fifth cardiac cycle), no His activation occurs; however, when A-V conduction fails to occur in **B** (during the third cardiac cycle), the His activation is present (*arrow*). Slow A-V conduction resumes at the end of both **A** and **B**. (From Wagner GS, Waugh RA, Ramo BW. Cardiac arrhythmias. New York: Churchill Livingstone, 1983:119, with permission)

INCIDENCES OF ARRHYTHMIAS IN NORMAL POPULATIONS

Many studies have documented high incidences of various arrhythmias in normal individuals of all ages.

In a study of 134 normal infants during the first 10 days of life,[13] the maximal heart rate reached 220 beats/min, while the minimal rate was 42 beats/min. Atrial premature beats (APBs) were found in 19 (14% of the infants), and sinus pauses occurred in 72%, with the longest pause reaching 1.8 s.

In a study of 92 healthy children aged 7 to11 years,[14] the fastest rate attained was 195 beats/min and the lowest rate was 37 beats/min. First-degree AV block was found in nine children and second-degree AV block in three. Atrial and ventricular premature beats were found in 21% and sinus pauses in two-thirds of the children.

In a third study, of 131 healthy boys aged 10 to 13 years,[15] waking maximal heart rates ranged between 100 and 200 beats/min, with minimal rates between 45 and 80 beats/min. Maximal heart rates during sleep were between 60 and 100 beats/min, with minimal rates between 30 and 70 beats/min. First-degree AV block was found in 8% and second degree AV block in 11% of the boys. Single atrial and ventricular premature beats (VPBs) were found in 13% and 26%, respectively.

In a study of 50 healthy women aged 22 to 28 years,[16] the waking maximal heart rate ranged from 122 to 189 beats/min, with minimal rates between 40 and 73 beats/min. Maximal heart rates during sleep ranged from 71 to 128 beats/min, with minimal rates between 37 and 59 beats/min. APBs occurred in 64% and VPBs in 54% of the women. One woman had one three-beat run of ventricular tachycardia and two women (4%) had periods of second-degree AV block.

In a study of 50 healthy male medical students,[17] the waking maximal heart rate ranged from 107 to 180 beats/min, with minimal rates between 37 and 65 beats/min. Maximal heart rates during sleep were between 70 and 115 beats/min, with minimal rates of 33 to 55 beats/min. Half of the students had sinus arrhythmia sufficient to cause a 100% change in consecutive cycles, and 28% had sinus pauses of more than 1.75 s. APBs were found in 56% of the students, while VPBs were found in 50%. Three students (6%) had periods of second-degree AV block.

An investigation of 98 healthy elderly subjects ranging from 60 to 85 years old and who had normal maximal treadmill tests[18] revealed sinus bradycardia in 91% of the subjects, supraventricular premature beats in 88%, supraventricular tachycardia in 13%, and atrial flutter in 1%. Ventricular arrhythmias included premature beats in 78% (many with pairs or multiform beats) and ventricular tachycardia in 4%.

A study of 20 male long-distance runners ranging in age from 19 to 29 years[19] found that all had APBs, 70% had VPBs, and 40% had periods of second-degree AV block.

Another study, of 101 healthy women,[20] disclosed VPBs in 34% and complex forms in 10%. Supraventricular premature beats were recorded in 28%, and VPBs were more frequent in women taking contraceptive pills or thyroid medication.

In a study of 50 healthy 80- to 89-year-old persons of both genders,[21] supraventricular premature beats were found in 100%, with 65% having more than 20 such beats per hour. Supraventricular tachycardia was found in 28%. More than 10 VPBs per hour were found in 32% of the subjects, with multifocal beats in 18%.

Among 147 healthy Swedish workers ranging in age from 15 to 65 years,[22] 95% of those under 40 years of age had less than three VPBs per hour, while in those over 40 years old, 95% had less than 36 VPBs per hour.

LADDER DIAGRAMS

Ladder diagrams are often helpful for understanding difficult arrhythmias. These diagrams have spaces for indicating atrial (A), atrial-to-ventricular junction (A-V), and ventricular (V) activation (Fig. 12.12). Additional spaces can be added as needed to diagram more complex arrhythmias. The ladder diagram should be constructed directly under or on a photocopy of the ECG recording, in two sequential stages, as follows:

1. Include what you can see (e.g., draw lines to represent the visible P waves and QRS complexes).
2. Add what you cannot see (e.g., connect the atrial and ventricular lines to represent AV or ventriculoatrial (VA) conduction, and draw lines to represent any missing P waves at regular PP intervals between visible P waves).

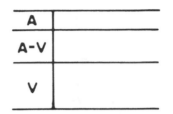

Figure 12.12. The format on which ladder diagrams can be constructed: spaces are provided for representing atrial (*A*), junctional (*J*), and ventricular (*V*) activation.

Figure 12.13 provides an illustration of the use of ladder diagrams to understand a cardiac arrhythmia with various PR intervals and varying QRS complex morphologies. In the first stage of the diagram, all visible P waves and QRS complexes have been represented. Note the reversed slope representing the premature, wide QRS complex, indicating the likelihood that it originated from the ventricles. When the lines representing AV conduction are added in the second stage, the prolonged PR interval following

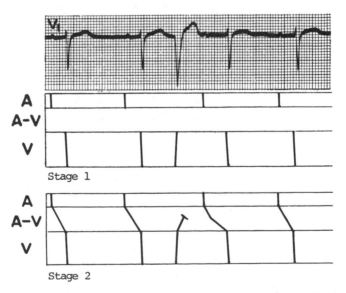

Figure 12.13. The two stages of construction of a ladder diagram: *Stage 1* involves the use of *slanted lines* to include the duration of the obvious waveforms representing both atrial and ventricular activation. The slanted lines indicate the presumed direction of spread of activation. *Stage 2* involves constructing lines in the A-V junctional space to connect the atrial and ventricular lines so as to represent the presumed direction of the spread of junctional activation. These lines are terminated and capped with short perpendicular lines to indicate the presumed failure of impulse conduction.

the third P wave is indicated by an angulation to represent a conduction disturbance. The VPB must have traveled retrogradely into the A-V junction, so that the next sinus impulse found the junction relatively refractory.

In subsequent chapters, ladder diagrams will be freely used as a visual aid to understanding mechanisms of arrhythmias. Figure 12.14A–D presents four examples to indicate how various symbols may be used to represent such phenomena as aberrant ventricular conduction (Fig. 12.14A), junctional rhythms (Fig. 12.14B), ventricular rhythms (Fig. 12.14C), and dissociation between atrial and ventricular rhythms (Fig. 12.14D).

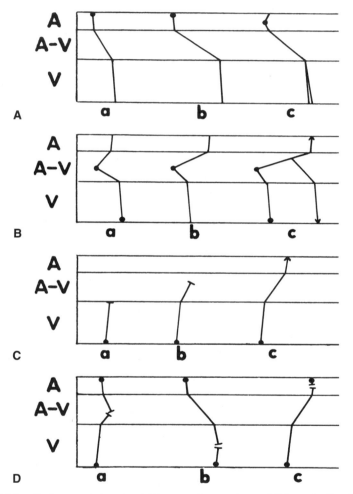

Figure 12.14. **A.** A normal sinus beat (a) encounters prolonged AV conduction (b) and is then replaced by an atrial beat that encounters both prolonged AV conduction and aberrant ventricular conduction (indicated by the *split line*) (c). *Solid circles* indicate the site of impulse formation. **B.** AV-junctional beats with progressively longer retrograde conduction times to the atria: in a, the P wave precedes the QRS complex, but in b it follows the QRS complex. In c, the retrograde conduction time is so long that a second QRS complex is generated. *Arrowheads* have been added to indicate the direction of impulse conduction (c), but the direction of the impulse is also indicated by the slopes of the lines. **C.** Ventricular beats with progressively greater penetration into the AV junction: no conduction (a), partial conduction (b), and complete retrograde VA conduction (c). **D.** In a, there is complete AV dissociation; in b, AV conduction results in "fusion" during the QRS complex; and in c, VA conduction results in fusion during the P wave.

GLOSSARY

Atrial flutter: the tachyarrhythmia at the slow end of the flutter/fibrillation spectrum, produced by macroreentry within a single circuit in the atria and characterized by regular uniform F waves.

Automaticity: the ability of specialized cardiac cells to achieve spontaneous depolarization and function as "pacemakers" to form new cardiac-activating impulses.

AV dissociation: a condition of independent beating of the atria and ventricles, caused either by block of the atrial-activating impulse in the AV junction or by interference with conduction of the atrial-activating impulse by a ventricular impulse.

Block: either a delay (first degree), partial failure (second degree), or total failure (third degree) of impulse conduction through a part of the heart.

Bradyarrhythmia: any rhythm with a ventricular rate of less than 60 beats/min.

Cardioversion: application of an electric shock in order to restore a normal heartbeat.

Dysrhythmia: a synonym (by usage) for arrhythmia.

Inhomogeneous conduction: the phenomenon in which the wave front of cardiac activation spreads unevenly through a part of the heart because of varying refractoriness from previous activation, creating the potential for impulse reentry.

Isorhythmic dissociation: AV dissociation, with the atria and ventricles beating at the same or almost the same rate.

Junctional: a term referring to the cardiac structures that electrically connect the atria and ventricles, and normally including the AV node and common (His) bundle, and abnormally including an accessory AV conduction (Kent) bundle.

Macroreentry: recycling of an impulse around a circuit that is large enough for its own activation to be represented on the surface ECG.

Microreentry: the recycling of an impulse around a circuit that is too small for its own activation to be represented on the surface ECG.

Pacemaker cells: specialized cardiac cells that are capable of automaticity.

Palpitation: a sensation felt in the chest as a result of the stronger ventricular contraction following a prolonged cardiac cycle.

Premature beat: a beat that occurs prior to the time when the next normal beat would be expected to appear.

Reentry circuit: a circular course traveled by a cardiac impulse, created by reentry, and having the potential for initiating premature beats and tachyarrhythmias.

Relative refractory: a terms referring to cells that have only partly recovered from their previous activation and are therefore capable of slow conduction of another impulse.

Spontaneous depolarization: the ability of a specialized cardiac cell to activate by altering the permeability of its membrane to a sufficient degree to attain threshold potential without any external stimulation.

Transtelephonic monitoring: cardiac monitoring in which the patient uses a pocket-sized transmitter to send a cardiac rhythm strip over the telephone when cardiac symptoms occur.

REFERENCES

1. Hoffman BF, Cranefield PF, Wallace AG. Physiological basis of cardiac arrhythmias. Mod Concepts Cardiovasc Dis 1966;35:103.

2. Marriott HJL, Fogg E. Constant monitoring for cardiac dysrhythmias and blocks. Mod Concepts Cardiovasc Dis 1970;39:103.

3. Holter NJ. New method for heart studies: continuous electrocardiography of active subjects over long periods is now practical. Science 1961;134:1214.

4. Zeldis SM, Levine BJ, Michelson EL, et al. Cardiovascular complaints: correlation with cardiac arrhythmias on 24-hour electrocardiographic monitoring. Chest 1982;78:456.

5. Michelson EL, Morganroth J. Spontaneous variability of complex ventricular arrhythmias detected by long-term electrocardiographic recording. Circulation 1980;61:690–695.

6. Grodman PS. Arrhythmia surveillance by transtelephonic monitoring; comparison with Holter monitoring in symptomatic ambulatory patients. Am Heart J 1979;98:459.

7. Judson P, Holmes DR, Baker WP. Evaluation of outpatient arrhythmias utilizing transtelephonic monitoring. Am Heart J 1979;97:759–761.

8. Cumbee SR, Pryor RE, Linzer M. Cardiac loop ECG recording: a new noninvasive diagnostic test in recurrent syncope. South Med J 1990;83:39–43.

9. Damato AN, Lau SH. Clinical value of the electrogram of the conduction system. Prog Cardiovasc Dis 1970;13:119–140.

10. Goldreyer BN. Intracardiac electrocardiography in the analysis and understanding of cardiac arrhythmias. Ann Intern Med 1972;77:117–136.

11. Vadde PS, Caracta AR, Damato AN. Indications of His bundle recordings. Cardiovasc Clin 1980;11:1–6.

12. Pick A. Mechanisms of cardiac arrhythmias; from hypothesis to physiologic fact. Am Heart J 1973;86:249–269.

13. Southall DP, Richards J, Mitchell P, et al. Study of cardiac rhythm in healthy newborn infants. Br Heart J 1980;43:14–20.

14. Southall DP, Johnston F, Shinebourne EA, et al. A 24-hour electrocardiographic study of heart rate and rhythm patterns in population of healthy children. Br Heart J 1981;45:281–291.

15. Scott O, Williams GJ, Fiddler GI. Results of 24-hour ambulatory monitoring of electrocardiogram in 131 healthy boys aged 10 to 13 years. Br Heart J 1980;44:304–308.

16. Sobotka PA, Mayer JH, Bauernfeind RA, et al. Arrhythmias documented by 24-hour continuous ambulatory electrocardiographic monitoring in young women without apparent heart disease. Am Heart J 1981;101:753–759.

17. Brodsky M, Wu D, Denes P, Kanakis C, et al. Arrhythmias documented by 24 hour continuous electrocardiographic monitoring in 50 male medical students without apparent heart disease. Am J Cardiol 1977;39:390–395.

18. Fleg JL, Kennedy HL. Cardiac arrhythmias in a healthy elderly population: detection by 24-hour ambulatory electrocardiography. Chest 1982;81:302–307.

19. Talan DA, Bauernfeind RA, Ashley WW, Kanakis C Jr, et al. Twenty-four hour continuous ECG recordings in long-distance runners. Chest 1982;82:19–24.

20. Romhilt DW, Choi SC, Irby EC. Arrhythmias on ambulatory monitoring in women without apparent heart disease. Am J Cardiol 1984;54:582–586.

21. Kantelip JP, Sage E, Duchene-Marullaz P. Findings on ambulatory monitoring in subjects older than 80 years. Am J Cardiol 1986;57:398–401.

22. Orth-Gomer K, Hogstedt C, Bodin L, et al. Frequency of extrasystoles in healthy male employees. Br Heart J 1986;55:259–264.

CHAPTER 13

Premature Beats

PREMATURE BEAT TERMINOLOGY

Normal sinus rhythm is commonly interrupted by a premature beat (PB). "Premature" in this terms refers to early occurrence and "beat" is short for heartbeat. A PB is recognized on the electrocardiogram (ECG) by the early appearance of a QRS complex; either normal or abnormal in configuration, and either preceded or not preceded by a P wave. Other terms are often substituted for the term "premature beat," including: premature contraction, early beat, extrasystole, premature systole, and *ectopic beat*.

The individual who has a PB may or may not experience a *palpitation*. This palpitation would be felt during the next on-time beat because of the increased ventricular contraction strength caused by the higher volume of blood that enters the ventricle during the delay following the PB. Figure 13.1 illustrates the following sequence of events that occur as a result of a single PB:

1. The PB occurs early in the cardiac cycle.
2. The presence of the PB prevents the occurrence of the next normal beat.
3. There is a pause following the PB until the next normal beat occurs.

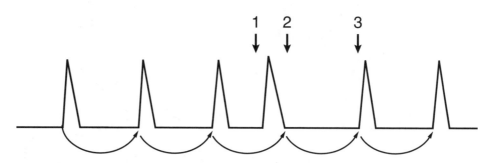

Figure 13.1. The timing of a regular underlying rhythm is indicated by the *curved lines* with *arrows*. A PB interrupts this rhythm **(1)**, preventing the occurrence of the next normal beat **(2)**; however, the following normal beat occurs at the expected time **(3)**.

A single PB is potentially the first beat of a sustained tachyarrhythmia (tach). It may be followed by any number of similarly appearing beats, to which the terms in the following two paragraphs are applied (Table 13.1).

Table 13.1. Terminology of Quantities of PBs

Number of Consecutive Beats	Term
1 beat	A premature beat
2 beats	A pair or a *couplet*
3 beats—1 minute continuation	Nonsustained tach
>1 minute continuation	Sustained tach

When a PB follows every normal beat, the term *bigeminy* is used, and when a PB follows every second normal beat, the term *trigeminy* is used. PBs may originate from any part of the heart other than the sinoatrial (SA) node. They are generally classified as *supraventricular premature beats* (*SVPBs*) or *ventricular premature beats* (*VPBs*), as indicated in Figure 13.2. This distinction is useful, because beats originating from anywhere above the branching of the common bundle (SVPBs) are capable of producing a normal or abnormal QRS complex, depending on whether they are conducted normally or aberrantly through the intraventricular conduction system. PBs originating from beyond the branching of the common bundle (VPBs), however, can produce only an abnormally prolonged QRS complex of more than 0.12 s, because they do not have equal access to both the right and left bundle branches. It should be emphasized that VPBs are always abnormally prolonged, but SVPBs are not always of normal duration.

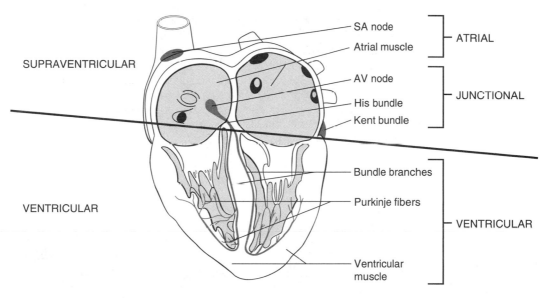

Figure 13.2. The parts of the supraventricular and ventricular areas are indicated. Note the *wide red band* connecting the left atrium and left ventricle on the epicardial surface, which represents a Kent bundle. (Modified from Netter FH. The Ciba collection of medical illustrations. vol 5. Heart. Summit, NJ: Ciba–Geigy, 1978:49.)

SVPBs may be either *atrial premature beats* (*APBs*) or *junctional premature beats* (*JPBs*). The term "junctional" is used instead of "nodal" because it is impossible to distinguish beats originating within the AV node from those originating in another structure located between the atria and the ventricles. Normally, the AV junction consists of only the AV node and the common bundle. Abnormally, however, an accessory AV conduction pathway (Kent bundle) may also be part of the AV junction.

DIFFERENTIAL DIAGNOSIS OF WIDE PREMATURE BEATS

When SVPBs have abnormally prolonged or wide QRS complexes (>0.12 s), identification of a supraventricular versus a ventricular origin for these beats may be facilitated by observing the effect on the regularity of the underlying sinus rhythm (Figure 13.3). A VPB typically does not disturb the sinus rhythm because it is not conducted retrogradely through the slowly conducting AV node into the SA node (Fig. 13.3A). Although the SA node discharges on time, the impulse cannot be conducted antegradely into the ventricles because of the refractoriness following the VPB. The pause between the VPB and the following conducted beat is termed a *compensatory pause* because it compensates for the prematurity of the VPB. The interval from the sinus beat prior to the VPB to the sinus beat following the VPB is equal to two sinus cycles.

In contrast to the case for a VPB (Fig. 13.3B), an SVPB does disturb the sinus rhythm. Unlike the VPB, the SVPB can be conducted retrogradely into the SA node, discharging it ahead of schedule and causing the following cycle to also occur ahead of schedule. The pause between the SVPB and the following sinus beat is therefore less than compensatory. This is apparent because the interval from the sinus beat prior to the SVPB to the sinus beat following the SVPB is less than the duration of two sinus cycles. However, when the SVPB prematurely discharges the SA node, it occasionally suppresses its automaticity. This *overdrive suppression* may delay the formation of the next sinus impulse for so long that the resulting pause is compensatory or even longer than compensatory. Thus, the compensatory pause must not be relied upon as the sole indicator of ventricular origin of a wide PB.

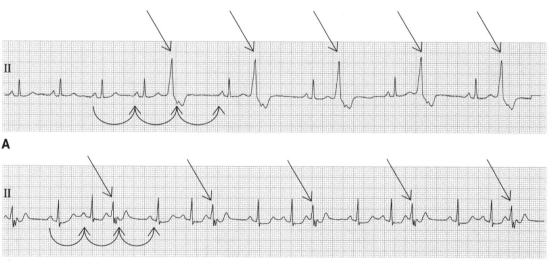

A

B

Figure 13.3. The *straight arrows* indicate the premature wide QRS complexes in **A** and **B**. The *curved arrows* marking the baseline PP interval indicate that the P waves following the PBs occur "on time" (at twice the normal PP interval) in **A** but not on time (at less than twice the normal PP interval) in **B**. Note that in **A** the P waves following the PB occurs at the same time as the *curved arrow*, but in **B** the P wave following the PB occurs prior to the time as the *curved arrow*.

MECHANISMS OF PRODUCTION OF PREMATURE BEATS

PBs may be caused by the two mechanisms indicated in Chapter 12 ("Introduction to Arrhythmias"): reentry or automaticity. It is usually difficult to determine the mechanism of causation of PBs unless two or more such beats occur in succession. Fortunately, the mechanism of causation of a PB is usually not clinically important unless consecutive abnormal beats are present. When identification of the mechanism for a PB is considered clinically important, the following observations of the coupling intervals between beats may be helpful (Fig. 13.4): reentry produces a constant relationship between normal and premature beats (Fig. 13.4A); automaticity produces a varying relationship between normal and abnormal beats but a constant relationship between abnormal beats (Fig. 13.4B) as in Table 13.2.

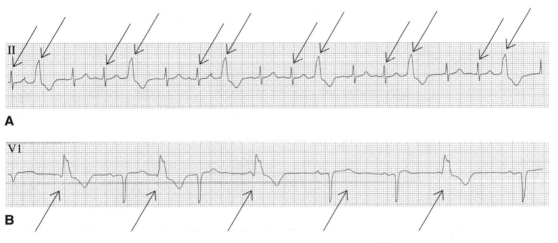

Figure 13.4. The *arrows* in the rhythm strips indicate the VPBs coupled to preceding normal beats **(A)** and related to each other **(B)**. In **B**, the *fourth arrow* indicates where a VPB would have occurred had the ventricles been receptive rather than refractory, as indicated by the presence of the T wave.

Table 13.2. Keys to Diagnosis of PB Mechanism

Observations	Mechanism
There are identical coupling intervals between each PB and the preceding normal beat (Fig. 13.4A).	Reentry
There are not identical coupling intervals between PBs and normal beats, but there are identical intervals between consecutive PBs (Fig. 13.4B).	Enhanced automaticity
There are neither identical coupling intervals between PBs and normal beats nor between consecutive PBs.	Either

ATRIAL PREMATURE BEATS

The usual APB has three features:

1. A premature and abnormal-appearing P wave.
2. A QRS complex similar to that of the normal sinus beats.
3. A following interval that is less than compensatory, owing to the retrograde activation of the SA node.

As a rule, all of these characteristics are obvious, but "deceptions" occur, so that no one characteristic is completely reliable. In Figure 13.5A, the premature P waves appear normal, and in Figure 13.5B the premature QRS complexes are not always similar to those of the normal sinus beats.

Some common ECG deceptions in recognizing APBs are:

1. The P wave may be unrecognizable because it occurs during the previous T wave (Fig. 13.5B and C).
2. The QRS complex may show aberrant ventricular conduction (Fig. 13.5B).
3. The pause between the APB and the following beat may appear to be compensatory or even longer because of overdrive suppression (Fig. 13.5C).

It is extremely rare to have all three of these deceptions appear at the same time. Therefore, with care, one usually has no trouble in identifying an APB.

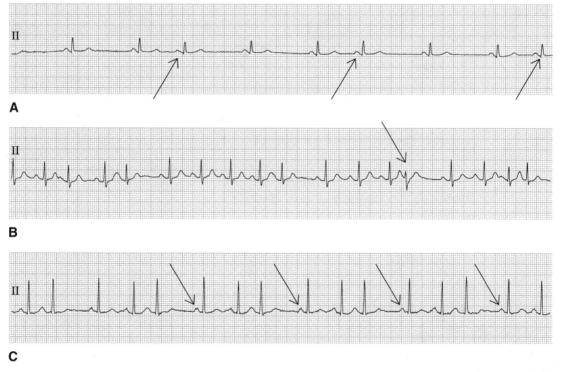

Figure 13.5. Three-lead II rhythm strips: *arrows* indicate normally appearing premature P waves in **A**, the third APB appearing abnormally in **B**, and the timing of the fully compensatory pause in **C**.

When an APB follows every sinus beat, the result is atrial bigeminy (Fig. 13.6A); when it follows every two consecutive sinus beats, the result is atrial trigeminy (Fig. 13.6B).

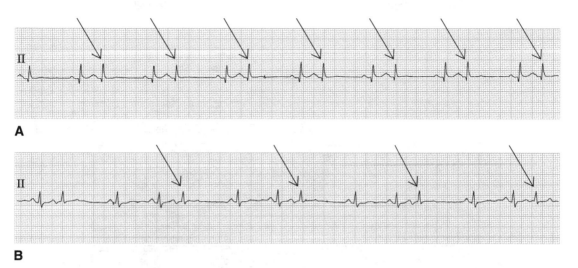

A

B

Figure 13.6. In A, every normal sinus beat and in B every second normal sinus beat is coupled through constant PP Intervals to APBs. The QRS complexes resulting from these APBs are indicated by the *arrows* in the lead II rhythm strips.

When APBs occur very early (a short coupling interval), some parts of the heart may not have had time to complete their recovery from the preceding normal activation. This may result in failure of the premature atrial activation to cause any ventricular activation. Indeed, the most common cause of an unexpected atrial pause is a nonconducted APB (Fig. 13.7). It is better to refer to such beats as "nonconducted" rather than "blocked" because by definition, block implies an abnormal condition. APBs fail to be conducted only because they occur so early in the cycle that the AV node is still in its normal refractory period. It is important to differentiate normal (physiologic) from abnormal (pathologic) nonconduction in order to avoid mistakenly initiating an antiarrhythmia treatment.

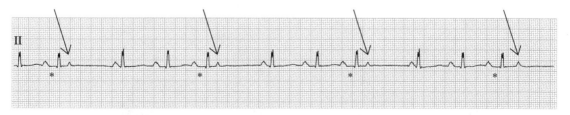

Figure 13.7. Nonconducted premature P waves are indicated by *arrows*, but even some on-time P waves have some conduction delay as indicated by prolonged PR intervals (*asterisks*).

Nonconducted APBs that occur in a bigeminal pattern are particularly difficult to identify (Fig 13.8). If the premature P waves are obscured by the T waves of the preceding normal beats, and if the earlier T waves during the regular sinus rhythm are not available for comparison, then the rhythm will usually be misdiagnosed as sinus bradycardia.

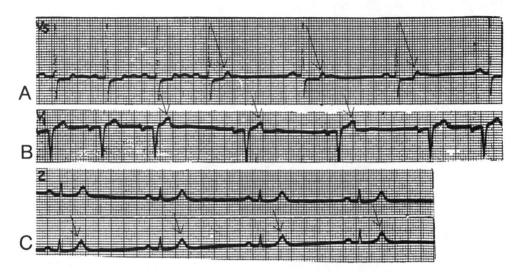

Figure 13.8. In **A** and **B**, the T waves preceding the pauses (*arrows*) appear different from usual. In **C**, there are suspicious peaks on the T waves (*arrows*), but there are no "usual" T waves available for comparison.

When APBs occur very early in the cardiac cycle of normal beats, they may have other effects on conduction to the ventricles, as illustrated in Figure 13.9. In Fig. 13.9*A*, there is prolonged AV conduction, while in Fig. 13.9*B* there is slightly prolonged AV conduction and also aberrant intraventricular conduction. In Fig. 13.9*B* there are varying coupling intervals (*PP intervals*) between normal sinus beats and APBs. When the PP interval is long, the premature P-to-R interval is normal, but when the PP interval is short, the premature P-to-R interval is prolonged. This inverse relationship occurs because of the uniquely long relative refractory period of the AV node: the longer the duration from its most recent activation, the better is the node able to conduct the following impulse, and vice versa. This concept is vital to use of the ECG to differentiate a nodal versus Purkinje location of AV block.

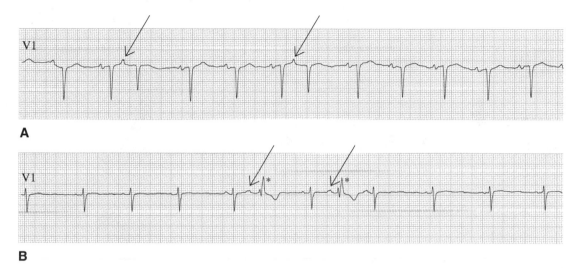

Figure 13.9. Recordings of lead V1 illustrate other varieties of physiologic conduction delays that may occur when the AV node alone **(A)** or both the AV node and the right bundle branch **(B)** have not had time to fully recover from their preceding normal activation. *Arrows* indicate prolonged AV-nodal conduction in **A** and **B**, and *asterisks* indicate RBB aberrancy in **B**.

When an early APB traverses the AV junction but encounters persistent normal refractoriness in one of the bundle branches or fascicles, aberrant ventricular conduction occurs, as in Fig. 13.9*B*. The morphology of the QRS complex is altered, and its duration may be so prolonged that it resembles a VPB. Detection of the preceding P wave and/or finding that the pause between the APB and the next sinus beat is less than compensatory will usually establish the diagnosis of an APB.

APBs may occur so early that even parts of the atria have not completed their refractory periods. During this time (the *vulnerable period*), the APB may initiate a reentrant atrial tachyarrhythmia, as illustrated in Figure 13.10. In this instance, the APB becomes the first beat of atrial flutter/fibrillation (Chapter 15, "Atrial Flutter/Fibrillation Spectrum"). Killip and Gault[1] developed the rule that when the PP interval is less than 50% of the previous PP interval, an APB is quite likely to initiate atrial flutter/fibrillation.

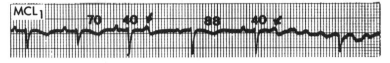

Figure 13.10. *Arrows* indicate two early APBs with PP intervals of 0.40 second (40 ms). The first PP interval is longer than half the preceding PP interval of 0.70 second (70 ms), but the second is shorter than half the preceding PP interval of 0.88 second (88 ms), initiating an atrial reentrant tachyarrhythmia (Chapter 15, "Reentrant Atrial Tachyarrhythmias—The Atrial Flutter/Fibrillation Spectrum").

JUNCTIONAL PREMATURE BEATS

 PBs arising in the AV junction may retrogradely activate the atria before, during, or after ventricular activation, and the retrograde P wave may therefore be seen preceding or following the QRS complex, or may be lost within the QRS complex. "Upper," "mid-," and "lower" are the terms, based on the position of the P wave in relation to the QRS complex, that have been used to signify the presumed site of origin of a JPB within the AV junction (Fig. 13.11A). However, as indicated in Fig. 13.11B, the P-to-QRS relationship also depends on the relative rates of conduction of the premature impulse from its origin to the atrial and ventricular myocardia. Therefore, the relationship between the P waves and QRS complexes in the ECG does not necessarily indicate the level within the AV junction from which JPBs originate, and the terms "upper," "mid-," and "lower" are no longer used.

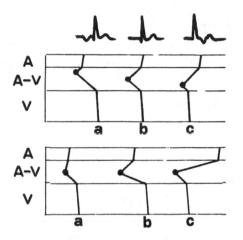

Figure 13.11. Three impulses (a, b, and c) are formed within the AV junction (A–V) in two ladder diagrams. In the **top** ladder diagram, the anatomic site of impulse formation (*solid circle*) varies, but the physiologic conduction velocity is constant, resulting in the P–QRS relationships shown at the top. The **bottom** ladder diagram illustrates the additional influence of variation of the velocity of conduction from the site of impulse formation to the atria and ventricles; however, the resultant P-QRS relationships are not illustrated.

The diagnosis of a junctional origin of PBs is easiest when a premature normal QRS complex is closely accompanied by an "upside down" P wave (Fig. 13.12). As would be expected, the morphology of the P waves associated with JPBs is markedly different from that of the P waves of normal sinus rhythm. The polarity of the P waves associated with JPBs is approximately opposite that of the P waves of normal sinus rhythm, as is best seen in a lead with base-to-apex orientation, such as lead II. A P wave originating from the AV junction is also inverted in the other inferiorly oriented leads (e.g., aVF), is upright in superiorly oriented leads aVR and aVL, and is almost flat in leftward-oriented leads I and V5.

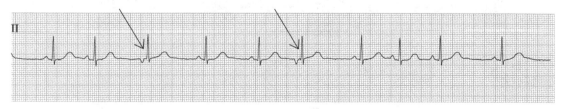

Figure 13.12. The contrasting appearances of P waves originating from the sinus node and the AV junction (*arrows*) are illustrated in this lead II rhythm strip.

A JPB may be confused with an APB when a premature normal QRS complex is not closely accompanied by an abnormal P wave (Fig. 13.13). In the top panel, the normally appearing and normally timed P wave following the premature normal QRS complex indicates a JPB. In the bottom panel, there are no accompanying P waves to provide clues to a junctional versus atrial origin of the PBs. Differentiation of these two sites of origin requires observation of the influence of the PB on the regularity of the underlying sinus rhythm. The sinus rhythm is typically reset by an APB, but may or may not be reset by a JPB. The pause following a JPB may therefore be fully compensatory.

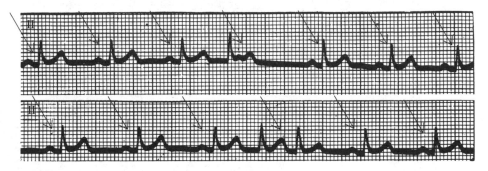

Figure 13.13. **Top** and **bottom** panels are recordings of lead II from the same individual. Note that the regular sinus rhythm (*arrows*) "marches through" or is "not reset" by the PBs.

A JPB may be confused with a VPB when the premature QRS complex is wide (>0.12 s). The various principles presented in Chapters 17 ("Ventricular Tachyarrhythmias") and 18 ("Supraventricular Tachyarrhythmias with Aberrant Ventricular Conduction") for differentiating supraventricular beats with aberrant intraventricular conduction from ventricular beats may be applied in such a case. Figure 13.14 shows JPBs with differing degrees of right bundle-branch (RBB) aberration. The retrograde atrial activation is apparent from the P waves following the premature QRS complexes. Although the first PB in each ECG strip cannot be distinguished from a VPB, the fact that the second PB manifests a lesser degree of the pattern of right bundle-branch block is a strong point in favor of the aberrant conduction coming from a JPB.

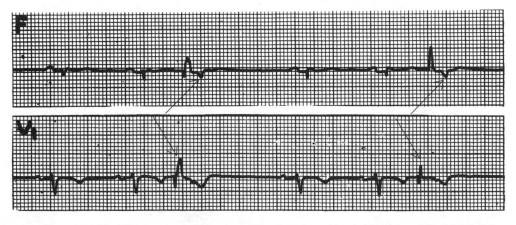

Figure 13.14. The long-axis (base-to-apex) orientation of lead aVF (*F*) provides the best view of the inverted P waves (*arrows*) in this case of JPBs with RBB aberration, and the short-axis (right versus left) orientation of lead *V1* provides the best view of the varying amounts of RBB aberrancy (*arrows*). The combined contributions of both leads confirm the junctional origin of the PBs.

VENTRICULAR PREMATURE BEATS

The characteristic VPB, as illustrated in Figure 13.15, is not preceded by a premature P wave, and is represented by a wide and bizarre QRS complex. It is followed by a compensatory pause because of its inability to conduct retrogradely through the AV node to reset the SA node.

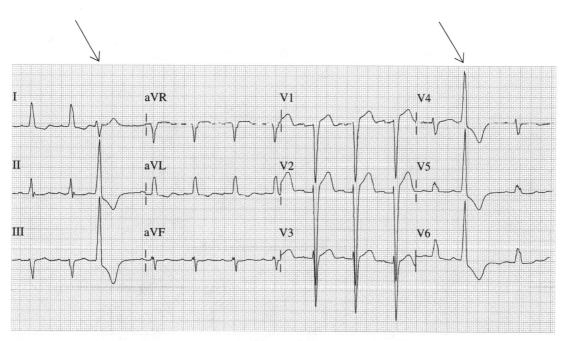

Figure 13.15. The views of typical VPBs (*arrows*) from multiple simultaneously recorded ECG leads. Note that VPBs occur only during displays of the first and fourth groups of leads.

However, the following exceptions to all of these characteristics may occur, thereby confounding the distinction of a ventricular from a supraventricular origin of the PB.

1. With regard to a preceding premature P wave, a VPB may be preceded by a premature P wave if both an APB and a VPB are present.
2. With regard to the appearance of the QRS complex, a VPB, although typically wider than 0.12 second, may appear to have a normal duration in any single lead because its initial or terminal component is isoelectric. A VPB may even, by coincidence, appear similar to the normal beats in a single lead, as illustrated in lead V1 in Figure 13.16. It is important to consider two or even three simultaneously recorded leads in determining the origin of a PB.

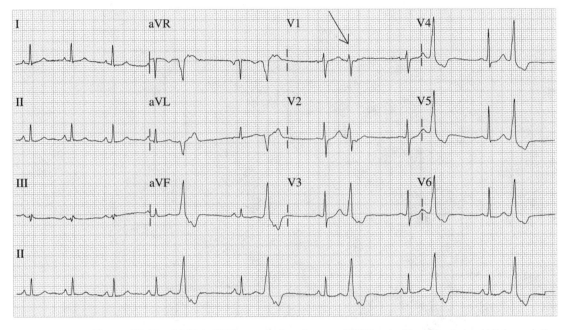

Figure 13.16. Multiple VPBs are obvious in many ECG leads. However, in lead V1 (*arrow*), the QRS complexes of the VPBs coincidentally appear very similar to those of the normal sinus beats. If only a lead V1 recording was available, the erroneous diagnosis of APBs might be made.

3. Regarding the pause following the VPB, if there is marked variation in the underlying sinus regularity because of sinus arrhythmia, it cannot be determined whether or not a pause is compensatory. When the sinus rhythm is regular, however, there are rare occurrences of a VPB that lacks a following compensatory pause.

A VPB that lacks a compensatory pause occurs for one of two reasons: (a) the VPB is interpolated between consecutive sinus beats; or (b) the VPB resets the sinus rhythm. These two possibilities are discussed below.

The Ventricular Premature Beat is Interpolated between Consecutive Sinus Beats

When a VPB is extremely premature (close to the time of the last sinus impulse), it cannot be conducted retrogradely through the still refractory AV node. However, when the sinus rate is slow, such a VPB occurs long before the following sinus impulse, and there is ample time for the AV node and ventricles to complete their refractory periods before the next normal sinus impulse is conducted anterogradely. The VPB is therefore "interpolated" between sinus beats, and there is no pause (Fig. 13.17).

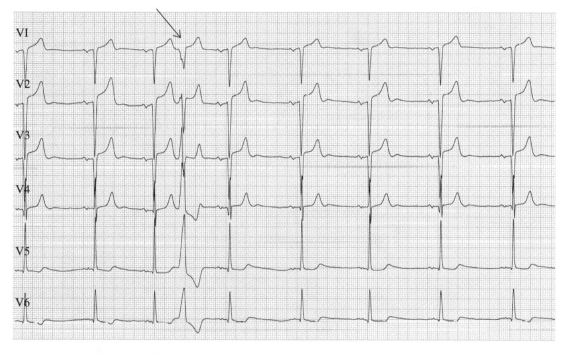

Figure 13.17. A single interpolated VPB occurs (*arrow*) between the third and fourth sinus beat. Note the slight sinus irregularity (sinus arrhythmia).

The PR interval of the sinus beat following the VPB is prolonged when the AV node is still partly refractory from its retrograde activation by the VPB. This is an example of "concealed conduction," because the absence of both a retrograde P wave and resetting of the sinus rhythm indicates that the impulse produced by the VPB never reached the atria. The continued bombardment of the AV node from both anterograde and retrograde directions prevents its complete recovery. If there is a recurrence of early VPBs, there may be progressively longer PR intervals (Fig. 13.18) until there is complete failure of conduction. Only then is the AV node able to completely recover, as indicated by the normal PR interval of the next sinus cycle. As was discussed earlier with regard to APBs, this represents a physiologic case of nonconduction, in contrast to pathologic AV block.

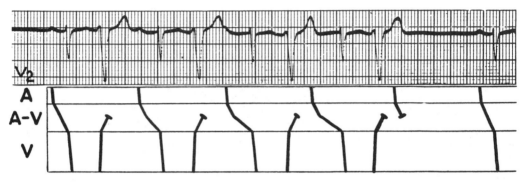

Figure 13.18. The ladder diagram indicates the relationships between the P waves and QRS complexes when both anterograde and retrograde activation prevent full recovery of the AV node.

The Ventricular Premature Beat Resets the Sinus Rhythm

When a VPB is only slightly premature (close to the time of the next sinus impulse), it can pass retrogradedly through the AV node, since this structure has recovered from the anterograde conduction of the previous sinus beat. The VPB can then enter the SA node and reset it in much the same way as does an APB. The retrograde P wave caused by this is usually obscured in the T wave of the VPB, but it may be detected in the ST segment of the VPB, as in Figure 13.19. The pause until the next sinus beat is therefore less than compensatory.

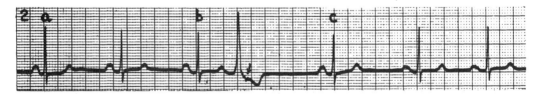

Figure 13.19. The *arrow* points to retrograde atrial activation by a VPB that resets the sinus node, as indicated by the less than compensatory pause (the *b–c* interval is less than the *a–b* interval).

When a VPB occurs so late that the next sinus P wave has already appeared (Fig. 13.20), the compensatory pause is hardly a pause at all. Only the short PR interval provides a clue that the wide QRS complex is indeed from a VPB. If the PR interval were normal, the diagnosis would most likely be intermittent bundle-branch block. The pattern of a normal P wave, short PR interval, and wide QRS complex could also be produced by ventricular preexcitation (Chapter 6, "Ventricular Preexcitation").

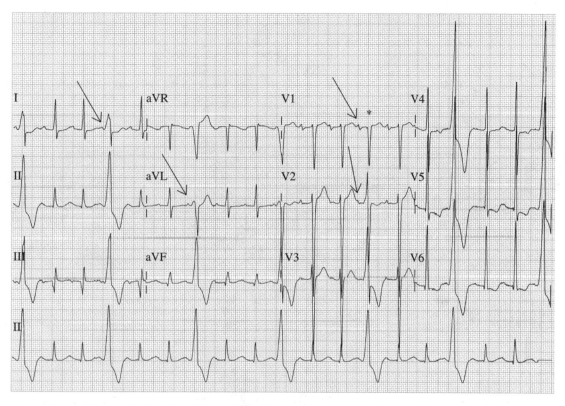

Figure 13.20. The VPBs in this ECG recording occur so late in the cycle that they follow the P waves of the normal sinus beats (*arrows*). Note, as in Figure 13.16, that the VPBs appear similar to the normal sinus beats in lead-V1 (*asterisk*).

THE RULE OF BIGEMINY

The occurrence of a long cardiac cycle (or pause) tends to precipitate reentry after the next normal beat. As discussed in Chapter 3 ("Interpretation of the Normal Electrocardiogram"), the ventricular recovery time, as measured by the QT interval, varies with the heart rate. Therefore, the normal beat that follows a compensatory pause has a longer recovery time than other normal beats. This longer recovery time increases the likelihood that adjacent myocardial cells are at different stages of the repolarization process. This greater difference in the cells' electrical potentials creates the possibility for current to "reenter" a recently recovered cell and to thus initiate another VPB.[2] A bigeminal pattern occurs with every normal beat followed by a VPB and with constant coupling intervals between each pair of normal sinus and VPBs, as illustrated in Figure 13.21. Ventricular bigeminy may not represent as much of a rhythm abnormality as it suggests. Preventing only the first VPB would prevent all subsequent VPBs.

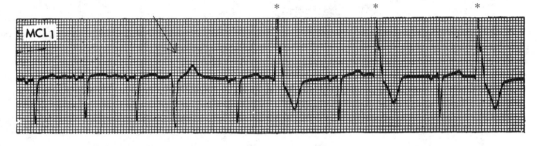

Figure 13.21. The use of lead MCL₁ provides identification of the ventricle of origin of the VPBs. The *arrow* shows the initial VPB (from the RV) producing a long cycle that precipitates another VPB (from the LV) which is shown by the *asterisk*. This pattern continues, resulting in a bigeminal rhythm.

RIGHT- VERSUS LEFT-VENTRICULAR PREMATURE BEATS

Figure 13.22 illustrates the contrast between VPBs originating in the right ventricle (*right VPBs*) and those originating from the left ventricle (*left VPBs*). The ventricle of origin of ectopic beats can best be recognized in lead V1, which is oriented to differentiate right- versus left-sided cardiac activity (Chapter 1, "Cardiac Electrical Activity"). If the VPB in lead V1 is predominantly positive (V1-positive), the impulse must be traveling anteriorly and rightward from its origin in the posteriorly located left ventricle (Fig. 13.22A). If the VPB in lead V1 is predominately negative (V1-negative), the impulse must be traveling posteriorly and leftward, usually from its origin in the anteriorly located right ventricle (Fig. 13.22B).[3] However, ischemic heart disease may produce left VPBs with V1-negative morphology (Chapter 17, "Ventricular Tachyarrythmias").

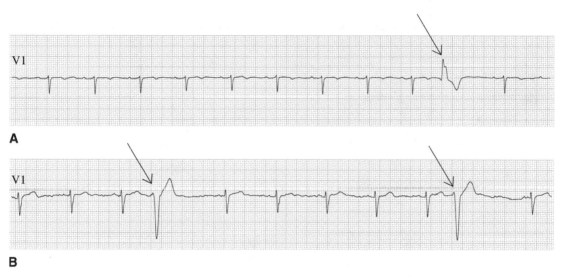

Figure 13.22. The contrasting appearances of V1-positive **(A)** and V1-negative **(B)** VPBs (*arrows*).

The differentiation between a right- and left-ventricular origin of VPBs is clinically useful for the following reasons:

1. Left VPBs are more often associated with heart disease, whereas right VPBs are commonly seen in individuals with normal hearts.[4,5]
2. Left VPBs are more likely than right VPBs to precipitate ventricular fibrillation during an acute myocardial infarction.[6]

A study of more than 1000 consecutive patients found no instances of ventricular fibrillation in the 249 patients who manifested only VPBs with a right-ventricular pattern in lead MCL_1. Patients with VPBs with a left-ventricular pattern, however, developed ventricular fibrillation 10.4% of the time (82 of 787 patients).

Morphologic features of left VPBs are:

1. Usually a monophasic (R) or diphasic (qR) complex in lead V1 and a diphasic (rS) or monophasic (QS) complex in lead V6 (Fig. 13.23).
2. An often greater amplitude of the first of two peaks (rabbit ears) in the QRS complex in lead V1, if this complex has two peaks. This is illustrated in Figures 13.21 and 13.22A.[7]

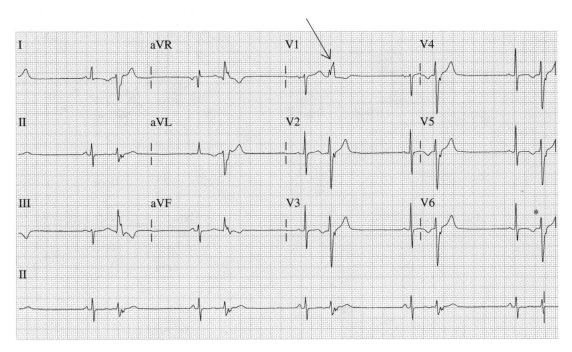

Figure 13.23. The monophasic V1 R wave (*arrow*) and diphasic V6 rS waves (*asterisk*) appearances that typify a left VPB. However, note that the first "rabbit ear" is atypically shorter than the right in the VPB in lead V1.

Morphologic features of right VPBs are:

1. An often typically positive morphology in lead V6, but a right-axis deviation in the frontal plane and a wide (>0.04 s) initial R wave in lead V1 (Fig. 13.24).[5,8]
2. A tendency to show a deeper (rS or QS) complex in lead V4 than in lead V1.[8]

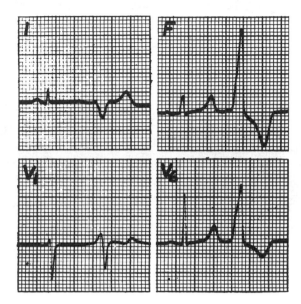

Figure 13.24. The typical morphology of a VPB originating from the right ventricle, viewed from limb leads I and aVF (*F*) and precordial leads *V1* and *V6*.

MULTIFORM VENTRICULAR PREMATURE BEATS

   When VPBs manifest different QRS-complex morphologies in the same lead (Fig. 13.25), they are termed *multiform VPBs*. Since such VPBs are assumed to arise from different foci, they are also called *multifocal VPBs*. It is possible, however, that the variation in QRS-complex morphology produced by VPBs may result from varying intraventricular conduction rather than from varying sites of origin. Indeed, varying patterns of VPBs have been produced from the same artificially stimulated focus.[9] Therefore, "multiform" is a more appropriate term than "multifocal" for VPBs showing different QRS-complex morphology.

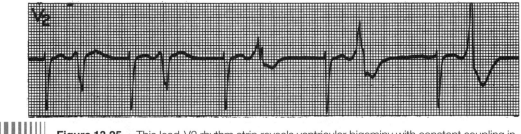

Figure 13.25.   This lead-V2 rhythm strip reveals ventricular bigeminy with constant coupling intervals but continually varying (multiform) VPB morphology.

GROUPS OF VENTRICULAR PREMATURE BEATS

 The definitions of the various groupings of VPBs was provided earlier in this chapter. Figure 13.26 illustrates the typical appearances of ventricular bigeminy (Fig. 13.26A), trigeminy (Fig. 13.26B), and couplets (Fig. 13.26C) of VPBs.

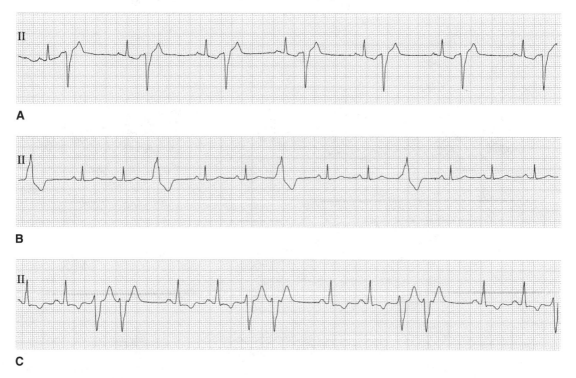

Figure 13.26. The contrasting appearances of the different sequences of VPBs in lead II rhythm strips.

In the typical form of bigeminy (Fig. 13.26A), a VPB is substituted for every alternate sinus beat, and each VPB is followed by a compensatory pause. However, when the VPBs are interpolated, a tachyarrhythmia with a bigeminal pattern is produced (Fig. 13.27).

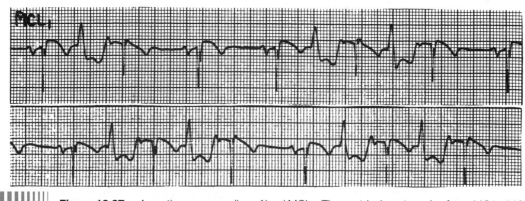

Figure 13.27. A continuous recording of lead MCL_1. The ventricular rate varies from 110 to 140 beats/min during the "tachycardia."

VENTRICULAR PREMATURE BEATS INDUCING VENTRICULAR FIBRILLATION

When VPBs occur so early that they interrupt the peak of the preceding T wave (Fig. 13.28), they may be ominous.[10] During this early phase of ventricular recovery, there is such inhomogeneity of receptiveness and refractoriness of conduction that the premature impulse may continue to encounter a receptive pathway. The impulse is able to repetitively reenter, thereby producing a tachyarrhythmia; which has been termed "ventricular tachycardia of the vulnerable period," "ventricular flutter," and "coarse ventricular fibrillation." The tachyarrhythmia may terminate spontaneously or progress to typical ventricular fibrillation.

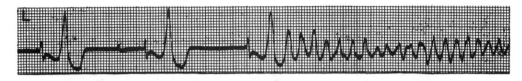

Figure 13.28. A lead-aVL (L) rhythm strip reveals a bigeminal rhythm produced by very closely coupled VPBs. The VPB that triggers the ventricular flutter has the same coupling interval and morphology as the other VPBs.

The peak of the T wave coincides with the vulnerable period in the cardiac cycle, and *R-on-T VPBs* are considered dangerous. Of a series of 48 patients who developed ventricular fibrillation outside the hospital, the initiating beat was an R-on-T VPB in more than two-thirds.[11] However, others have questioned the threat of R-on-T VPBs as compared with later VPBs.[12] One study that carefully documented the VPBs that initiated fibrillation in 20 consecutive patients demonstrated that in more than half, the culpable VPBs occurred after completion of the T wave.[13] Therefore, ventricular fibrillation can be initiated by late VPBs. Surawicz summarizes the situation by concluding that R-on-T VPBs pose a risk of inducing ventricular fibrillation only in the early stages of myocardial infarction, in hypokalemia, and in the presence of a long QT interval.[14]

PROGNOSTIC IMPLICATIONS OF VENTRICULAR PREMATURE BEATS

VPBs are ubiquitous. Most people have them more or less frequently, and even continuous ventricular bigeminy is sometimes found in apparently normal hearts. Usually, VPBs are a benign nuisance. During the acute phase of infarction, they appear in 80 to 90% of patients, but are also found in the majority of actively employed middle-aged men.[15] Benign VPBs commonly disappear when the sinus rate increases, such as during exercise. The prognostic significance of exercise-induced VPBs is uncertain. VPBs have been reported to occur more readily with isometric than with isotonic (dynamic) exercise.[16]

Many studies have been directed at evaluating the prognostic significance of VPBs during and after acute myocardial infarction. In patients who have survived myocardial infarction, complex VPBs (multiform, couplets, etc.) have been shown to increase the risk of sudden death.[17,18] This is in marked contrast to the prognostic importance of similarly appearing VPBs outside the setting of myocardial infarction. In a 7-year follow-up of 72 asymptomatic subjects with frequent and complex VPBs, none died, although a number had angiographically proven significant coronary disease.[19]

Lown's grading system for VPBs[20,21] (Table 13.3) has become a popular frame of reference for gauging the risk of death after myocardial infarction. There is increased risk as the numerical grade advances from 0 to 5. A subsequent study found that consecutive VPBs (Grade 4) were associated with a worse prognosis than were early, single VPBs (Grade 5).[22]

Table 13.3. Lown's Grading System of Ventricular Premature Beats

Grade	Description of VPBs
0	None
1	Less than 30/hour
2	30 or more/hour
3	Multiform
4A	Two consecutive
4B	3 or more consecutive
5	R-on-T

Moss has proposed a simplified, two-level system for grading the prognostic significance of VPBs after acute myocardial infarction, as follows[23]:

Uniform morphology and late cycle	Low risk	(2-year mortality 10%)
Multiform and/or early cycle	High risk	(2-year mortality 20%)

A study by Califf and colleagues has documented the relationship between VPBs and left-ventricular function in patients with ischemic heart disease.[24] A subsequent study by these same authors failed to find a subgroup of patients with VPBs of any description and good left ventricular function that had a high risk of sudden death.[25] Therefore, VPBs do not appear to be independent predictors of a high risk of mortality in patients with ischemic heart disease.

GLOSSARY

Aberrantly: being conducted abnormally (usually through the ventricular conduction system).

Atrial premature beat (APB): a P wave produced by an impulse that originates in the atria and appears before the expected time of the next P wave generated from the sinus node.

Bigeminy: a rhythm pattern in which every sinus beat is followed by a premature beat.

Compensatory pause: the long cycle length (pause) following a PB completely "compensates for" the short cycle length preceding the PB. This is identified when the interval between the beginning of the P waves of the sinus beats preceding and following a PB is equal to two PP intervals of sinus beats not associated with PBs.

Couplet: two consecutive premature beats.

Coupling intervals: the periods between normal sinus beats and PBs. With APBs, the PP′ is the coupling interval, and with JPBs and VPBs the QRS–QRS′ is the coupling interval.

Ectopic beat: A beat arising in any location other than the sinus node.

Interpolated: occurring between normal beats.

Junctional premature beat (JPB): a P wave and QRS complex produced by an impulse that originates in the AV node or His bundle and appears before the expected time of the next P wave and QRS complex generated from the sinus node.

Left VPBs: premature beats originating from the left ventricle, usually with a V1-positive morphology, but sometimes with a V1-negative morphology when associated with ischemic heart disease.

Multifocal VPBs: VPBs originating from two or more different ventricular locations.

Multiform VPBs: VPBs with two or more different morphologies in a single ECG lead.

Overdrive suppression: a decrease in the rate of impulse formation resulting from premature activation of the pacemaking cells.

Palpitation: the physical awareness of a heartbeat.

PP interval: the interval between consecutive P waves.

R-on-T VPB: a VPB that occurs so prematurely that it occurs during the T wave of the previous beat.

Right VPBs: premature beats originating from the right ventricle, always with a V1-negative morphology.

Supraventricular premature beat (SVPB): either an APB or a JPB.

Trigeminy: a rhythm pattern in which every second sinus beat is followed by a premature beat.

V1-negative QRS complex: an abnormally wide QRS complex that is predominantly negative in lead V1; sometimes called a "left-bundle-branch-block–like" QRS complex.

V1-positive QRS complex: an abnormally wide QRS complex that is predominantly positive in lead V1; sometimes called a "right-bundle-branch-block–like" QRS complex.

Ventricular premature beat (VPB): a QRS complex produced by an impulse originating from the ventricles and appearing before the expected time of the next QRS complex generated from the sinus node or other basic underlying rhythm.

Vulnerable period: the time in the cardiac cycle, before complete repolarization, when a reentrant tachyarrhythmia may be induced by the introduction of a premature impulse.

REFERENCES

1. Killip T, Gault JH. Mode of onset of atrial fibrillation in man. Am Heart J 1965;70:172.
2. Langendorf R, Pick A, Winternitz M. Mechanisms of intermittent ventricular bigeminy. I. Appearance of ectopic beats dependent upon length of the ventricular cycle, the "rule of bigeminy." Circulation 1955;11:422–430.
3. Kaplinsky E, Ogawa S, Kmetzo J, et al. Origin of so-called right and left ventricular arrhythmias in acute myocardial ischemia. Am J Cardiol 1978;42:774–780.
4. Lewis S, Kanakis C, Rosen KM, et al. Significance of site of origin of premature ventricular contractions. Am Heart J 1979;97:159–164.
5. Rosenbaum MB. Classification of ventricular extrasystoles according to form. J Electrocardiol 1969;2:289–297.
6. O'Bryan C. Personal communication to Dr. Marriott, 1981.
7. Gozensky C, Thorne D. Rabbit ears: an aid in distinguishing ventricular ectopy from aberration. Heart Lung 1974;3:634–636.
8. Swanick EJ, LaCamera F Jr, Marriott HJL. Morphologic features of right ventricular ectopic beats. Am J Cardiol 1972;30:888–891.
9. Booth DC, Popio KA, Gettes LS. Multiformity of induced unifocal ventricular premature beats in human subjects: electrocardiographic and angiographic correlations. Am J Cardiol 1982;49:1643–1653.
10. Smirk FH, Palmer DDG. A myocardial syndrome, with particular reference to the occurrence of sudden death and of premature systoles interrupting antecedent T waves. Am J Cardiol 1960;6:620.
11. Adgey AJ, Devlin JE, Webb SW, et al. Initiation of ventricular fibrillation outside hospital in patients with ischemic heart disease. Br Heart J 1982;47:55.
12. Engel TR, Meister SG, Frankl WS. "The R-on-T" phenomenon; an update and critical review. Ann Intern Med 1978;88:221–225.
13. Lie KI, Wellens HJ, Downar E, et al. Observations on patients with primary ventricular fibrillation complicating

acute myocardial infarction. Circulation 1975;52:755–759.

14. Surawicz B. R-on-T phenomenon: dangerous and harmless. J Appl Cardiol 1986;1:39.

15. Hinkle LE Jr, Carver ST, Stevens M. The frequency of asymptomatic disturbances of cardiac rhythm and conduction in middle-aged men. Am J Cardiol 1969;24:629–650.

16. Atkins JM, Matthews OA, Blomqvist CG, Mullins CB. Incidence of arrhythmias induced by isometric and dynamic exercise. Br Heart J 1976;38:465–471.

17. Moss AJ, Davis HT, DeCamilla J, et al. Ventricular ectopic beats and their relation to sudden and nonsudden cardiac death after myocardial infarction. Circulation 1979;60:998–1003.

18. Ruberman W, Weinblatt E, Goldberg JD, et al. Ventricular premature beats and mortality after myocardial infarction. N Engl J Med 1977;297:750–757.

19. Horan MJ, Kennedy HL. Characteristics and prognosis of apparently healthy patients with frequent and complex ventricular ectopy: evidence for a relative benign syndrome with occult myocardial and/or coronary disease. Am Heart J 1981;102:809–810.

20. Lown B, Wolf M. Approaches to sudden death from coronary heart disease. Circulation 1971;44:130–142.

21. Lown B, Graboys TB. Management of patients with malignant ventricular arrhythmias. Am J Cardiol 1977;39:910–918.

22. Bigger JT, Weld FJ. Analysis of prognostic significance of ventricular arrhythmias after myocardial infarction. Shortcomings of the Lown grading system. Br Heart J 1981;45:717–724.

23. Moss AJ. Clinical significance of ventricular arrhythmias in patients with and without coronary artery disease. Prog Cardiovasc Dis 1980;23:33–52.

24. Califf RM, Burks JM, Behar VS, et al. Relationships among ventricular arrhythmias, coronary artery disease, and angiographic and electrocardiographic indicators of myocardial fibrosis. Circulation 1978;57:725–732.

25. Califf RM, McKinnis RA, Burks J, et al. Prognostic implications of ventricular arrhythmias during 24 hour ambulatory monitoring in patients undergoing catheterization for coronary artery disease. Am J Cardiol 1982;50:23–31.

CHAPTER 14

Accelerated Automaticity

The arrhythmias presented in this chapter have gradual onsets and terminations because they result from acceleration of automaticity in the cells of the pacemaking and conduction systems. This is apparent on the electrocardiogram (ECG) as a gradual decrease in the interval between cardiac cycles (the RR interval) during the period of onset and a gradual increase during the period of termination of a tachyarrhythmia caused by accelerated automaticity. In Figure 14.1, there is a tachyarrhythmia during exercise at a heart rate of 140 beats/min with no visible P waves and wide (V1-negative) QRS complexes (0.14 s). When the exercise is stopped, the heart rate gradually slows and P waves emerge from the ends of each of the T waves, indicating that the rhythm is sinus tachycardia with left bundle-branch block (LBBB).

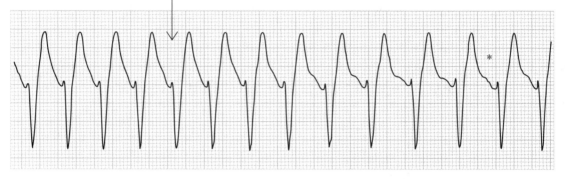

Figure 14.1. Lead-V1 rhythm strip: *arrow* indicates the time at which exercise was stopped, and *asterisk* indicates the P wave emerging from the T wave. (From Wagner GS, Waugh RA, Ramo BW. Cardiac arrhythmias. New York: Churchill Livingstone, 1983:145, with permission.)

Cells termed *pacemakers* (Chapter 1, "Cardiac Electrical Activity"), and located in the SA node, at various sites in the atria, and throughout the His–Purkinje system, have the capacity for spontaneous depolarization. Atrial and ventricular muscle cells and AV-nodal cells have not been shown to have pacemaking capabilities. The rate of impulse formation by pacemaker cells is determined by the rate of their spontaneous depolarization, and the more superior the location of the pacemaking cell, the more rapidly this depolarization occurs. Accelerated automaticity is considered to be a tachyarrhythmia only when the heart rate exceeds the arbitrary limit of 100 beats/min. Since the upper limit of normal automaticity of the SA-nodal and atrial cells is 100 beats/min, any acceleration in the rate of automaticity of these cells is considered a tachyarrhythmia. The upper limit of normal automaticity is 60 beats/min in the common bundle and 50 beats/min in the bundle branches. The rhythm produced is simply called an *accelerated rhythm* until it reaches 100 beats/min. The pacemaking sites, the terms used for the arrhythmias produced by their acceleration, and their rate ranges are presented in Table 14.1.

Table 14.1. Sites, Terms, and Rates of Pacemaker Tachs

Site	Term	Rate Range (beats/min)
Sinus node	Sinus tachycardia	100–200
Atria	Atrial tachycardia	100–200
Common bundle	Accelerated junctional rhythm (AJR)	60–130
Bundle branches	Accelerated ventricular rhythm (AVR)	50–110

Examples of arrhythmias due to accelerated atrial, junctional, and ventricular automaticity are presented in Figure 14.2. In Figure 14.2A, the *accelerated atrial rhythm (AAR)* is apparent from the frequent, regular (evenly spaced), but "different from sinus" P waves. In Figure 14.2B, the accelerated junctional rhythm (AJR) is apparent from the frequent, regular, normally appearing QRS complexes not preceded by P waves. In Figure 14.2C, the accelerated ventricular rhythm (AVR) is apparent from the frequent, regular, abnormally appearing QRS complexes not preceded by P waves.

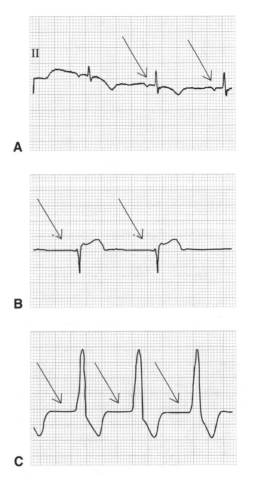

Figure 14.2. Lead-II rhythm strip with *arrows* indicating abnormally directed P waves **(A)**, and absence of P waves **(B** and **C)**.

Usually, the cardiac rhythm is controlled by the SA node. However, there are several reasons why the rhythm becomes dominated by the accelerated pacing activity from a nonsinus site. These include:

1. A pharmacologic agent that selectively increases automaticity in lower pacemakers.
2. Blockage of sinus impulses in the AV conduction system, permitting an escape focus in the common bundle to control the ventricular rhythm.
3. Local pathology (especially ischemia) that induces automaticity in lower areas with pacemaking capability.
4. Local pathology that decreases automaticity within the SA node.

SINUS TACHYCARDIA

The rate of cardiac impulse formation is regulated by the balance between the parasympathetic and sympathetic divisions of the autonomic (or involuntary) nervous system. The more superior the location of pacemaking cells, the greater is the degree of their autonomic regulation. An increase in parasympathetic activity decreases the rate of impulse formation, while an increase in sympathetic activity increases the rate. The sympathetic nervous system becomes activated by any condition that requires "flight or fight." Sinus tachycardia that results from this is therefore a physiologic response to the body's needs, rather than a pathologic cardiac condition. By this principle, treatment of a tachyarrhythmia should be directed at correcting the underlying condition, and not at suppression of the SA node itself. Maximal sympathetic stimulation can increase the heart rate produced by the SA node to 200 beats/min or, rarely, 220 beats/min in younger individuals. The generally accepted formula for maximal sinus rate is: 220 beats/min – age. The rate rarely exceeds 160 beats/min in nonexercising adults.

In sinus tachycardia there is normally one normal P wave for every QRS complex, but coexisting abnormalities of AV conduction may alter this relationship. The PR interval is shorter than during normal sinus rhythm because the increased *sympathetic tone* that produces the sinus tachycardia also speeds up AV-nodal conduction. The QRS complex is usually normal in appearance, but can be abnormal either because of a fixed intraventricular conduction disturbance (such as bundle-branch block, hypertrophy, or myocardial infarction) or because the rapid rate of activation does not permit time for full recovery of the intraventricular conduction system before the arrival of the next impulse (Chapter 5, "Intraventricular Conduction Abnormalities"). Figure 14.3 demonstrates sinus tachycardia with LBBB. Conduction block is proven to be due to rate-related aberrancy when it disappears during sinus slowing induced by carotid sinus massage and returns when the rate gradually increases following the massage.

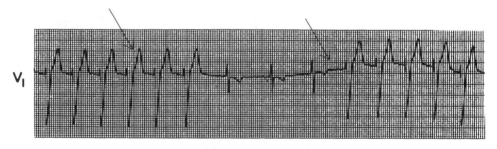

V_I

Figure 14.3. Lead-V1 rhythm strip with *arrows* indicating the beginning and ending of carotid sinus massage. (From Wagner GS, Waugh RA, Ramo BW. Cardiac arrhythmias. New York: Churchill Livingstone, 1983:140, with permission.)

Although the other tachyarrhythmias caused by accelerated automaticity and discussed in this chapter do not mimic sinus tachycardia, a common clinical problem is the differentiation of sinus tachycardia from various reentrant tachyarrhythmias, which are discussed in later chapters. If discrete P waves (with antegrade orientation), a short PR interval, and a normal QRS-complex duration are present, the diagnosis of sinus tachycardia is most likely. True sinus tachycardia is shown in Figure 14.4A, and two reentrant supraventricular tachyarrhythmias that appear similar to sinus tachycardia are shown in Figure 14.4B and C. When apparent sinus tachycardia is associated with a prolonged PR interval, one should suspect that it is not really a sinus tachycardia. Figure 14.4B presents an example of the reentrant atrial tachyarrhythmia termed atrial flutter (Chapter 15, "Reentrant Atrial Tachyarrhythmias—The Atrial Flutter/Fibrillation System") with only every other flutter wave conducted to the ventricles (2:1 AV conduction) and masquerading as sinus tachycardia. An abnormal frontal-plane P wave axis also suggests a nonsinus origin of the tachyarrhythmia. Figure 14.4C presents an example of reentrant junctional tachycardia (Chapter 16, "Reentrant Junctional Tachyarrhythmias"), with inverted P waves following each QRS complex.

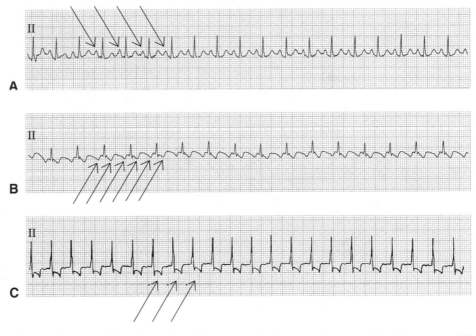

Figure 14.4. Lead-II rhythm strips with *arrows* indicating sinus P waves **(A)**, flutter waves **(B)**, and retrograde P waves **(C)**. (From Wagner GS, Waugh RA, Ramo BW. Cardiac arrhythmias. New York: Churchill Livingstone, 1983:176, with permission.)

When the appearance of atrial activity fails to provide the foregoing clinical differentiation of the source of a tachyarrhythmia, it may be necessary to observe the onset and termination of the tachyarrhythmia: A gradual change in rate establishes the diagnosis of sinus tachycardia (Fig. 14.5A). The sudden block in AV conduction allows visualization of the typical sawtoothlike atrial activity of flutter (Fig. 14.5B). The sudden termination of the tachyarrhythmia establishes the diagnosis of reentrant junctional tachycardia (Fig. 14.5C). If the beginning or ending of the tachyarrhythmia does not appear spontaneously, a diagnostic maneuver or pharmacologic intervention to increase parasympathetic nervous activity, such as a vagal maneuver, may be necessary. The absence of any change in the ECG during the *vagal maneuver* does not permit any diagnostic conclusion. A transesophageal or intraatrial recording may be required when no diagnosis can be made from surface ECG recordings (Fig. 12.9). A summary of the progressive steps toward the diagnosis of an unknown tachyarrhythmia would include:

1. Note the P-wave morphology and the PR and QRS intervals in the ECG.
2. Observe either the onset or the termination of the tachyarrhythmia in the ECG.
3. Perform a maneuver to increase parasympathetic activity.
4. Record the atrial activity from the esophagus or right atrium.

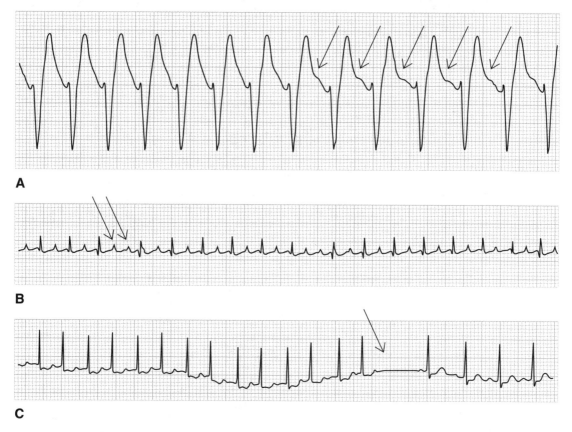

Figure 14.5. Lead II rhythm strips with arrows indicating gradual emergence of P waves from T waves **(A)**, sudden appearance of consecutive flutter waves **(B)**, and sudden termination of the tachyarrhythmia **(C)**. (From Wagner GS, Waugh RA, Ramo BW. Cardiac arrhythmias. New York: Churchill Livingstone, 1983:144,179, with permission.)

ATRIAL TACHYARRHYTHMIAS: ACCELERATED ATRIAL RHYTHM, PAROXYSMAL ATRIAL TACHYCARDIA WITH BLOCK, AND MULTIFOCAL ATRIAL TACHYCARDIA

Enhanced automaticity causes three varieties of atrial tachycardias: AAR, *paroxysmal atrial tachycardia (PAT) with block*, and *multifocal atrial tachycardia (MAT)*. Normal individuals may have periods when a lower atrial-pacing site dominates the SA node producing an AAR; *digitalis toxicity* is the only common cause of PAT with block; and MAT almost always occurs with chronic pulmonary disease.

The presence of AAR is apparent when the morphology of the QRS complex is normal in the presence of a ventricular rate in the range of 60 to130 beats/min and there are preceding abnormal P waves caused by atrial activation originating in a site other than the SA node (Fig 14.2A). The PR interval may be normal or decreased, depending on the distance from the atrial pacing site to the AV node.

The term *paroxysmal* is actually inaccurate with regard to PAT with block, because it implies the sudden onset and termination of a cardiac rhythm. The atrial rate gradually accelerates as digitalis is added (or potassium is depleted), and then gradually decelerates when the digitalis is withheld (or potassium is replaced) as in Figure 14.6.[1,2] Digitalis has a parasympathetic effect on both the SA and AV nodes, resulting in sinus slowing and AV block. However, digitalis has a sympathetic effect on other sites with pacemaking capability, and thereby enhances automaticity. If the site of this enhancement is above the AV node, the result is the combination of atrial tachycardia with AV block.

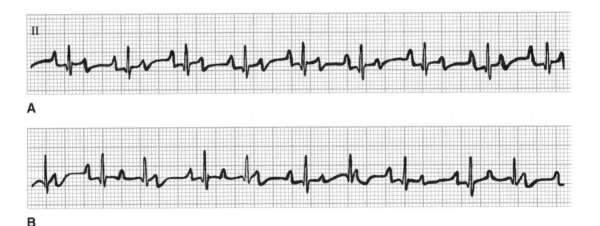

A

B

Figure 14.6. Lead-II rhythm strips from a 75-year-old woman with congestive heart failure treated with digitalis and diuretics. **A**. A "paroxysmal atrial tachycardia" caused by digitalis toxicity in the setting of hypokalemia ($K^+ = 3.1$ mEq/L). The atrial rate is 180 beats/min and there is 2:1 AV block. **B.** Digitalis had been withheld and potassium given ($K^+ = 4.6$ mEq/L), resulting in the slowing of the atrial rate to 168 beats/min. (From Wagner GS, Waugh RA, Ramo BW. Cardiac arrhythmias. New York: Churchill Livingstone, 1983:138, with permission.)

MAT is a rapid, irregular atrial tachyarrhythmia with multiple, differently appearing P waves that has also been termed *chaotic atrial tachycardia*[3] (Fig. 14.7). In contrast to the atrial acceleration that occurs with digitalis toxicity, there is no enhancement of the parasympathetic effect on the AV node in MAT, and therefore every P wave is conducted to the ventricles (1:1 AV conduction). MAT is typically a transitional arrhythmia between frequent atrial premature beats (APBs) and atrial flutter/fibrillation. In a series of 31 patients reported by Lipson and Naimi, 20 had preceding APBs and 17 progressed to atrial flutter/fibrillation.[3]

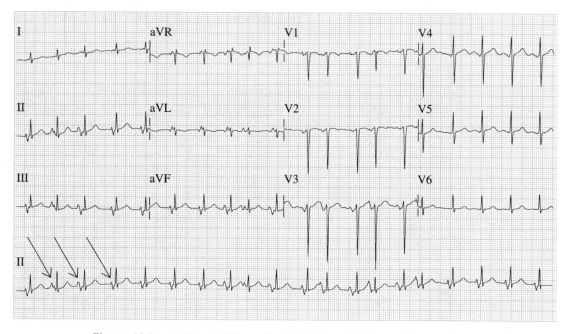

Figure 14.7. A 12-lead ECG and lead-II rhythm strip from a 53-year-old woman with severe pulmonary emphysema. *Arrows* indicate marked variation in P-wave morphology in the rhythm strip.

ACCELERATED JUNCTIONAL RHYTHM

AJR is produced by enhanced automaticity in the AV node or common bundle of the ventricular Purkinje system. As in AAR, acceleration of impulse formation in the AV junction occurs in AJR as a normal variation in cardiac rhythm. The presence of AJR is easily diagnosed when the morphology of the QRS complex is normal, the ventricular rate is in the range of 60 to 130 beats/min, and there are no preceding P waves (Fig. 14.2B). Retrogradely conducted atrial activation is present during or after anterograde ventricular activation, but the inverted P waves may be obscured by the larger QRS complexes or may be hidden in T waves (Fig. 14.8). When inverted P waves are visible but the heart rate is rapid, it is difficult to determine whether the P wave is associated with the preceding QRS complex (AJR) or with the following QRS complex (sinus tachycardia with a prolonged PR interval). If P waves can be seen clearly on a 12-lead ECG, their direction in the frontal plane should provide differentiation of these conditions.

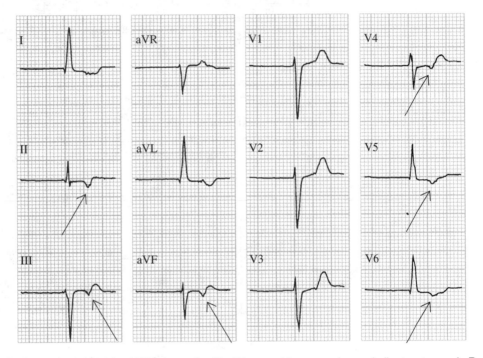

Figure 14.8. A 12-lead ECG from a healthy 51-year-old woman. *Arrows* indicate retrograde P waves associated with junctional beats.

Other forms of AJR may produce normal P waves before the QRS complex, but with varying PR intervals because the SA node is activating the atrium and an accelerated junctional pacing site is activating the ventricles. This is an example of dissociation between atrial and ventricular activity (called AV dissociation) (Fig. 14.9). It may be nec-

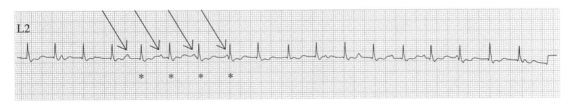

Figure 14.9. A lead-II (L2) rhythm strip from a 72-year-old woman with digitalis toxicity. *Arrows* indicate the antegrade (sinus) P waves dissociated from the junctional beats (*asterisks*).

essary to observe a long rhythm strip to document this dissociation, because the atrial and ventricular rates may be similar (isorhythmic), with a constant PR interval.

A regular ventricular rate of more than 60 beats/min with normally appearing QRS complexes in the presence of atrial fibrillation (Chapter 15, "Reentrant Atrial Tachyarrhythmias—The Atrial Flutter/Fibrillation System") is diagnostic of AJR. There is another example of dissociation between a tachyarrhythmia resulting from reentry above the AV node and a tachyarrhythmia resulting from acclerated automaticity below the AV node (Fig. 14.10). This combination of decreased conduction in the AV node and enhanced automaticity in the common bundle is usually caused by digitalis toxicity (Chapter 22, "Dr. Marriott's Systematic Approach to the Diagnosis of Arrhythmias"). If this condition is unrecognized, additional digitalis will further accelerate the AJR.

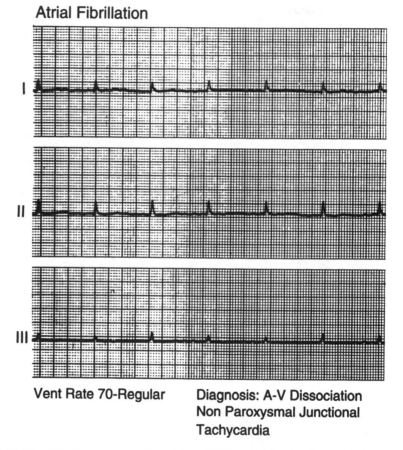

Atrial Fibrillation

I

II

III

Vent Rate 70-Regular

**Diagnosis: A-V Dissociation
Non Paroxysmal Junctional
Tachycardia**

Figure 14.10.   Simultaneous recording of three ECG leads, showing the undulating baseline of atrial fibrillation dissociated from the regular narrow QRS complexes of AJR. Nonparoxysmal junctional tachycardia is another term used for AJR. (From Wagner GS, Waugh RA, Ramo BW. Cardiac arrhythmias. New York: Churchill Livingstone, 1983:149, with permission.)

ACCELERATED VENTRICULAR RHYTHM

AVR is produced by enhanced automaticity in the bundle branches or the fascicles of the ventricular Purkinje system. As in AAR and AJR, this acceleration of impulse formation in the ventricles occurs as a normal variation in cardiac rhythm. The presence of AVR is easily diagnosed when the morphology of the QRS complex is abnormal in the presence of a heart rate in the range of 50 to 110 beats/min and there are no preceding P waves (Fig. 14.2C). In AVR, retrogradely conducted atrial activation is present during or after anterograde ventricular activation, but the inverted P waves may be obscured by the larger QRS complexes or T waves.

AVR is often given other names, such as accelerated idioventricular rhythm or *slow ventricular tachycardia*. Since the pacing rate of the cells causing AVR, which are located at the distal end of the pacemaking and conduction system, is normally very slow, AVR is diagnosed when the ventricular rate exceeds 50 beats/min. The most rapid rate of AVR is 110 beats/min, and the heart rate in this condition rarely exceeds 100 beats/min. AVR most commonly occurs during the early hours of an acute myocardial infarction, with reported incidences ranging from 8% to 46%. AVR is also a common manifestation of digitalis toxicity.

AVR occurs either because the sinus rhythm slows and permits the AVR to reveal itself or because the ventricular rhythm accelerates so much that it usurps control from a normally functioning SA node (Fig. 14.11). These precipitating sources of AVR can therefore be differentiated by observing the pattern of sinus rhythm preceding the onset of the AVR.

When AVR is present, the rates of sinus and ventricular impulse formation are usually similar. The dominance of the ventricular pacemaker may begin (Fig. 14.11A) and terminate (Fig. 14.11B) with one or more QRS complexes formed partly by a sinus-originated impulse and partly by a ventricular originated impulse (fusion beats).

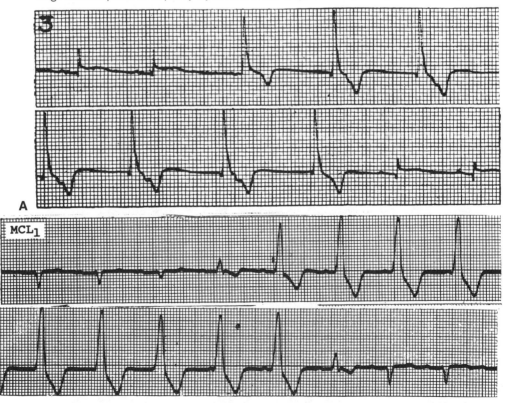

Figure 14.11. The contrasting appearances of the onset of an AVR that results from an increased discharge rate of the ventricular pacemaker **(A)** and its termination that results from slight acceleration of the sinus rate **(B)**.

AVR, like AJR, commonly occurs when atrial fibrillation is accompanied by decreased AV-nodal conduction. These combined effects often result from digitalis toxicity. Once the AVR caused by these effects gets under way, it usually proceeds as a perfectly regular rhythm, although it sometimes shows progressive acceleration or progressive slowing until it spontaneously ceases.

In some instances of AVR, there is retrograde conduction to the atria (Fig. 14.12) rather than dissociation between the atria and ventricles. AVR is usually benign, even when multiform, and neither affects the blood pressure nor leads to more serious ventricular arrhythmias.[4,5] However, since the normal sequence of atrial and ventricular activation is absent, and there is loss of the normal atrial contribution to ventricular filling, AVR may be accompanied by a feeling of weakness or unsteadiness.

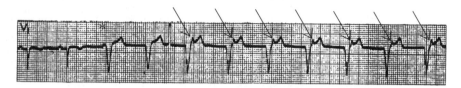

Figure 14.12. In this ECG, AVR appears after two beats of sinus rhythm. It is initially dissociated from the atrial activity (*asterisk*), and the causative impulse is then conducted retrogradely to capture the atrial rhythm (*arrows*).

GLOSSARY

Accelerated atrial rhythm (AAR): a tachyarrhythmia that is caused by an increase of automaticity in atrial pacemaking cells.

Accelerated junctional rhythm (AJR): a tachyarrhythmia that is caused by an increase of automaticity in the pacemaking cells of the His bundle.

Accelerated rhythm: an increase in a particular cardiac rhythm above its normal limit.

Accelerated ventricular rhythm (AVR): a tachyarrhythmia that is caused by an increase of automaticity in pacemaking cells of the bundle branches and their fascicles.

Carotid sinus massage: manual stimulation of the area of the neck that overlies the bifurcation of the carotid artery, to increase parasympathetic nervous activity.

Chaotic atrial tachycardia: another term used for multifocal atrial tachycardia.

Digitalis toxicity: an arrhythmia produced by the drug digitalis.

Multifocal atrial tachycardia (MAT): a rapid rhythm produced by increased automaticity in pacemaking cells located at multiple sites within the atria.

Pacemaker: A cell in the heart or an artificial device that is capable of forming or generating an electrical impulse.

Paroxysmal: a term referring to an arrhythmia of sudden occurrence.

Paroxysmal atrial tachycardia (PAT) with block: a tachyarrhythmia, commonly caused by digitalis toxicity, in which a rapid atrial rhythm is accompanied by failure of some of the atrial impulses to be conducted through the AV node to the ventricles.

RR Interval: the interval between consecutive R waves.

Slow ventricular tachycardia: another term used for an accelerated ventricular rhythm.

Sympathetic tone: the relative amount of sympathetic nervous activity as compared to the amount of parasympathetic activity.

Vagal maneuver: an intervention that increases parasympathetic activity in relation to the amount of sympathetic activity.

REFERENCES

1. Lown B, Wyatt NF, Levine HD. Paroxysmal atrial tachycardia with block. Circulation 1960;21:129–143.
2. Geer MR, Wagner GS, Waxman M, et al. Chronotropic effect of acetylstrophanthidin infusion into the canine sinus nodal artery. Am J Cardiol 1977;39:684–689.
3. Lipson MJ, Naimi S. Multifocal atrial tachycardia (chaotic atrial tachycardia): clinical associations and significance. Circulation 1970;42:397–407.
4. Denes P, Kehoe R, Rosen KM. Multiple reentrant tachycardias due to retrograde conduction of dual atrioventricular bundles with atrioventricular nodal-like properties. Am J Cardiol 1979;44:162–170.
5. Epstein ML, Stone FM, Benditt DG. Incessant atrial tachycardia in childhood: association with rate-dependent conduction in an accessory atrioventricular pathway. Am J Cardiol 1979;44:498–504.

CHAPTER 15

Reentrant Atrial Tachyarrhythmias—The Atrial Flutter/Fibrillation Spectrum

The supraventricular tachyarrhythmias in the *atrial flutter/fibrillation spectrum* are caused by the continuing reentry of an electrical impulse within the atrial myocardium. Figure 15.1 schematically contrasts this mechanism with the tachyarrhythmias caused by accelerated automaticity and described in Chapter 14 ("Accelerated Automaticity") and those caused by junctional reentry and described in Chapter 16 "Reentrant Junctional Tachyarrhythmias"). Since the reentrant circuit includes a large area of atrial myocardium, the reentry mechanism responsible for atrial flutter/fibrillation should be considered macroreentry, as discussed in Chapter 12 ("Introduction to Arrhythmias"). (Atrial microreentrant tachyarrhythmias also occur, but are very uncommon, and are also diagrammed in Figure 15.1.)

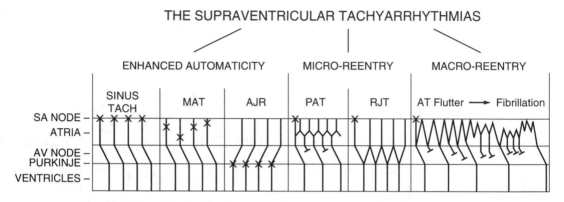

THE SUPRAVENTRICULAR TACHYARRHYTHMIAS

Figure 15.1. In the ladder diagrams, *x* indicates the site of impulse formation, a *vertical line* indicates normal conduction through atria or ventricles, a *diagonal line* indicates normal conduction though the AV node and conduction around a reentry circuit, and a *short perpendicular line* indicates the site of block of impulse conduction. *MAT*, multifocal atrial tachycardia; *AJR*, accelerated junctional rhythm; *PAT*, paroxysmal atrial tachycardia; *RJT*, reentrant junctional tachycardia.

Atrial flutter and *atrial fibrillation* are at the two extremes of a spectrum. At the flutter end of the spectrum, the causative reentering impulse cycles around a single circuit (within the right atrium); producing slower, regular, uniform, and sharp ("sawtoothlike") waves (*F waves*). At the fibrillation end of the spectrum, the causative reentering impulse proceeds around multiple circuits; producing more rapid, irregular, multiform, and rounded waves (*f waves*). As a result of the macroreentry mechanism responsible for both atrial flutter and fibrillation, P waves are replaced either by F waves representing the continuous activation within the flutter circuit or by f waves representing the continuous activation within the fibrillation circuit.

PAROXYSMAL ATRIAL TACHYCARDIA

Although atrial microreentrant tachycardia (paroxysmal atrial tachycardia [PAT]) occurs rarely, it is useful to present an example because of its clearly identifiable characteristics (Fig. 15.2). In Figure 15.2*A*, a microreentrant tachycardia masquerades as a typically appearing sinus tachycardia (110 beats/min) with first-degree atrioventricular (AV) block (0.26 s). However, in Figure 15.2*B*, the true atrial rate of 220 beats/min is revealed by the vagal stimulation provided by carotid sinus massage. In the case shown in Figure 15.2, sinus rhythm emerged after electrical cardioversion, confirming the reentrant mechanism of the tachycardia. The similar P-wave morphologies during paroxysmal atrial tachycardia and sinus rhythm indicate that the microreentrant circuit is in or near the sinus node, high in the right atrium.

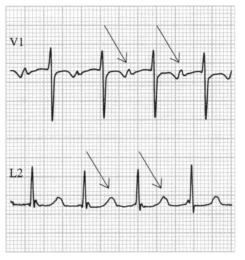

A

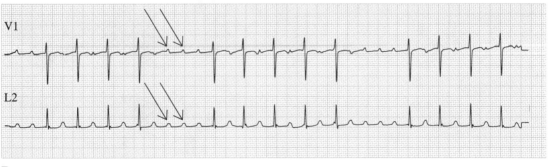

B

Figure 15.2. Lead-II (L2) and V1 rhythm strips from a 43-year-old woman presenting with shortness of breath who was found to have idiopathic cardiomyopathy. *Arrows* indicate similar-appearing P waves in L2 and V1 in the presenting condition **(A)**, and during carotid sinus massage **(B)**.

ATRIAL RATE AND REGULARITY IN ATRIAL FLUTTER/ FIBRILLATION

 The F waves of atrial flutter occur at rates between 200 and 350 beats/min (Fig. 15.3*A*).[1,2] As the atrial rate increases above 350 beats/min, either the atrial waves have some characteristics of both flutter and fibrillation at a single point in time (Fig. 15.3*B*) or there are alternations between F and f waves, with the appropriate term being *atrial flutter–fibrillation*. Fibrillation varies from coarse to fine. In *coarse fibrillation*, prominent f waves are clearly visible in many leads of the electrocardiogram (ECG) (Fig. 15.3*C*), but in *fine fibrillation* either there are small f waves or no visible atrial activity at all (Fig. 15.3*D*).

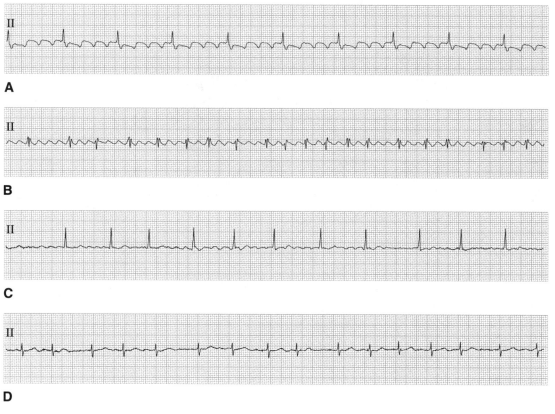

Figure 15.3. The contrasting appearances of four points in the atrial flutter/fibrillation spectrum: flutter **(A)**, flutter–fibrillation **(B)**, coarse fibrillation **(C)**, and fine fibrillation **(D)**.

Some patients' atrial rhythms may spontaneously undergo a change from flutter to fibrillation, while others have such variation only when certain drugs are administered. Digitalis increases the atrial rate toward the fibrillation end of the spectrum by shortening the refractory periods of atrial myocardial cells within the reentry circuit (Fig. 15.4A). Conversely, drugs such as quinidine and procainamide (Vaughn Williams Class IA) and flecanide (Class IC) decrease the atrial rate toward the flutter end of the spectrum by lengthening the refractory periods of these atrial myocardial cells (Fig. 15.4B).

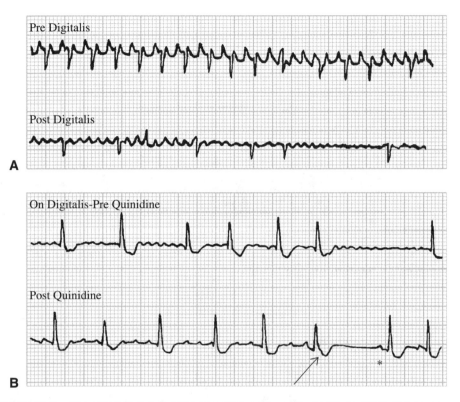

Figure 15.4. The effect of digitalis **(A)** and quinidine **(B)** on the atrial flutter/fibrillation spectrum in two patients. The *arrow* in **B** indicates the quinidine-induced termination of atrial reentry, and the *asterisk* indicates the onset of sinus rhythm. (From Wagner GS, Waugh RA, Ramo BW. Cardiac arrhythmias. New York: Churchill Livingstone, 1983:159, with permission.)

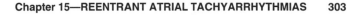

VENTRICULAR RATE AND REGULARITY IN ATRIAL FLUTTER/FIBRILLATION

Atrial flutter produces a ventricular rhythm that varies from precisely regular to *irregularly irregular*; however, fibrillation always produces an irregularly irregular ventricular rhythm. Therefore, when atrial fibrillation is accompanied by a regular ventricular rate, there is dissociation between the atrial and ventricular rhythms.

Since the atrial rate may vary dramatically within the flutter/fibrillation spectrum, the ventricular rate may also vary. At times, it may change abruptly from rapid and regular to slow and irregular, incorrectly suggesting a change in the basic underlying atrial rhythm (Fig. 15.5). After two beats of sinus rhythm, an atrial premature beat (APB) initiates a supraventricular tachyarrhythmia that is initially regular and then becomes irregular. The regular phase is most likely caused by flutter at a rate of 200 beats/min with 1:1 atrioventricular (AV) conduction, after which the irregular phase occurs because the atrial rate accelerates into the flutter/fibrillation spectrum at 300 beats/min, with a resultant slower, irregular ventricular rate.

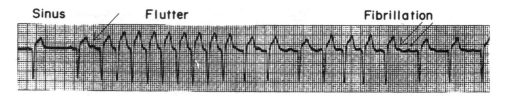

Figure 15.5. A lead-V1 rhythm strip from an 82-year-old woman with chronic heart failure and a history of recurrent "rapid heart beats." The first *arrow* indicates the APB that initiates the atrial reentrant tachycardia, and the second and third *arrows* indicate the f waves when the ventricular rate slows. (From Wagner GS, Waugh RA, Ramo BW. Cardiac arrhythmias. New York: Churchill Livingstone, 1983:155, with permission.)

During atrial flutter, the ratio of atrial to ventricular waveforms may vary from 1:1 to 2:1 to 6:2 to 4:1 (Fig. 15.6A-E) so that the ventricles may or may not have a rapid rate of contraction. The ratio of atrial to ventricular waveforms depends on the capability of the slowly conducting AV node to transport the atrial impulses to the common bundle. When ratios of atrial to ventricular waveforms of 1:1, 2:1, or 4:1 remain constant (Fig. 15.6A,B, and E), the ventricular rhythm is regular. When the ratio is 6:2 (because the atrial impulses are blocked at two levels within the AV node), the ventricular rhythm is regularly irregular. When the AV conduction ratio is variable (e.g., switching between 2:1 and 6:2 conduction), the ventricular rhythm is irregularly irregular.

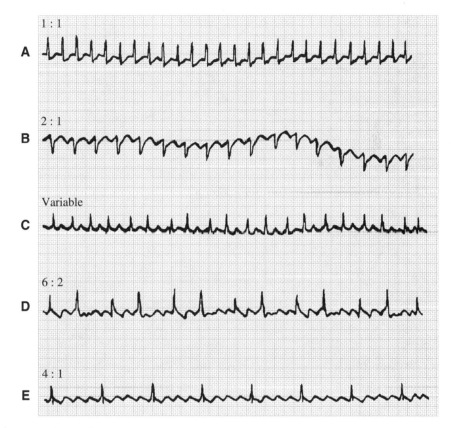

Figure 15.6. **A–E:** are lead-II rhythm strips from five patients with atrial flutter. Various typical patterns of AV conduction in atrial flutter are shown. **A.** There is 1:1 conduction with a rate of 200 beats/min. **B.** The atrial rate is 250 beats/min and there is a regular ventricular rate of 125 beats/min with a constant relationship between the flutter waves and the QRS complexes. **C.** The atrial rate is 300 beats/min (note the typical flutter waves during periods of increased AV block), and there is a variable, irregular ventricular response. **D.** The atrial rate is 270 beats/min, and there is a regularly irregular ventricular response in a pattern of six flutter waves for every two QRS complexes. **E.** The atrial rate is 240 beats/min, and there is a 4:1 ventricular response, again with a constant relationship between atrial activity and each ventricular complex. (From Wagner GS, Waugh RA, Ramo BW. Cardiac arrhythmias. New York: Churchill Livingstone, 1983:156, with permission.)

When atrial fibrillation is present, the innumerable f waves compete for penetration of the AV node, making it most difficult for any impulse to reach the common bundle. Therefore, the ventricular rhythm is slower at the fibrillation end of the flutter/fibrillation spectrum (Fig. 15.7).[3–5] Typically, a 1:1 AV relationship persists to the upper limit of the atrial rate during exercise or with other conditions that enhance sympathetic stimulation. However, when the atrial rate increases through other mechanisms (such as artificial atrial pacing or a reentrant tachyarrhythmia), the 1:1 AV relationship persists only until the atrial rate reaches 150 to 160 beats/min. Above this atrial rate, the physiologic delay in AV-nodal conduction prevents some atrial impulses from reaching the ventricles. As the atrial rate increases further, the ventricular rate decreases because of the competition within the AV node. The nonconducted atrial impulses are blocked only after they have been able to penetrate some distance into the node. Their concealed conduction depolarizes a part of the AV node, making it refractory to the following atrial impulse.[6] Changes in the sympathetic-to-parasympathetic balance can either facilitate (sympathetic) or further inhibit (parasympathetic) AV-nodal conduction.

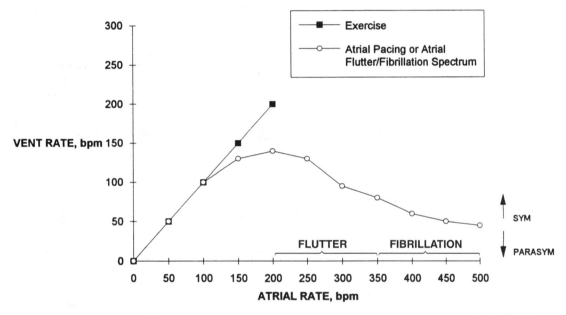

Figure 15.7. Ventricular rate regulation by the balance between sympathetic (*SYM*) and parasympathetic (*PARASYM*) tone is indicated by *arrows*. Note that the ventricular rate follows the atrial rate to about 100 beats/min regardless of the mechanism of increase in atrial rate as indicated by the *open squares*. (From Wagner GS, Waugh RA, Ramo BW. Cardiac arrhythmias. New York: Churchill Livingstone, 1983:9, with permission.)

ONSET OF ATRIAL FLUTTER/FIBRILLATION

Both spontaneous and electrically induced atrial flutter/fibrillation may typically be produced when APBs occur within a narrow range of the atrial refractory period. Thus, flutter/fibrillation is typically sudden in onset, as are all reentrant arrhythmias (Fig. 15.8).

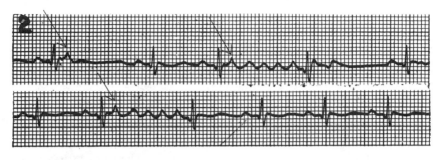

Figure 15.8. A lead-II (2) continuous rhythm strip from a 57-year-old man with complaint of recurrent "palpitations." *Arrows* indicate three APBs, two of which initiate brief runs of atrial flutter.

Like the ventricles, the atria have a vulnerable period: a point in the atrial cycle at which an APB is most likely to precipitate atrial flutter/fibrillation (Fig. 15.9). Killip and Gault have formulated the situation as follows: if the interval from the normal P wave to the premature P wave is less than half of the preceding interval between normal P waves, the premature P wave is within the atrial vulnerable period and may induce flutter/fibrillation.[7]

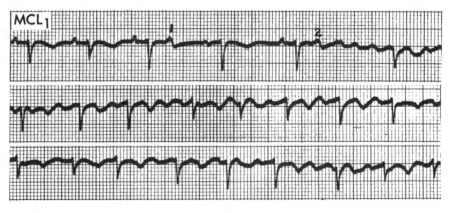

Figure 15.9. A lead-MCL$_1$ recording from an 88-year-old woman with pulmonary emphysema. The *1* indicates the APB occurring just outside and the *2* indicates the APB occurring just inside the atrial vulnerable period.

TERMINATION OF ATRIAL FLUTTER/FIBRILLATION

As illustrated in Figure 15.8, atrial flutter/fibrillation may terminate spontaneously. Presumably, the reason for this is that the recycling impulse fails to encounter receptive cells and thus has nowhere to go. When the reentry persists and creates either acute cardiac dysfunction or a chronic clinical problem, some medical intervention may be required. There are two possible treatment strategies:

1. Enhance the AV block to slow the ventricular rate.
2. Attempt to terminate the flutter/fibrillation.

Terminating or "breaking" this atrial reentrant tachycardia may be accomplished either with drugs or through electrical stimulation. A drug can effect termination of a tachyarrhythmia either by increasing the speed of the recycling impulse so that it encounters only cells that are still refractory, or by prolonging the refractory periods of the involved cells. No drugs yet exist that both speed conduction and prolong the refractory period. The primary therapeutic effect of available drugs is prolongation of refractoriness. An electrical stimulation can terminate a tachyarrhythmia by suddenly depolarizing all cardiac cells that are not already in the depolarized state (Fig. 15.10A). This eliminates the receptivity to reentry that is required to maintain the tachyarrhythmia. As illustrated in Figure 15.10B, such an electrical stimulation cannot break a tachyarrhythmia produced by accelerated automaticity; instead the rapidly discharging site continues to maintain the tachyarrhythmia after the brief interruption.

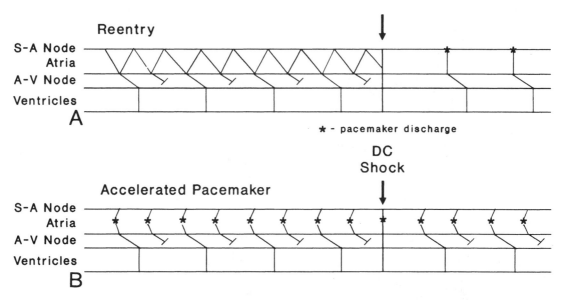

Figure 15.10. Ladder diagrams used to contrast the expected responses of tachyarrhythmias caused by atrial macroreentry **(A)** with those caused by enhanced atrial automaticity **(B)**. *Asterisks* indicates the site of automaticity and the *arrow* indicates the time of the precordial direct-current shock. (From Wagner GS, Waugh RA, Ramo BW. Cardiac arrhythmias. New York: Churchill Livingstone, 1983:25, with permission.)

When the atrial reentry of an impulse causing a tachyarrhythmia is orderly, as at the flutter end of the flutter/fibrillation spectrum, it can be suddenly terminated by intra-atrial electrical stimulation from an external pacemaker. Maintenance of the orderly reentry of the impulse requires that particular areas of atrial myocardium have completed their refractory periods and are receptive to the advancing wave of depolarization. A properly timed stimulus, delivered via a properly positioned pacing electrode, produces premature activation of such receptive areas, and the advancing wavefront encounters no cells that it can depolarize.

When the reentry is disorderly, as at the fibrillation end of the spectrum, it cannot be terminated by intraatrial stimulation, since no particular areas of atrial myocardium are essential for maintenance of a disorderly reentry. Therefore, electrical termination requires that stimuli be applied simultaneously to the entire atrial myocardium (Fig. 15.10A). Such premature activation of all potentially receptive areas leaves the advancing wavefronts with nothing available to depolarize. A body-surface electrical shock (electrical cardioversion) can terminate tachyarrhythmias of the entire flutter/fibrillation spectrum.

Table 15.1 summarizes many of the characteristics of the atrial flutter/fibrillation spectrum.

Table 15.1. Characteristics of the Atrial Flutter/Fibrillation Spectrum[a]

Atrial rate	200	220	300	360	400	500+
Ventricular rate	200	180	150	120	100	70
Ventricular rhythm	Regular	Regularly irregular	Regular	Regularly irregular	Irregular	
Name	Flutter		Flutter-fibrillation		Fibrillation	
Stability	Minimal		Moderate		Maximal	
Digitalis decreases AV conduction	Seldom		Sometimes		Usually	
DC shock terminates	Low energy		Intermediate		High energy	
Pacing terminates	Usually		Sometimes		Never	

[a] Modified from Wagner GS, Waugh RA, Ramo BW. Cardiac arrhythmias. New York: Churchill Livingstone, 1983: 154.

ATRIAL FLUTTER

Atrial flutter is much less common in adults than is atrial fibrillation. It is most often found in patients with *ischemic heart disease*, and is particularly rare in *mitral valve disease*. Flutter may complicate any form of heart disease, may be precipitated by any acute illness, and often occurs transiently after cardiac surgery. In the first few years of life, flutter is much more common than fibrillation, presumably because fibrillation requires a greater mass of atrial muscle.

In the usual variety of atrial flutter, the typical sawtooth pattern of F waves is typically best seen in the inferiorly oriented leads of the ECG (Fig. 15.11). Indeed, the F-wave deflections are positive in leads V1 and V2 and negative in leads V5 and V6, and there may be no evidence of atrial activity in the laterally oriented leads such as I and aVL. In the precordial leads, the F waves commonly mimic discrete P waves.

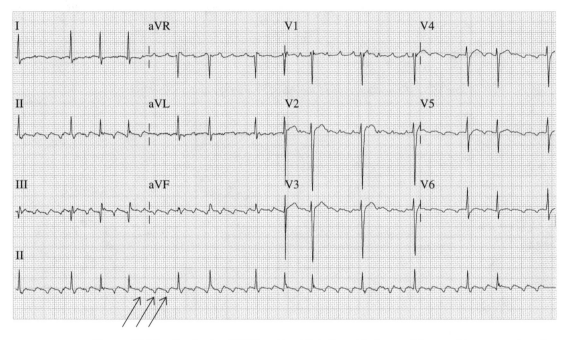

Figure 15.11. Twelve-lead ECG and lead-II rhythm strip from a 68-year-old man one day after cholecystectomy. The patient had a long history of poorly treated hypertension. *Arrows* indicate the typical "sawtooth" appearance of F waves in the lead-II rhythm strip.

In a rare variety of atrial flutter, however, the F waves may be inconspicuous in the limb leads and seen clearly only in precordial leads V1–V3 (Fig. 15.12).

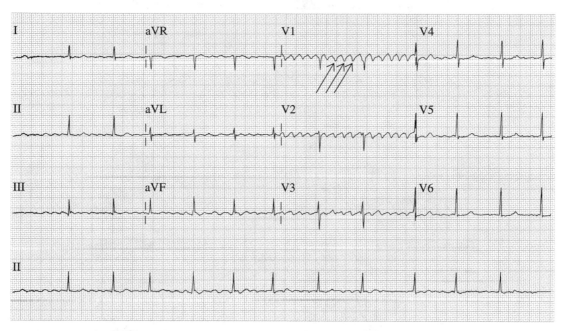

Figure 15.12. Twelve-lead ECG and lead-II rhythm strip from an 81-year-old woman during a routine health evaluation. No cardiac-related symptoms were present. *Arrows* indicate the "sawtooth" appearance of the F waves in lead V1.

PATTERNS OF ATRIOVENTRICULAR CONDUCTION

When atrial flutter is untreated, the usual AV conduction ratio is 2:1 (Fig. 15.13*A*), due to the normal refractoriness in the AV node. This rhythm should be termed "atrial flutter with 2:1 conduction" rather than "2:1 block" because the AV node is playing its normal physiologic role as a shield that protects the ventricles from the rapid atrial rate. It may be difficult to recognize either of the F waves in each cardiac cycle in atrial flutter because one of the waves is partly or completely masked by the QRS complex and the other is masked by the T wave. The diagnosis becomes obvious only when an increase in the AV-nodal block produces a slowing of the ventricular rate (Fig. 15.13).

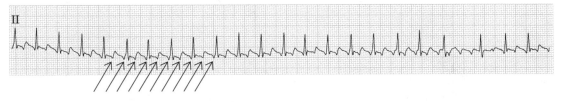

Figure 15.13. A lead-II rhythm strip from a 71-year-old woman with mitral valve disease who presented with acute shortness of breath. *Arrows* indicate the F waves during 2:1 conduction, which then became obvious during later 3:1 conduction.

Odd-numbered AV conduction ratios (1:1, 3:1, etc.) are rare. Figure 15.14 presents an example of 1:1 conduction with both atrial and ventricular rates of about 250 beats/min. Such abnormally rapid AV conduction is rarely possible unless an accessory pathway is present (discussed Chapter 6, "Ventricular Preexcitation"). In the case of such conduction, the regular wide QRS complexes without obvious atrial activity often lead to an erroneous diagnosis of ventricular tachycardia (Chapter 17, "Reentrant Ventricular Tachyarrhythmias").

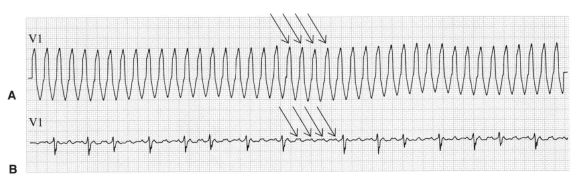

Figure 15.14. Lead-V1 rhythm strips from a 32-year-old woman who had undergone repair of an atrial septal defect as a child and who presented to the hospital emergency department with profound dyspnea and weakness. No atrial activity is visible during the presenting, wide QRS-complex tachyarrhythmia **(A)**, but *arrows* indicate the flutter waves in **B** occurring at the identical rate as the QRS complexes in **A**, recorded after several days of intensive treatment of congestive heart failure.

Figure 15.15 presents atrial flutter with the rare 3:1 AV ratio. The diagnosis is obvious in lead II, but the recording in lead V1 has the appearance of sinus tachycardia. Instead of one P wave, there are three F waves during each cardiac cycle. The first F wave mimics a P wave, the second is obscured by the QRS complex, and the third appears as a peak in the T wave.

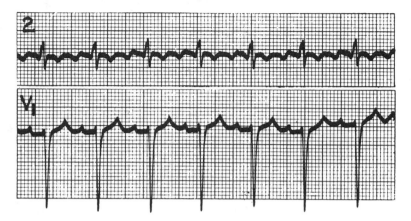

Figure 15.15. A two-channel rhythm strip (II and V1) from a 62-year-old woman with chronic obstructive lung disease.

An interesting feature of atrial flutter is the variety of conduction patterns that may develop because of the interplay at various levels within the AV node.[6] These may produce a regularly irregular ventricular rhythm with a bigeminal pattern. Although all of the atrial impulses enter the AV node, as indicated by the ladder diagram, only two of every three reach the ventricles. A supraventricular tachyarrhythmia (Fig. 15.16A) is proven to be atrial flutter with a 2:1 AV conduction ratio by pharmacologic sympathetic blockade (Fig. 15.16B). The intervention causes a second level of block within the node. The regularly irregular ventricular rhythm has six F waves for every two QRS complexes (6:2 AV conduction ratio).

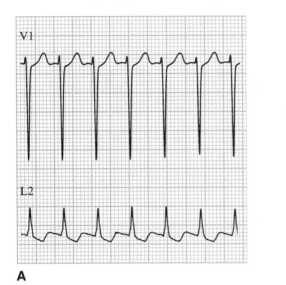

A

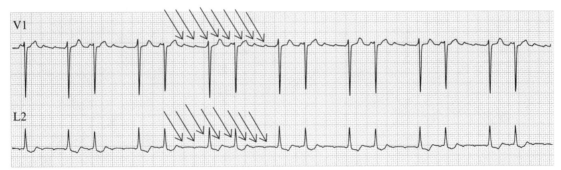

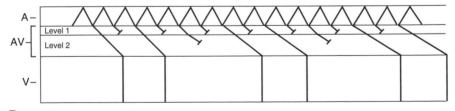

B

Figure 15.16. Leads V1 and II (L2) rhythm strips from a 44-year-old man who presented to the emergency department with weakness and a feeling of his "heart fluttering" **(A)** and after β-adrenergic blocking treatment was begun **(B)**. No atrial activity is visible in **A**, but *arrows* indicate the locations of the F waves in **B**. The ladder diagram beneath the rhythm strip in **B** illustrates 2:1 conduction in Level 1 of the AV node and 3:2 conjunction in Level 2. The size of the diagram has been increased to approximately twice that of the rhythm strip in **B** in order to enhance clarity.

Conduction ratios of 6:1 and higher are sometimes produced when atrial flutter is accompanied by an AV-nodal conduction abnormality, as can be seen in Figure 15.17. In this situation, it may be difficult to distinguish between some AV conduction (termed second-degree block) and no AV conduction (termed third- degree block) (Chapter 20, "Atrioventricular Block"). Some AV conduction may be assumed when, as in Figure 15.17A, a constant ventricular rate (RR intervals) is accompanied by a constant relationship between atria and ventricles (FR intervals). In contrast, the rhythm strip shown in Figure 15.17B presents an example of atrial flutter with complete (third-degree) AV block, as indicated by constant RR intervals accompanied by varying FR intervals.

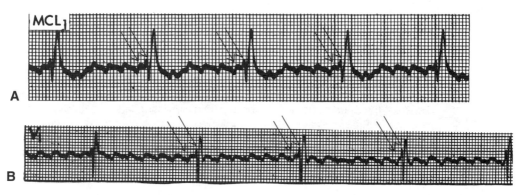

Figure 15.17. A QRS complex with RSR' configuration in lead MCL$_1$ in **A** is due to right bundle-branch block RBBB and that in lead V1 in **B** is due to an escape focus in the left bundle branch. *Arrows* in **A** indicate constant F to QRS intervals, and in **B** indicate varying intervals.

As discussed above, the atrial rate in the flutter/fibrillation spectrum may be greatly influenced by drugs: the rate may be accelerated by digitalis and decelerated by quinidine, procainamide (Class IA), and flecanide (Class IC). In Figure 15.18, the top strip was taken on a day while the patient was receiving digitalis alone. The bottom strip was obtained one day later, 24 hours after quinidine was begun. The atrial rate slowed from 270 to 224 beats/min, but the ventricular rate increased from 96 to 108 beats/min. This inverse relationship between atrial and ventricular rates (Fig. 15.7) occurs because the more beats that enter the AV node, the fewer are able to completely traverse it and reach the ventricles.

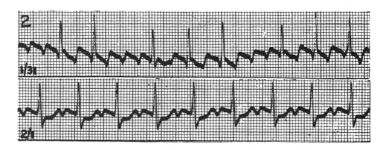

Figure 15.18. Lead-II rhythm strips from a 73-year-old man receiving chronic digitalis therapy for heart failure before (January 31) and 1 day after quinidine therapy was begun in an attempt to convert the patient's cardiac rhythm to sinus rhythm.

ATRIAL FIBRILLATION

Atrial fibrillation may complicate any cardiac disease, and is sometimes seen in the absence of any apparent cardiac disease (*lone fibrillation*).[8] The five most common conditions that produce atrial fibrillation are[9,10]:

1. Rheumatic heart disease.
2. Ischemic heart disease.
3. Hypertensive heart disease.
4. Heart failure of any cause.
5. Thyrotoxicosis.

Advancing age and increased left-atrial size are also related to the development of atrial fibrillation.[11,12] Chronic atrial fibrillation in the elderly often conceals an underlying *sick sinus node*, and such patients frequently have postmortem evidence of narrowing of the sinus node artery with atrophy of the sinus node cells.[13] It is not known whether dysfunction of the sinus node leads to the atrial fibrillation in such cases, or whether disuse of the sinus node during chronic atrial fibrillation leads to its dysfunction.

Chronic atrial fibrillation, once established, usually lasts for life. However, it may occasionally revert to sinus rhythm after surgical replacement of a stenotic mitral valve.[14] Atrial fibrillation appears during two stages of ischemic heart disease: acute myocardial infarction and chronic heart failure.

CHARACTERISTICS OF THE f WAVES OF ATRIAL FIBRILLATION

    Atrial fibrillation is recognized by irregular undulation of the ECG baseline, with an irregularly irregular ventricular rhythm. The undulation may be gross and distinct (Fig. 15.19A), intermediate in form (15.19B), or barely perceptible (15.19C). For descriptive purposes, the fibrillations may be called coarse, medium, and fine, respectively. Although the size of the f waves in atrial fibrillation has not been found to correlate with the size of the atria or the type of the heart disease in which fibrillation occurs,[15] large f waves are unlikely to occur in the presence of a normal-sized left atrium.[16]

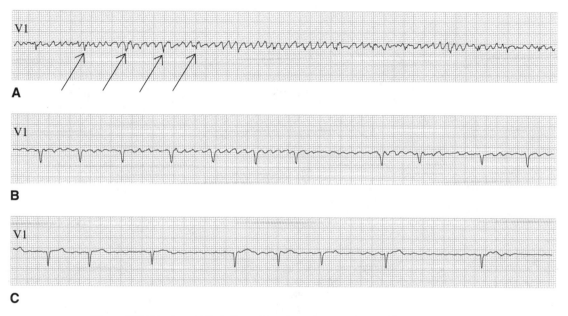

Figure 15.19.   Lead-V1 rhythm strips from three patients with atrial fibrillation. *Arrows* indicate the hidden QRS complexes in **A–C**.

When there is no recognizable deflection of the baseline, atrial fibrillation may be inferred from an irregularly irregular ventricular response (Fig. 15.20A). In fine fibrillation, some baseline undulation may be seen in leads V1 to V3 (Fig. 15.20B).

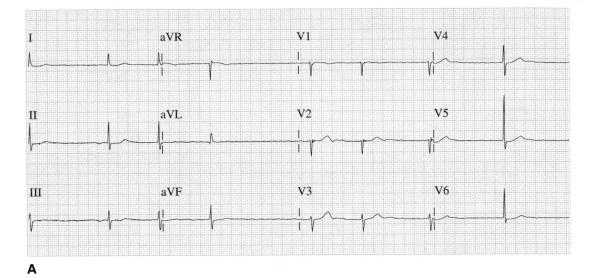

A

B

Figure 15.20. Twelve-lead ECGs from an 89-year-old woman with a previous anterior myocardial infarction **(A)** and a 57-year-old woman with chronic obstructive pulmonary disease **(B)**.

PATTERNS OF ATRIOVENTRICULAR CONDUCTION

    The ventricular rate during atrial fibrillation is variable. If the AV node is normal and its conduction has not been suppressed by digitalis (a β-adrenergic receptor blocker) or a calcium antagonist, rates as high as 200 beats/min may develop (Fig. 15.21A). However, if the AV node is diseased or markedly suppressed by drugs, the ventricular rate may be markedly reduced (Fig. 15.21B).

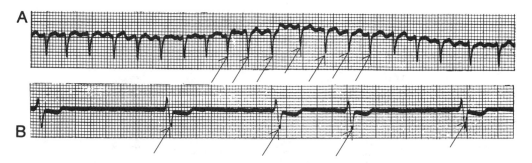

Figure 15.21.   Lead-V1 rhythm strips from two patients with atrial fibrillation. *Arrows* indicate irregularly irregular ventricular rhythm.

Unlike the slower, more orderly atrial flutter, atrial fibrillation is not capable of producing a regular ventricular rhythm. Therefore, when both atrial fibrillation and a regular ventricular rhythm coexist, they are independent of each other. Such AV dissociation may occur for two reasons:

1. There is excessive AV block, which creates the need for emergence of impulse formation from a site in the ventricular Purkinje system (Chapter 20, "Atrioventricular Block").
2. There is normal AV conduction, but interference has developed from enhanced automaticity in the ventricular Purkinje system (Chapter 14, "Accelerated Automaticity").

In Figure 15.22, the ventricular rhythm is regular and the rate varies from accelerated (65 beats/min) (Fig. 15.22A) to within the typical escape range (50 beats/min) (Fig. 15.22B) to a rate in the slow escape range (40 beats/min) (Fig. 15.22C). The proper terminology for each of these conditions would be atrial fibrillation with: AV dissociation due to high-degree AV block and accelerated junctional rhythm (Fig. 15.22A), complete AV block with right-ventricular escape rhythm (Fig. 15.22B), and complete AV block with left-ventricular escape rhythm (Fig. 15.22C). At times, the escape site may be below the branching of the common bundle, producing a widened QRS complex.

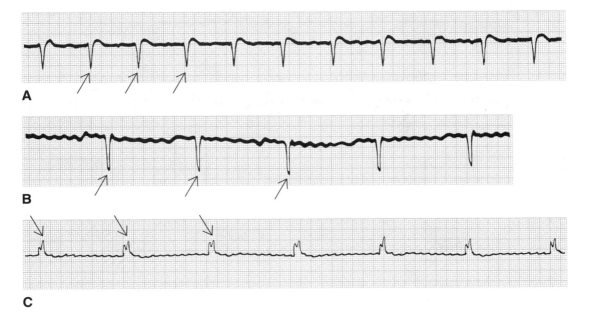

Figure 15.22.   Lead-V1 rhythm strips from three patients with atrial fibrillation. *Arrows* indicate regular ventricular rhythms.

Whenever atrial fibrillation is accompanied by a regular ventricular rate, and the patient is receiving digitalis, one should consider the possibility of digitalis toxicity.[17] In such a case, additional digitalis could cause acceleration of the junctional or ventricular rhythm, producing accelerated junctional rhythm (AJR) or accelerated ventricular rhythm (AVR) (Chapter 14, "Accelerated Automaticity"). In this situation, the atrial fibrillation is accompanied by a regular ventricular rhythm at an accelerated rate. The proper terminology would be "atrial fibrillation with AV dissociation due to AJR or AVR."

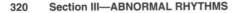

ATRIAL FLUTTER/FIBRILLATION WITH VENTRICULAR PREEXCITATION

  Normally, the AV node is the only electrical pathway connecting the atria and the ventricles. However, as discussed in Chapter 6 ("Ventricular Preexcitation"), some individuals have the congenital abnormality of an accessory AV conduction pathway (Bundle of Kent). Since this pathway is composed of myocardial cells, these individuals have a bypass of the AV-nodal protection that is so important when atrial flutter/fibrillation occurs. The normal inverse relationship between the atrial and ventricular rates illustrated in Figure 15.7 is lost. Instead, the preexcitation pathway permits a direct relationship between the two rates, and thereby allows for particularly rapid ventricular rates at the fibrillation end of the spectrum. The refractory period of the accessory pathway determines the ventricular rate, and rates as high as 300 beats/min sometimes occur (Fig. 15.23A and B).[18,19] In such cases there is a serious risk of ventricular fibrillation, either because the descending impulse arrives during the vulnerable phase of the ventricular cycle, or because the rapid ventricular rate causes such a low cardiac output that myocardial ischemia results.

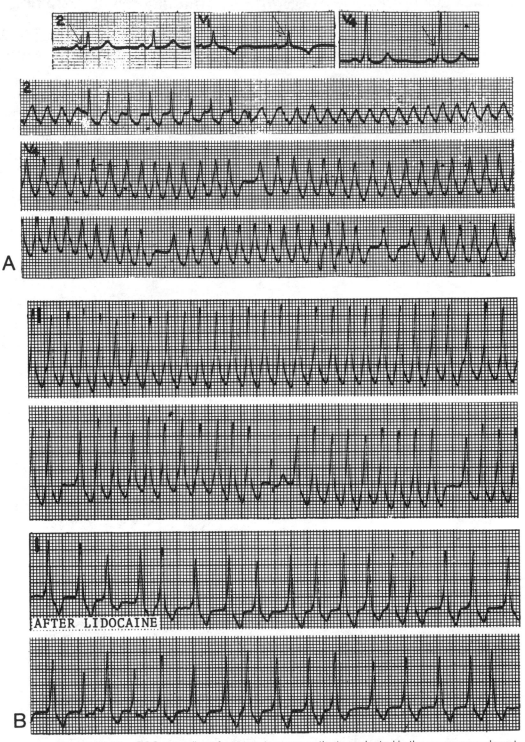

Figure 15.23. ECG recordings from two teenage patients evaluated in the emergency department with complaints of palpitations and weakness. A previous ECG during sinus rhythm **(A)** documented ventricular preexcitation (leads 2, V1, and V4). Lead II (2) and V4 rhythm strips in **A** and a lead I rhythm strip in **B** document the rapid irregularly irregular wide QRS tachycardias. Note the marked slowing of the ventricular rate following Lidocaine administration in **B**.

It can be extremely difficult, and sometimes impossible, to differentiate atrial flutter/fibrillation with preexcitation from a ventricular tachycardia. At the flutter end of the spectrum, there is often a 1:1 AV ratio and a regular ventricular rhythm (Figs. 15.14 and 15.23*A* and *B*, top). Intermittent irregularity or normal-appearing QRS complexes (second strip in Fig. 15.23*B*) are also indicative of atrial flutter. At the fibrillation end of the spectrum, there is less than a 1:1 ratio accompanied by an irregular ventricular rhythm (bottom two strips in Fig. 15.23*A*). Throughout the atrial flutter/fibrillation spectrum, a slow QRS upstroke may indicate the delta wave of ventricular preexcitation.

When atrial fibrillation and ventricular preexcitation coexist:

1. The ventricular cycle length may be as short as 0.20 second, the equivalent of a rate of 300 beats/min (Fig. 15.23*A* and *B*, top rhythm strips).
2. Some ventricular cycles may be more than twice as long as the shortest cycles (bottom two rhythm strips in Fig. 15.23*A*).

This latter variation of more than 100% in cycle length would represent an extremely unusual degree of irregularity in a reentrant ventricular tachycardia (Chapter 17, "Ventricular Tachyarrhythmias").

Failure to recognize the presence of a preexcitation pathway in the presence of atrial fibrillation may lead to a serious error in treating this tachyarrhythmia. This is because digitalis has the opposite effect on the ventricular rate when a preexcitation pathway is present than when only the AV node is available for conduction. When atrial fibrillation is present, the ventricular rate is determined by the length of the refractory period of the AV conduction pathway. As noted above, digitalis prolongs the refractory period of the AV node. However, as discussed in Chapter 11 ("Miscellaneous Conditions"), digitalis shortens the refractory period of myocardial cells. As a result, digitalis can paradoxically increase the ventricular rate and induce ventricular fibrillation when a preexcitation pathway is present.[20]

GLOSSARY

Atrial fibrillation: the tachyarrhythmia at the rapid end of the flutter/fibrillation spectrum; it is produced by macroreentry within multiple circuits in the atria, and is characterized by irregular multiform f waves.

Atrial flutter: the tachyarrhythmia at the slow end of the flutter/fibrillation spectrum; it is produced by macroreentry within a single circuit in the atria, and is characterized by regular uniform F waves.

Atrial flutter–fibrillation: the tachyarrhythmia in the middle of the flutter/fibrillation spectrum; it has some aspects of flutter and some of fibrillation.

Atrial flutter/fibrillation spectrum: a range of tachyarrhythmias caused by macroreentry in the atria, and which extends from flutter with an atrial rate of 200 beats/min through flutter-fibrillation and coarse fibrillation to fine fibrillation without atrial activity detectable on the body surface.

Calcium antagonist: a drug that diminishes calcium entry into cells and slows conduction through the AV node.

Coarse fibrillation: fibrillation marked by prominent f waves in some of the ECG leads.

Concealed conduction: nonconducted atrial impulses that depolarize part of the AV node and thereby make it refractory to following impulses.

Electrical cardioversion: use of transthoracic electrical current to terminate a reentrant tachyarrhythmia, such as those in the atrial flutter/fibrillation spectrum.

F waves: the regular, uniform, sawtoothlike atrial activity characteristic of flutter.

f waves: the irregular multiform atrial activity characteristic of fibrillation.

Fine fibrillation: either minute f waves or no atrial activity at all in any of the ECG leads.

Irregularly irregular: a term describing an irregular rhythm with no discernible pattern to the sequence of ventricular beats.

Ischemic heart disease: a cardiac abnormality caused by decreased blood flow to the myocardium, usually because of atherosclerosis with or without superimposed thrombosis in the coronary arteries.

Lone fibrillation: atrial fibrillation occurring in an individual who shows no evidence of cardiac disease.

Mitral valve disease: a condition marked either by an abnormally tight (stenotic) or leaky (insufficient) valve between the left atrium and left ventricle.

Rheumatic heart disease: active or inactive disease of the heart resulting from rheumatic fever and characterized by inflammatory changes in the myocardium or by scarring of the valves that reduces the functional capacity of the heart.

Sick sinus syndrome: a term that is loosely used clinically to describe any abnormally low sinus rate. These bradyarrhythmias are more likely to be caused by increased parasympathetic nervous activity than by disease in the sinus node.

REFERENCES

1. Waldo AL, Henthorn RW, Plumb VJ. Atrial flutter—recent observations in man. In: Josephson ME, Wellens HJJ, eds. Tachycardias: mechanisms, diagnosis, treatment. Philadelphia: Lea & Febiger, 1984:113–127.
2. Wells JL Jr, MacLean WAH, James TN, et al. Characterization of atrial flutter: studies in man after open heart surgery using fixed atrial electrodes. Circulation 1979;60:665–673.
3. Langendorf R, Pick A, Catz LN. Ventricular response in atrial fibrillation: role of concealed conduction in the atrioventricular junction. Circulation 1965;32:69–83.
4. Lau SH, Damato AN, Berkowitz WD, et al. A study of atrioventricular conduction in atrial fibrillation and flutter in man using His bundle recordings. Circulation 1969;40:71–78.
5. Moore EN. Observations on concealed conduction in atrial fibrillation. Circ Res 1967;21:201–211.
6. Besoain-Santander M, Pick A, Langendorf R. A-V conduction in auricular flutter. Circulation 1950;2:604.
7. Killip T, Gault JH. Mode of onset of atrial fibrillation in man. Am Heart J 1965;70:172.
8. Peter RH, Gracey JG, Beach TB. A clinical profile of idiopathic atrial fibrillation. Ann Intern Med 1968;68:1296–1300.
9. Kannel WB, Abbott RD, Savage DD. Coronary heart disease and atrial fibrillation: the Framingham study. Am Heart J 1983;106:389–396.
10. Morris DC, Hurst JW. Atrial fibrillation. Curr Probl Cardiol 1980;5:1–51.
11. Henry WL, Morganroth J, Pearlman AS, et al. Relation between echocardiographically determined left atrial size and atrial fibrillation. Circulation 1976;53:273–279.
12. Probst P, Goldschlager N, Selzer A. Left atrial size and atrial fibrillation in mitral stenosis: factors influencing their relationship. Circulation 1973;48:1282–1287.
13. Davies MJ, Pomerance A. Pathology of atrial fibrillation in man. Br Heart J 1972;34:520–525.
14. Zimmerman TJ, Basta LL, January LE. Spontaneous return of sinus rhythm in older patients with chronic atrial fibrillation and rheumatic mitral valve disease. Am Heart J 1973;86:676–680.
15. Morganroth J, Horowitz LN, Josephson ME, Kastor JA.

Relationship of atrial fibrillatory wave amplitude to left atrial size and etiology of heart disease. Am Heart J 1979;97:184–186.

16. Bartall H, Desser KB, Benchimol A, et al. Assessment of echocardiographic left atrial enlargement in patients with atrial fibrillation. An electrovectorcardiographic study. J Electrocardiol 1978;11:269–272.

17. Kastor JA. Digitalis intoxication in patients with atrial fibrillation. Circulation 1973;47:888–896.

18. Klein GJ, Bashore TM, Sellers TD, et al. Ventricular fibrillation in the Wolff-Parkinson-White syndrome. Circulation 1976;11:187.

19. Grant RP, Tomlinson FB, Van Buren JK. Ventricular activation in the pre-excitation syndrome (Wolff-Parkinson-White). Circulation 1958;18:355.

20. Sellers TD Jr, Bashore TM, Gallagher JJ. Digitalis in the pre-excitation syndrome. Analysis during atrial fibrillation. Circulation 1977;56:260–267.

CHAPTER 16

Reentrant Junctional Tachyarrhythmias

The *reentrant junctional tachyarrhythmias* (*RJT*) usually occur in young people without underlying heart disease. The occurrence of RJT has been related to periods of anxiety, excess caffeine intake, and fatigue. Reentry within the atrioventriocular (AV) junction can result in a single junctional premature beat (JPB) or in sustained RJT. These tachyarrhythmias may be more difficult to understand and identify than those originating in the atria and ventricles because the AV junction is not represented by any waveform in the electrocardiogram (ECG).

In the normal heart, the only electrically conducting structures of the junction between the atria and ventricles are the AV node and the common (His) bundle. However, congenitally anomalous accessory AV (Kent) bundles, either located centrally in the region of the AV node and His bundle or peripherally, may serve as part of the circuit of RJTs. Usually, the accessory pathway is identified by ECG evidence of ventricular preexcitation during sinus rhythm (Chapter 6, "Ventricular Preexcitation"). The combination of ventricular preexcitation and RJT is called the Wolff-Parkinson-White (WPW) syndrome, as discussed in Chapter 6 ("Ventricular Preexcitation") (Fig. 16.1).[1] The younger the individual with RJT, the more likely that an accessory AV conduction pathway is present.

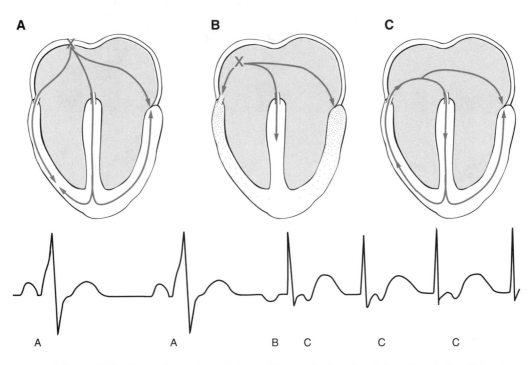

Figure 16.1. Formation and conduction of the cardiac impulse during sinus rhythm **(A)** and an APB **(B)**, and impulse conduction through the various parts of the heart during a sustained tachyarrhythmia **(C)** are shown anatomically **(top)** and electrocardiographically **(bottom)**. Sites of impulse formation are indicated by *x*, the directions of impulse conduction by *arrows*, the AV node by an open channel at the summit of the ventricular septum, the Kent bundle by an *open channel* between the right atrium and ventricle, and persistent refractoriness in the ventricles and Kent bundle by *stippling*. (Modified from Wagner GS, Waugh RA, Ramo BW. Cardiac arrhythmias. New York: Churchill Livingstone, 1983:13, with permission.)

In most individuals, the accessory pathway is capable of conduction in both the anterograde and retrograde directions. However, in some individuals, the accessory pathway may be capable of conduction only in one direction, causing either ventricular preexcitation or RJT, as follows.

1. If only anterograde conduction is possible along an accessory AV pathway, there is preexcitation during sinus rhythm without RJT.
2. If only retrograde conduction is possible along an AV accessory pathway, there is no preexcitation during sinus rhythm but there is the potential for RJT. In this instance, a *concealed AV-bypass pathway* is present.

VARIETIES OF REENTRANT JUNCTIONAL TACHYARRHYTHMIAS

The mechanism that produces RJT may be either microreentry occurring totally within the AV node (*AV-nodal tachycardia*) (Fig. 16.2*A*) or macroreentry involving one atrium, an accessory pathway, one ventricle, and the AV node (*AV-bypass tachycardia*) (Fig. 16.2*B* and *C*). The presence of an accessory AV conduction pathway creates the potential for the development of reentry circuits in which the impulses travel in either the normal or reverse direction through the AV node and ventricular Purkinje system. Although its reentry circuit also includes atrial and ventricular myocardium, AV-bypass tachyarrythmia is included as an RJT because its existence depends on the presence of a congenital anomaly in the junction between the atria and ventricles. The term *orthodromic (AV-bypass) tachycardia* is used when the impulse proceeds in the normal direction (Figs. 16.1*C* and Fig. 16.2*B*), and the term *antidromic (AV-bypass) tachycardia* is used when the impulse proceeds in the reverse direction (Fig. 16.2*C*). (This reverse impulse direction results from a premature beat [PB] that occurs in close proximity to the AV node and therefore finds the node still in its refractory phase.) A concealed AV-bypass pathway is capable only of participating in an orthodromic tachycardia.

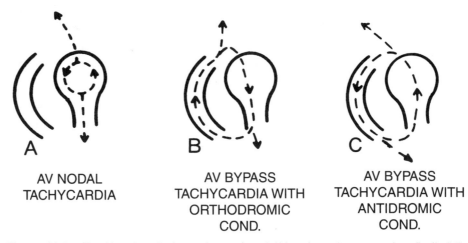

AV NODAL TACHYCARDIA	AV BYPASS TACHYCARDIA WITH ORTHODROMIC COND.	AV BYPASS TACHYCARDIA WITH ANTIDROMIC COND.
A	B	C

Figure 16.2. The Kent bundle (*curved space*) and AV node and common bundle (*bulblike space*) are represented to indicate the anatomic sites **(A–C)** of the three varieties of RJT. *Dashed lines* indicate the locations of and *arrows* indicate the directions of conduction within the three reentry circuits.

The different terms used to characterize an RJT fall into three categories:

1. Those that apply to the clinical behavior of the RJT: persistent, permanent, incessant, sustained, nonsustained, chronic, relapsing, and repetitive.
2. Those that describe the site of origin of the RJT: supraventricular, atrial, AV-nodal, AV-bypass, and junctional.
3. Those that describe the mechanism of the RJT: reentrant, reciprocating, paroxysmal, circus movement, slow–fast, fast–slow, orthodromic, and antidromic.

Table 16.1 presents the types of RJT that are discussed in this chapter.

Table 16.1.   Common Types of RJT

AV-Nodal Tachycardia	AV-Bypass Tachycardia
Slow–fast AV-nodal tachycardia	Orthodromic AV-bypass tachycardia
Fast–slow AV-nodal tachycardia	Antidromic AV-bypass tachycardia

CONDUCTION THROUGH THE ATRIA AND VENTRICLES

Since the AV junction is distal to the atria, RJT produces retrograde atrial activation resulting in inversion of the P waves in the ECG, as illustrated in Figure 16.1. The P waves are therefore negative in the long-axis-oriented leads (e.g., lead II).

Two of the varieties of RJT—AV-nodal tachycardia (Fig. 16.3B) and orthodromic AV-bypass tachycardia (Fig. 16.3C)—produce anterograde ventricular activation that can result in normal-appearing QRS complexes, and and these two varieties of RJT are therefore considered supraventricular tachyarrhythmias. Like all supraventricular tachyarrhythmias, however, an RJT can result in abnormal QRS complexes if it encounters aberrant conduction within the bundle branches or fascicles. Conversely, antidromic AV-bypass tachycardia (which originates when a PB occurs in such close proximity to the interatrial septum that the AV node and/or the His bundle are still refractory) can produce only abnormal QRS complexes, because its impulses are aberrantly conducted to the ventricles via an accessory AV conduction pathway (Fig. 16.3D). Note the normal P wave appearance and timing in Figure 16.3A, the absence of a P wave because atrial activation occurs during the QRS complex in Figure 16.3B, the inverted P wave immediately following the QRS complex in Figure 16.3C, and the inverted P wave immediately preceding the QRS complex in Figure 16.3D.

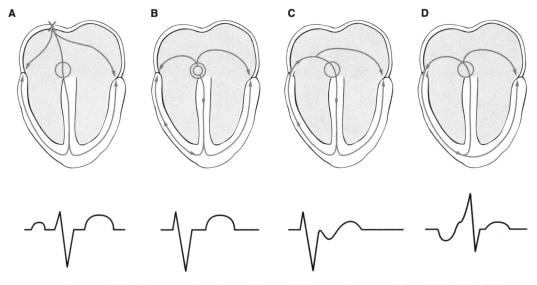

Figure 16.3. The same format as in Figure 16.1 is used to present the relationships between intracardiac impulse conduction and the surface ECG during sinus rhythm **(A)**, AV-nodal reentrant tachycardia **(B)**, orthodromic AV-bypass tachycardia **(C)**, and antidromic AV-bypass tachycardia **(D)**. The *circle* above the summit of the interventricular septum represents the AV node, and the *small circle* within this larger circle in **B** represents the microreentry circuit shown in Figure 16.2A.

NATURAL HISTORY OF REENTRANT JUNCTIONAL TACHYARRHYTHMIAS

 Several studies have been done on the follow-up of children and young adults with RJT with and without evidence of ventricular preexcitation.[2-3] A high percentage of neonates with RJT have evidence of ventricular preexcitation, but many of these infants spontaneously lose their accessory pathway during the first year of life. Some lose only the capability for anterograde conduction through their accessory AV pathway, but retain the capability for retrograde conduction, as evident from recurrent episodes of RJT. There is a decreasing incidence of evidence of preexcitation among progressively older groups of patients with RJT.

 One study reported that 85% of adults with RJT did not have evidence of an accessory pathway, and that those without accessory pathways were older than those with such pathways (a mean of 55 versus 40 years old).[4] There was also a higher incidence of underlying heart disease in adults without accessory pathways (50% versus 10%).

DIFFERENTIATION FROM OTHER TACHYARRHYTHMIAS

 When the QRS complex is normal, RJT superficially resembles both sinus tachycardia and atrial flutter (with a 2:1 AV conduction ratio). If atrial activity is visible in the ECG, its appearance should be diagnostic, since it differs markedly in RJT, sinus tachycardia, and atrial flutter, as shown in Table 16.2.

Table 16.2. Characteristic Atrial Activity

Arrhythmia	Atrial Activity
RJTs	Discrete retrograde P waves
Sinus tachycardia	Discrete anterograde P waves
Atrial flutter	Regular F waves

However, there may be no visible atrial activity in any of the ECG leads, as in the example shown in Figure 16.4. The ventricular rate may also be diagnostically helpful, because sinus tachycardia rarely exceeds 150 beats/min in a nonexercising adult, whereas RJT almost always exceeds this rate (about 155/min in Fig. 16.4). The effect of an atrial premature beat on the tachycardia also may be diagnostically helpful, since it would be expected to reset the sinus rate during sinus tachycardia but to either have no effect or to terminate an RJT, as will be illustrated later in this chapter.

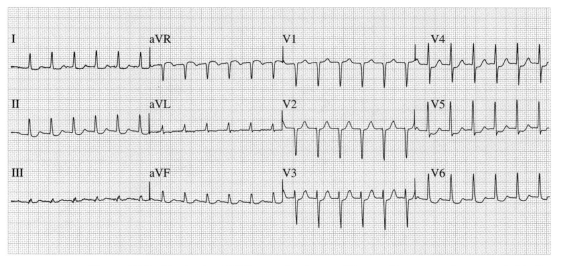

Figure 16.4. Twelve-lead ECG recording from a 20-year-old woman who presented to the emergency department with a sudden onset of weakness and palpitations.

Observance of the onset or termination should differentiate sinus tachycardia from RJT because the enhanced automaticity of sinus tachycardia gradually accelerates and decelerates, in contrast to the abrupt behavior of reentrant tachyarrhythmias. This characteristic, however, does not differentiate RJT from atrial flutter with 2:1 AV conduction, since the ventricular rates in both of these arrhythmias are similar, and both are caused by reentry. Further observation of the rhythm may, however, help in differentiating these two arrhythmias because the 2:1 conduction pattern of atrial flutter tends to be unstable and alternates with a 4:1 pattern, thereby providing a clear view of the F waves. On the other hand, no differentiating features between atrial flutter with 2:1 conduction, and RJT may be apparent even on a full 12-lead ECG, as shown in Figure 16.4. Figure 16.5 illustrates typical abrupt termination of an RJT. Note, however, that there may be slight slowing of the tachyarrhythmia just before the abrupt termination. The period of asystole following termination of the reentry causing the RJT is quickly ended by reemergence of the normal sinoatrial-node (SA) pacemaker. In this instance, an escape pacemaker also emerges, so that the initial QRS complex following the RJT is a fusion beat. This coincidental occurrence masquerades as ventricular preexcitation, but the subsequent sinus beats have no delta wave.

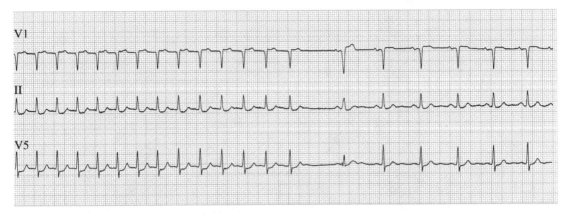

Figure 16.5. A three-lead rhythm strip from the patient in Figure 16.4 during spontaneous termination of the tachyarrhythmia.

When an arrhythmia fails to terminate spontaneously, a vagal maneuver may provide the differential diagnosis of its nature. A classic review by Lown and Levine provides a comprehensive review of the techniques for safely and effectively performing this intervention.[5] The typical responses of paroxysmal atrial tachycardia, atrial flutter, and RJT to vagal maneuvers are presented in Figure 16.6. All three tacharrhythmias have a supraventricular appearance (QRS-complex duration <0.12 s) with atrial activity either apparent following the T waves (Fig. 16.6A and B) or absent (Fig. 16.6C). The paroxysmal atrial tachycardia (Fig. 16.6A) and the atrial flutter (Fig. 16.6B) are unaffected by the maneuver, but the diagnosis is provided by the increased AV-nodal block. The abrupt termination of the arrhythmia seen in Figure 16.6C is a typical response of RJT. The increase in parasympathetic activity terminates RJT by prolonging the AV-nodal refractory period, thereby eliminating the receptive pathway for the recycling impulse. When the arrhythmia fails to respond to the parasympathetic stimulation, the diagnosis remains uncertain, and transesophageal or intraatrial recording may be indicated.

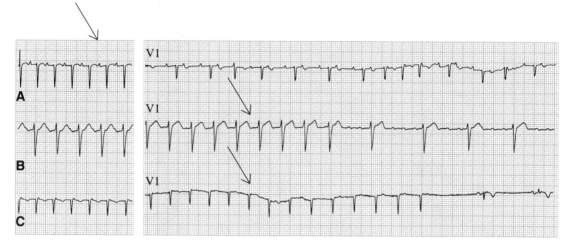

Figure 16.6. Lead-V1 rhythm strips from three patients with various supraventricular tachyarrhythmias. All three appear as undifferentiated SVT at the left and then differentiated as a particular entity at the right. *Arrows* above the rhythm strips indicate the onset of carotid sinus massage in these typical examples of the responses of paroxysmal atrial tachycardia **(A)**, atrial flutter **(B)**, and RJT **(C)**.

When the QRS complex is abnormal because of aberrant conduction via the accessory pathway in antidromic AV-bypass tachycardia or via the Purkinje system in either orthodromic AV-bypass tachycardia or AV-nodal tachycardia, the differential diagnosis becomes more difficult, because ventricular tachycardia must also be considered. Clues to this differentiation are presented in Chapters 17 and 18 ("Ventricular Tachyarrhythmias" and "Supraventricular Tachyarrhythmias with Aberrant Ventricular Conduction," respectively).

DIFFERENTIATION BETWEEN ATRIOVENTRICULAR NODAL AND ATRIOVENTRICULAR BYPASS TACHYCARDIA

 The differentiation between AV-nodal and AV-bypass tachycardias becomes most important when the arrhythmia is resistant to conservative treatment and catheter ablation is being considered. The diagnosis of antidromic AV-bypass tachycardia is facilitated by the presence of delta waves at the onset of the QRS complexes in the ECG, since the impulses causing this type of tachycardia enter the ventricles via the accessory pathway, as illustrated in Figure 16.7.

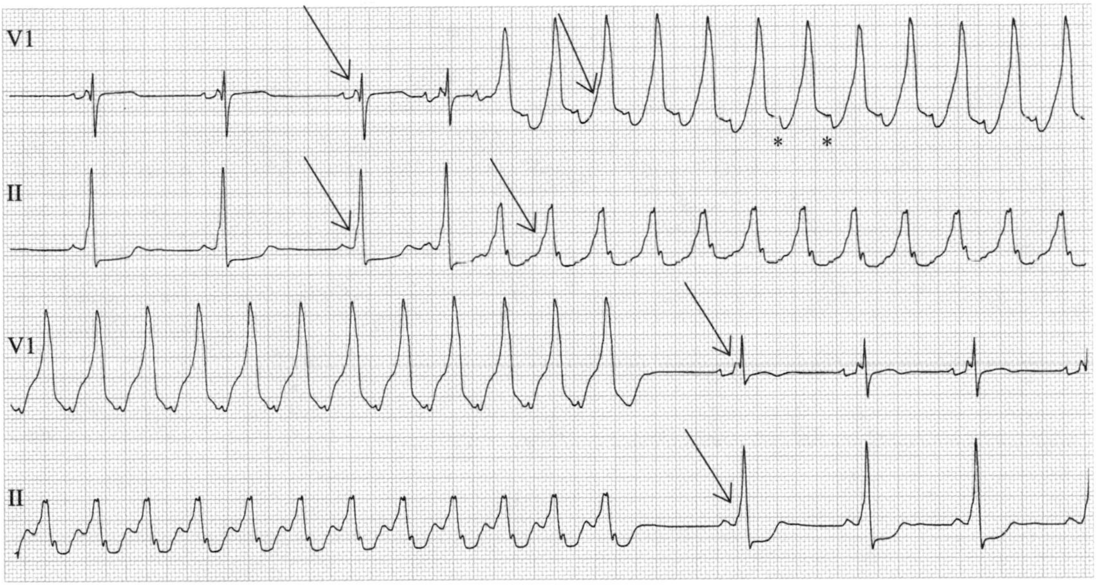

Figure 16.7. Continuous two-lead (V1 and II) rhythm strips from a patient who developed a wide-QRS-complex tachycardia **(top)** that could have been atrial flutter with 1:1 conduction, antidromic AV-bypass tachycardia, or ventricular tachycardia. The slur on the initial QRS waveform suggests either the flutter or the antidromic tachycardia, and this is confirmed by observing return of the prominent delta wave after sinus rhythm **(bottom)**. *Arrows* indicate delta waves present before, during, and after the tachycardia. *Asterisks* indicate abnormally appearing P waves preceding each wide QRS complex.

Differentiation between the other two types of RJT is more difficult. Orthodromic AV-bypass tachycardia may be assumed when there has been preexcitation during sinus rhythm (Fig. 16.1A). However, the accessory pathway may be concealed in sinus rhythm if it is incapable of anterograde conduction. The diagnosis of orthodromic AV-bypass tachycardia is facilitated by observing the following characteristics, which are uniquely present because of the location of the macroreentry circuit[6]:

1. A negative P wave in lead I, which suggests that both the left atrium and a left-sided accessory pathway are components of a macroreentry circuit.
2. A sudden decrease in the rate of the tachycardia coincident with the development of aberrant conduction. This suggests that both the bundle branch in which the aberrancy has occurred and an accessory pathway on the same side of the heart are components of a macroreentry circuit.

The relationship of the P wave to the QRS complex is also helpful in distinguishing AV-nodal from orthodromic AV-bypass tachycardia, as illustrated in Figure 16.8. Since the macroreentry circuit in orthodromic AV-bypass tachycardia includes both an atrium and a ventricle, the P waves and QRS complexes in this type of tachycardia cannot occur simultaneously (Fig. 16.8A), and because of the direction of the reentry circuit, the P wave cannot immediately precede the QRS complex (Fig. 16.8C). Conversely, since the microreentry circuit of AV-nodal tachycardia is contained within the AV node, the P waves and QRS complexes must occur either completely simultaneously (Fig. 16.8A) or almost simultaneously (Fig. 16.8B and C). Therefore, differentiation between AV-nodal and orthodromic AV-bypass tachycardia is only difficult when P waves immediately follow the QRS complexes (Fig. 16.8B). However, the retrograde P wave in AV-nodal tachycardia typically appears as a "pseudo-S wave" of the QRS complex, whereas the QRS complex and retrograde P wave in orthodromic AV-bypass tachycardia are separated from one another.

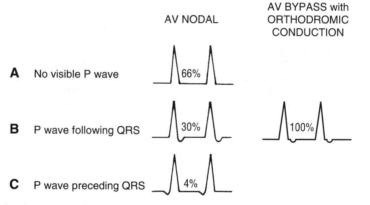

Figure 16.8. Instances of occurrence of the various P wave-to-QRS-complex relationships during these two RJTs is indicated between the consecutive cardiac cycles in **A–C**.[6]

Figure 16.9 presents examples of the three varieties of the relationship between the P wave and QRS complex that may occur with AV-nodal tachycardia (Fig. 16.9A–C), and the typical relationship of the P wave and QRS complex in orthodromic AV-bypass tachycardia (Fig. 16.9D). Lead-II rhythm strips have been selected for illustrating these examples when available (Fig. 16.9A-C), because this long-axis-oriented view provides the inverted appearance of the retrogradely conducted atrial activation (P waves) in these two types of tachyarrhythmia. Note that these P waves could be mistaken for either the S wave (Fig. 16.9B) or Q wave (Fig. 16.9C) of a wider QRS complex. Sometimes, this narrow-QRS-complex tachyarrhythmia even masquerades as a wide-QRS-complex (duration = 0.12 s) tachyarrhythmia.

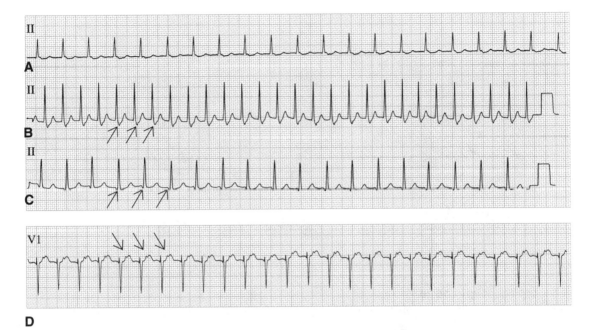

Figure 16.9. The contrasting P-wave-to-QRS-complex relationships during the three varieties of AV-nodal tachycardia, presented in the same order as in Figure 16.8 **(A–C)**, and the P-wave-to-QRS-complex relationship in orthodromic AV-bypass tachycardia **(D)**. *Arrows* indicate the retrograde P waves appearing as pseudo S waves **(B)**, pseudo Q waves **(C)**, and notched T waves **(D)**.

Because of the decreased duration of the QT interval during a tachyarrhythmia (Chapter 3, "Interpretation of the Normal Electrocardiogram"), the following retrograde P wave may be concealed in the T wave during orthodromic AV-bypass tachycardia, as shown in Figure 16.10. The multiple views provided by simultaneous ECG leads may be required for recognition of the P waves in orthodromic AV-bypass tachycardia when they occur simultaneously with the T waves. In Figure 16.10, the diagnosis of orthodromic AV-bypass tachycardia is clearly established by the presence of delta waves during the baseline sinus rhythm and abrupt onset of the arrhythmia initiated by an inverted P wave. However, of the three leads presented, the P waves during the tachycardia are clearly visible only in long-axis-oriented lead II.

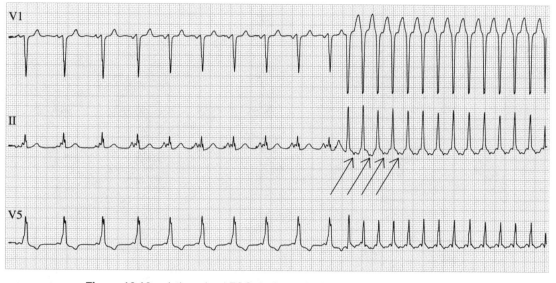

Figure 16.10. A three-lead ECG rhythm strip during sinus rhythm and the abrupt onset of orthodromic AV-bypass tachycardia. *Arrows* indicate the retrograde P waves visible in lead II.

THE TWO VARIETIES OF ATRIOVENTRICULAR-NODAL TACHYCARDIA

 Investigators have shown that the AV node may contain two parallel and independent conduction pathways, one characterized by slow anterograde conduction but faster retrograde conduction, and the other by fast anterograde conduction but slower retrograde conduction.[7] As illustrated in Figure 16.11, these two pathways form the limbs of the microreentry circuit in the following two varieties of AV-nodal tachycardia:

1. Slow–fast AV-nodal tachycardia: The impulse proceeds down the slow pathway and up the fast pathway (Fig. 16.11A).
2. Fast–slow AV-nodal tachycardia: The impulse proceeds down the fast pathway and up the slow pathway (Fig. 16.11B).

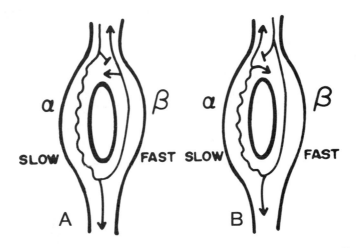

Figure 16.11.   A and B. Schematic diagrams illustrating the contrasting routes of impulse conduction within the slow (α) and fast (β) AV-nodal pathways. The slower conduction is represented by a *wavy line*.

The clinical and ECG characteristics of each of these two forms of AV-nodal tachycardia are listed in Table 16.3.

Table 16.3.   Dual Pathways in the AV Node

	Slow–Fast	Fast–Slow
Synonyms	Paroxysmal	Persistent, etc.
Initial P-R	Prolonged	Normal
Incidence	Usual form in adults	Especially in children
Triggered by	APB	Spontaneous; APB; VPB
P-to-QRS relations	P coincides or immediately follows QRS	R-P > P-R

 The distinguishing relationships of the P wave to the QRS complex illustrated in the "nodal" half of Figure 16.8. *A* and *B* are typical of the slow–fast form of AV-nodal tachycardia, while the relationship shown in Figure 16.8*C* is typical of the fast–slow form.

SLOW–FAST ATRIOVENTRICULAR-NODAL TACHYCARDIA

The slow–fast form of AV-nodal tachycardia is common in adults, and may be congenital, but often results either from diseases or drugs that impair AV-nodal conduction. The AV-nodal reentry is usually started by an APB associated with a prolonged PR interval (Fig. 16.12). The premature impulse finds the faster pathway still refractory but the slower pathway available for its conduction to the ventricles. By the time the impulse reaches the distal AV node, the fast pathway has completed its refractory period and reentry is possible. This process may result in a single junctional premature beat (an *echo beat*) or in either nonsustained or sustained slow–fast AV-nodal tachycardia. The retrograde P wave is often hidden by the QRS complex, since activation of the atria occurs via the fast pathway at the same time that activation of the ventricles occurs via the Purkinje system. The P wave is either entirely invisible on the surface ECG, as in Figure 16.8*A*, or is seen just emerging from the terminal part of the QRS complex, as in Figure 16.8*B* and Figure 16.12.

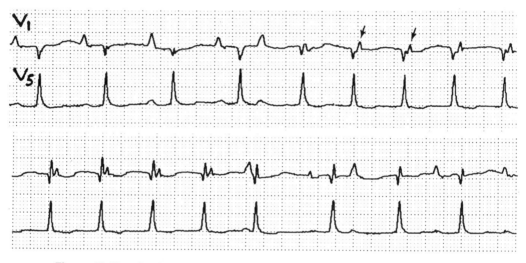

Figure 16.12. Continuous recordings of simultaneous leads V1 and V5. The slow–fast variety of AV-nodal tachycardia, with its closely following retrograde P waves (*arrows*), is initiated and terminated by APBs. Note the premature P wave following the fourth QRS complex in the top strip that initiates the tachycardia and the premature P wave preceding the fifth QRS complex in the bottom strip that terminates it.

FAST–SLOW ATRIOVENTRICULAR-NODAL TACHYCARDIA

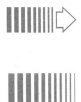

The fast–slow form of AV-nodal tachycardia is the least common variety of RJT in adults, and is therefore called the "atypical" form of AV-nodal tachycardia. Since fast–slow AV-nodal tachycardia proceeds in an anterograde direction down the fast pathway, it does not begin with a prolonged PR interval. The use of the slow pathway for the retrograde limb of the circuit allows ventricular activation (and even recovery) to be completed before atrial activation. As a result, it is very easy to see the retrograde P wave between the T wave and the next QRS complex (Fig. 16.8C and 16.9C).

GLOSSARY

Antidromic tachycardia: an RJT of the AV-bypass variety, produced by macroreentry in which the causative impulse recycles sequentially through an accessory AV-bypass pathway, a ventricle, the AV node, and an atrium.

AV-bypass tachycardia: an RJT produced by macroreentry, which includes the AV node along with an atrium, a ventricle, and an accessory AV-bypass pathway.

AV-nodal tachycardia: an RJT produced by microreentry within the AV node.

Concealed AV-bypass pathway: a Kent bundle that is capable only of VA conduction, and is therefore incapable of producing ventricular preexcitation.

Echo beat: an APB produced by reentry within the AV node.

Fast–slow AV-nodal tachycardia: An RJT of the AV-nodal variety, produced by microreentry in which the impulse travels down the fast pathway and up the slow pathway.

Orthodromic tachycardia: an RJT of the AV-bypass variety produced by macroreentry in which the impulse recycles sequentially through the AV node, a ventricle, an accessory AV-bypass pathway, and an atrium.

Reentrant junctional tachyarrhythmias (RJT): any of the tachyarrhythmias (RJTs) produced by continual recycling of an impulse through structures that are present either normally or abnormally between the atria and the ventricles.

Retrograde atrial activation: spread of an activating impulse from the AV junction through the atrial myocardium and toward the SA node.

Slow–fast AV-nodal tachycardia: an RJT of the AV-nodal variety, produced by microreentry in which the impulse travels down the slow pathway and up the fast pathway.

REFERENCES

1. Wolff L. Syndrome of short P-R interval with abnormal QRS complexes and paroxysmal tachycardia (Wolff-Parkinson-White syndrome). Circulation 1954;10:282.
2. Lundberg A. Paroxysmal tachycardia in infancy. Follow-up study of 47 subjects ranging in age from 10 to 26 years. Pediatrics 1973;51:26–35.
3. Giardinna ACV, Ehlers KH, Engle MA. Wolff-Parkinson-White syndrome in infants and children. Br Heart J 1972;34:839–846.
4. Wu D, Denes P, Amat-y-Leon F, et al. Clinical, electrocardiographic and electrophysiologic observations in patients with paroxysmal supraventricular tachycardia. *Am J Cardiol* 1978;41:1045–1051.
5. Lown B, Levine SA. The carotid sinus: clinical value of its stimulation. Circulation 1961;23:766.
6. Farre J, Wellens HJJ. The value of the electrocardiogram in diagnosing site of origin and mechanism of supraventricular tachycardia. In: Wellens HJJ, Kulbertus HE, eds. What's new in electrocardiography. Boston: Martinus Nijhoff, 1981:131.
7. Sung RJ, Castellanos A. Supraventricular tachycardia: mechanisms and treatment. Cardiovasc Clin 1980;11:27–34.

CHAPTER 17

Reentrant Ventricular Tachyarrhythmias

A ventricular tachyarrhythmia can result from enhanced automaticity in Purkinje cells (Chapter 14, "Accelerated Automaticity") or from reentry occurring either in a localized area (microreentry) or in a wider area of myocardium (macroreentry).[1-5] Only an extremely accelerated ventricular rhythm (AVR) caused by enhanced automaticity can achieve a rate greater than 100 beats/min, and thereby actually qualify for the term "tachyarrhythmia." The great majority of what are called ventricular tachyarrhythmias are instead caused by reentry (Chapter 12, "Introduction to Arrhythmias").

Figure 17.1 presents ladder diagrams that illustrate the mechanisms of the different ventricular tachyarrhythmias. The arrhythmia commonly called *ventricular tachycardia* (*VT*) is analogous to the atrioventricular (AV)-nodal variety of junctional tachyarrhythmia (Fig. 16.2) in that it originates from a reentry circuit so small that it is not represented on the electrocardiogram (ECG). VT can be easily differentiated from AVR on the basis of rate (>120/min vs <120/min, respectively). The macroreentry mechanism of *ventricular flutter/fibrillation* is analogous to that of the atrial flutter/fibrillation spectrum presented in Chapter 15 ("Reentrant Atrial Tachyarrhythmias—The Atrial Flutter/Fibrillation Spectrum"). This mechanism produces no discrete QRS complexes or T waves, just as the atrial flutter/fibrillation mechanism produces no discrete P waves. Torsades de pointes is an atypical form of reentrant ventricular tachyarrhythmia that is difficult to classify. There is no analogy to this tachyarrhythmia occurring in other parts of the heart. Torsades de pointes is probably caused by macroreentry: "macro-" because the ECG shows no discernible QRS complexes or T waves, and "reentry" because the arrythmia both appears and terminates abruptly.

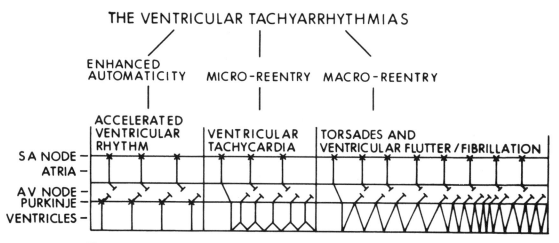

Figure 17.1. In the ladder diagrams, an *X* indicates the site of impulse formation, a *vertical line* indicates normal conduction through the atria or ventricles, a *diagonal line* indicates conduction through the AV node and conduction around a reentry circuit, and a *short perpendicular line* indicates the site of block. (Modified from Wagner GS, Waugh RA, Ramo BW. Cardiac arrhythmias. New York: Churchill Livingstone, 1983:189.)

VENTRICULAR TACHYCARDIA

By definition, VT consists of at least three consecutive QRS complexes originating from the ventricles and recurring at a rapid rate (over 120 beats/min). Like other tachyarrhythmias, VT is considered either nonsustained or sustained, depending on whether it persists for a specified time, as defined below. The rhythm of VT is either regular or only slightly irregular.

In this chapter, the term "the ventricles" refers to any area distal to the branching of the common bundle (Bundle of His), and includes both the Purkinje cells of the pacemaking and conduction system and the ventricular myocardial cells. The reentry circuit in VT is confined to a localized region, and the remainder of the myocardium receives the electrical impulses, just as it would if they were originating from the slower automatic (pacemaking) focus (Fig. 17.1). The QRS complexes and T waves that appear on the ECG in VT are generated from the regions of ventricular myocardium not involved in the reentry circuit.

During VT, the atria may be associated with the ventricles via retrograde activation, or may be dissociated from the ventricles, with their own independent rhythm (usually sinus rhythm), as seen in Figure 17.2. Because wide QRS complexes or T waves are occurring constantly in either of these situations, the P waves are often lost in the barrage of ventricular cycles. Sometimes, however, the P waves may be recognized as bumps or notches in the ventricular cycles. When atrial and ventricular activation are associated, there is a particular ventricular-to-atrial ratio, such as 1:1, 2:1, 3:2, and so on. More commonly, there is AV dissociation, without a relationship between the ventricular and atrial rhythms.

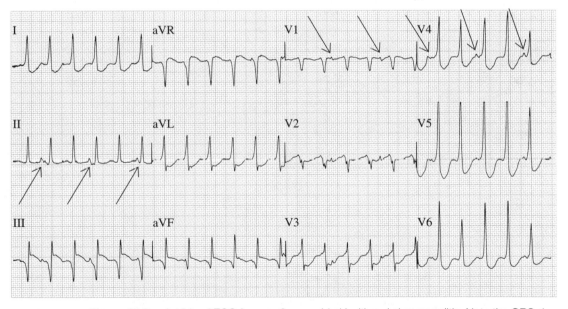

Figure 17.2. A 12 lead ECG from an 8-year-old girl with a viral myocarditis. Note the QRS duration is slightly less than 0.12 second because of the patient's age. *Arrows* indicate the P waves occurring without a fixed relationship to the QRS complexes. The P waves are clearly visible only in leads II, III, and V1 to V4.

ETIOLOGY

VT usually occurs as a complication of severe heart disease, but may occasionally appear in otherwise healthy individuals, in whom it may originate either from the right-ventricular outflow tract or the posterior fascicle of the left bundle branch.[6–10] VT originating from both of these regions can usually be "cured" by radiofrequency catheter ablation.

Many antiarrhythmic drugs also have proarrhythmic effects that are manifested either by VT or torsades de pointes.[11,12] Those drugs that slow conduction (such as flecainide) may prolong the QRS complex and convert nonsustained VT into sustained VT; those that prolong recovery time (such as quinidine or sotalol) may prolong the QTc interval and produce torsades de pointes (Chapter 22, "Drug Toxicity"). VT is most likely to occur as a proarrhythmic effect in patients with poor ventricular function caused by ischemic heart disease.[3]

VT is a major complication of ischemic heart disease, acutely during the early hours of myocardial infarction and chronically following a large infarction. VT may appear almost immediately after complete proximal obstruction of a major coronary artery, when there is epicardial injury but not yet infarction. It tends to be unstable, often leading to ventricular fibrillation. However, during the weeks to months after a large infarction, a more stable form of VT may appear. Chronically arrhythmogenic infarcts are typically large enough to decrease left ventricular function, and may have other typical anatomic characteristics.[13] One study has reported that in patients with a wide-QRS-complex tachyarrhythmia, two aspects of the clinical history consistently predicted a ventricular site of origin[14]:

1. A previous myocardial infarction.
2. No previous tachyarrhythmia.

VT also occurs as a complication of various nonischemic cardiomyopathies,[1] including the "idiopathic dilated," "hypertrophic obstructive," and "arrhythmogenic right ventricular" forms.

DIAGNOSIS

The diagnosis of VT would be an easy task if the impulses causing all supraventricular tachyarrhythmias (SVTs) were conducted normally through the ventricles. However, aberrant conduction of supraventricular impulses, via the bundle branches and fascicles or an accessory pathway, occurs frequently (Chapter 18, "Supraventricular Tachyarrhythmias with Aberrant Ventricular Conduction"). The importance of differentiating VT from SVTs was emphasized in one study by the adverse responses of VT to the calcium-channel-blocking drug verapamil. In this study, half of a group of patients were given verapamil because of an erroneous diagnosis of SVT, and as a result, many of these patients promptly deteriorated and some required resuscitation.[14]

The most common sources of error in the diagnosis of VT are listed in Table 17.1 and are explained below.

Table 17.1. Common Sources of Error in Diagnosis of VT

1. Believing that VT cannot be well tolerated
2. Depending on a single lead, especially lead II
3. Depending on independent atrial activity
4. Putting faith in irregularity
5. Ignoring or neglecting QRS morphology

Believing That VT Cannot Be Well Tolerated

It is commonly believed that VT is associated with a greater alteration of hemodynamics than are SVTs, but a study by Morady and colleagues showed this to be a misconception.[15] Moreover, a study by Tchou and colleagues found that all patients with proven VT were hemodynamically stable when first seen.[14] The main factors that determine a patient's tolerance to a tachyarrhythmia of any origin are (a) the ventricular rate, (b) the size of the heart; and (c) the severity of the underlying clinical problem and associated conditions.

Depending on a Single Lead

When no P waves are revealed on a standard 12-lead ECG, the details of the morphology of the QRS complex may provide differentiation between VT and SVTs.[16-20] When observing QRS-complex morphology in order to differentiate VT from an SVT with aberrancy, it is important to consider the relative values of different ECG leads. Figure 17.3 illustrates the superiority of using lead V1 (with its right-versus-left orientation) rather than lead II (with its base-to-apex orientation) for differentiating VT from an SVT. When abnormally wide QRS complexes have a V1-positive morphology, the differential diagnosis is between VT from the left ventricle (left-ventricular tachycardia: LVT) and SVT with right bundle-branch block (RBBB) (Fig. 17.3A). When abnormally wide QRS complexes have a V1-negative morphology, the differential diagnosis is between VT from the right ventricle (right-ventricular tachycardia: RVT) and SVT with left bundle-branch block (LBBB) (Fig. 17.3B). The ECG in lead II may have a similar appearance in all of these arrhythmias, as in the examples shown in Figure 17.3A and B. This is one of several reasons why a right chest lead (V1 or MCL₁) is superior to an inferiorly oriented limb lead (lead II) for rhythm monitoring.

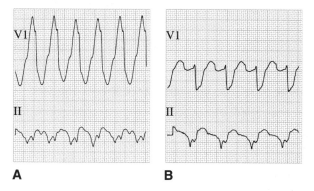

A   **B**

Figure 17.3. Simultaneous lead-V1 and -II rhythm strips from two patients with wide-QRS-complex tachyarrhythmias.

Depending on Independent Atrial Activity

Identification of independent atrial activity (AV dissociation) eliminates the possibility of an SVT originating from the atria or depending on an accessory pathway, but it does not exclude an SVT originating within the AV node. Figure 17.4 presents an example of an AV-nodal tachycardia with left bundle-branch (LBB) aberrancy, confirmed by observing the similar QRS morphology occurring during sinus rhythm. However, this is the exception. When there is AV dissociation with a wide-QRS-complex tachycardia, the diagnosis of VT is highly probable. In a study by Wellens and colleagues, AV dissociation was identified on the ECG in 32 of 70 patients with VT proven by intracardiac recording, and in none of 70 patients with an aberrantly conducted SVT.[20]

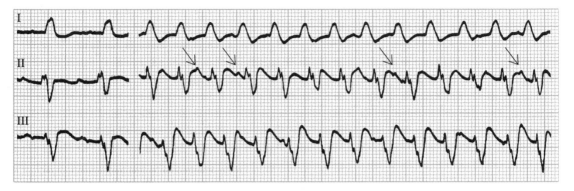

Figure 17.4. Recordings of limb leads I, II, and III during sinus rhythm **(left)** and AV-nodal tachycardia **(right)**. *Arrows* indicate the normally directed P waves visible in lead II without constant PR intervals.

Putting Faith in Irregularity

VT has been said to be characterized by slight irregularities of both ventricular rate and ECG waveform morphology. However, like all reentrant tachyarrhythmias, VT is usually almost regular. In the study by Wellens and colleagues, there was complete regularity in 55 of the 70 patients with VT and in 65 of the 70 with an SVT.[20] Therefore, the degree of regularity does not help the differential diagnosis between VT and SVT.

Since the ECG waveform morphology of VT is usually consistent from beat to beat, the term *monomorphic* is applied. When an intermittent irregularity appears in the morphology of the QRS complex, either on time or slightly early, the most likely cause is a breakthrough of conduction of the atrial rhythm to the ventricles. If the atrial breakthrough occurs during a ventricular beat, the result is a fusion beat. If the breakthrough occurs before a ventricular beat has begun, the result is a capture beat, as in beats 5 and 18 in Figure 17.5. Fusion describes a hybrid QRS-complex morphology, in which a portion of the QRS complex represents the areas of the ventricles activated by the VT while the other portion of the complex represents the areas activated by a competing atrial impulse, as in Figure 17.5, beats 10 and 15. Capture means that the entire QRS complex represents activation of the ventricles by a competing atrial impulse. If either fusion or capture beats are proven to be present, the diagnosis is almost certainly VT. However, fusion and/or capture beats are seldom seen in VT, and then only at the less rapid rates (<160 beats/min). Indeed, they appeared in only four of a series of 33 reported patients with sustained VT.[20]

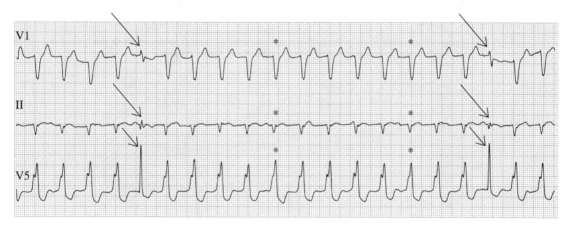

Figure 17.5. A three-lead rhythm strip from a 62-year-old man who presented with acute shortness of breath 2 months after an inferior–posterior MI. *Arrows* indicate capture beats and *asterisks* indicate fusion beats.

Ignoring or Neglecting QRS Morphology

The diagnostic weaknesses of the methods discussed above have been documented.[19,20] During the past 25 years, electrophysiologic studies have provided the capability for using intracardiac recordings to differentiate VT from an SVT with aberrancy. The development of drugs such as verapamil, which are often therapeutic in an SVT but life-threatening in VT, have made the accurate bedside diagnosis of VT more critical.[21–23] As better clues were sought, it became evident that subtle differences in the shape of the QRS complexes often afforded a reliable indication of their source.[15,20,24,25] The use of clues based on the morphology of the QRS complex for the differential diagnosis of VT versus an SVT with aberrancy is discussed in detail below, and with the addition of certain important aspects in Chapter 18 ("Ventricular Versus Supraventricular with Aberrant Conduction").

The simple measurement of the duration of wide QRS complexes may provide important diagnostic information, particularly if a recording is available of the patient's

QRS-complex morphology during sinus rhythm. Wellens and colleagues found that a QRS-complex duration of longer than 0.14 second is a good indicator of VT, since in their study, all 59 patients with this duration had electrophysiologic confirmation of VT.[19] However, an exception to this "rule of thumb" could occur, because as indicated in Chapter 5 ("Intraventricular Conduction Abnormalities"), complete LBBB or RBBB may increase the duration of the QRS complex to longer than 0.14 second. A less wide (0.12 to 0.14 sec) QRS complex is not necessarily indicative of SVT with aberrancy, since only about 50% of patients with confirmed VT had QRS complexes with durations in this range.[19]

In LVT, the lead-V1-positive QRS complex usually includes either a monophasic R wave or a diphasic qR complex, and only occasionally a triphasic RSR′ complex. When the QRS complex in right-sided chest leads such as V1 or MCL₁ has two positive peaks (an R and an R′, with or without an S wave between these two peaks), the peaks have been termed "rabbit ears." The relative heights of these "ears" have been used to differentiate LVT from SVT with right bundle-branch (RBB) aberrancy.[26] A taller R than R′ wave (taller first "ear") suggests the presence of LVT (Fig. 17.6), because RBB aberration is characterized by a taller R′ than R wave (taller second "ear") (Chapter 5, "Intraventricular Conduction Abnormalities"). In this example of LVT, note also the diagnostic QS morphology in lead V6.

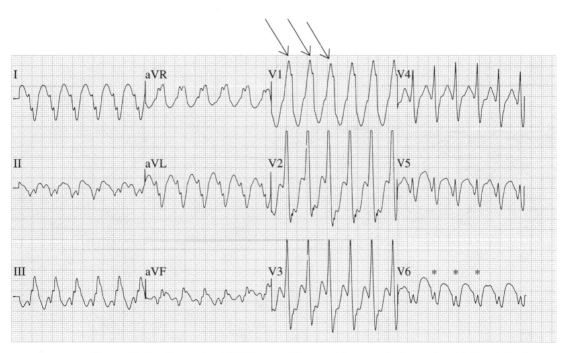

Figure 17.6. Twelve-lead ECG from a 59-year-old man with chronic heart failure following an extensive anterior myocardial infarction. *Arrows* indicate the taller first "rabbit ear" in lead V1. *Asterisks* indicate the QS pattern in lead V6.

Vera and coworkers[24] evaluated 1,100 wide QRS complexes during atrial fibrillation, and found that the triphasic rsR′ configuration in lead V1 offered 24-to-1 odds in favor of ventricular aberration, whereas a monophasic R wave or diphasic qR complex provided 9-to-1 odds in favor of VT.

A complete or almost complete absence of any positive deflection (QS or rS complexes) in lead V6 is almost diagnostic of VT originating from either ventricle, since these patterns could not be produced by either RBBB or LBBB. Such patterns in lead V6 appear with LVT in Figure 17.6 and with RVT in Figure 17.7. Conversely, a triphasic qRs morphology in lead V6, is virtually diagnostic of SVT with aberrancy. Note the unusually slow rate (110 beats/min) and long QRS-complex duration (0.2 sec) in Figure 17.7, caused by pharmacologic treatment with propafenone.

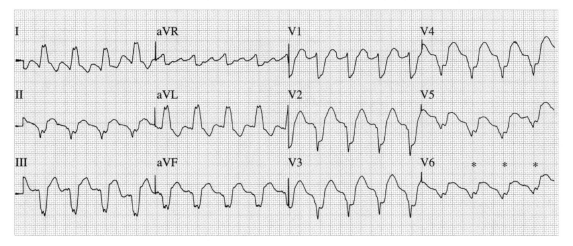

Figure 17.7. Twelve-lead ECG from a 63-year-old man with recurrent VT and heart failure awaiting cardiac transplantation while being maintained on propafenone therapy. *Asterisks* indicate the QS appearance in lead V6.

Wellens and colleagues analyzed the morphologic features of the ECGs of 100 patients with proven VT and those of 100 patients with SVT and aberration.[19,20] They confirmed the value of the triphasic rsR′ pattern in lead V1 and qRs pattern in lead V6 in recognizing RBBB aberration. They also confirmed a monophasic R or diphasic qR morphology, and the rS and QS configurations in lead V6, as hallmarks of VT. In addition, they introduced several new ECG clues that favored VT, including the single, symmetrical peak in lead V1, and an equiphasic QR complex in lead V1 or V6. Wellens and colleagues also observed that left-axis deviation and a QRS-complex duration exceeding 0.14 second favored VT. Like Vera and coworkers, Gulamhusein and associates[25] examined anomalous beats during atrial fibrillation, and again confirmed many of the previously recognized clues. Some of the most important findings in the studies by Wellens and Gulamhusein and their colleagues are listed in Tables 17.2 and 17.3.

Table 17.2. QRS Contours Favoring Ventricular Tachycardia[a]

	Wellens[19, 20]	Gulamhusein[25]
V1	15/15 (100%)	84/86 (98%)
V1	7/7 (100%)	177/187 (95%)
V6	27/31 (87%)	189/190 (100%)
V6	17/17 (100%)	38/40 (94%)

[a] In each pair of numbers, denominator is number of times contour was encountered; numerator is number of times it was ventricular in origin.

Table 17.3. QRS Contours Favoring Ventricular Aberration

	Wellens[19, 20]	Gulamhusein[25]
V1	38/41 (93%)	55/55 (100%)
V6	44/47 (94%)	27/27 (100%)

Concordance of the predominant direction of wide precordial QRS complexes is another useful ECG clue in evaluating for possible VT. When all of the ventricular complexes from leads V1 to V6 are either negative (concordant precordial negative) or positive (concordant precordial positive), the diagnosis is most likely VT, since these patterns would be highly atypical of either RBBB or LBBB. Concordant negativity, as presented in Figure 17.8A, is virtually diagnostic of RVT, and concordant positivity (Fig. 17.8B) is virtually diagnostic of LVT.

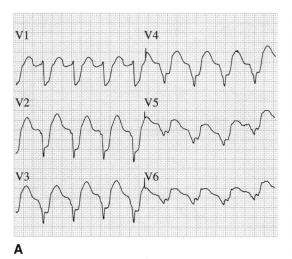

Figure 17.8. The ECG recordings in the six precordial leads from Figure 17.7 **(A)** are contrasted with those from a 62-year-old man who returned with acute chest pain 1 month after a posterolateral MI **(B)**.

Brugada and associates[27] developed the following two additional morphologic criteria for the diagnosis of VT from the precordial leads of the ECG (Fig. 17.9):

1. None of the precordial leads has an RS morphology (Fig. 17.9A).
2. If an RS morphology is present, the interval from the onset of the QRS to the nadir of the S wave exceeds 0.10 second (Fig. 17.9B).

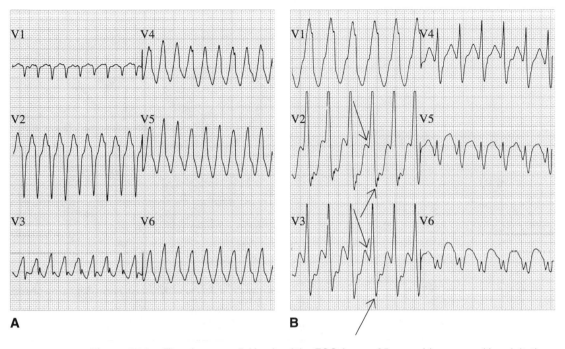

Figure 17.9. The six precordial leads of the ECG from a 25-year-old woman with palpitations of sudden onset **(A)** illustrate VT with no lead (V1 to V6) having an RS morphology, and those from the patient whose ECG is shown in Figure 17.6 **(B)**, illustrating VT with a prolonged interval from onset of the QRS complex to the nadir of the S wave. *Arrows* in **B** indicate the period of 0.12 second from QRS onset to S nadir in leads V2 and V3.

Rosenbaum[28] described a pattern of QRS morphology that is commonly present in healthy young individuals with RVT. The location of the reentry circuit is in the RV outflow tract. As illustrated in Figure 17.10, there is the typical pattern of LBBB except for:

1. Right-axis deviation in the frontal plane (Fig. 17.10A).
2. A broad initial R wave in lead V1 (Fig. 17.10B).

With true LBBB, there is neither the greater delay in the posterior than in the anterior fascicle that would be required to produce RAD, nor the left-to-right septal activation that would be required to produce a prominent R wave in lead V1.

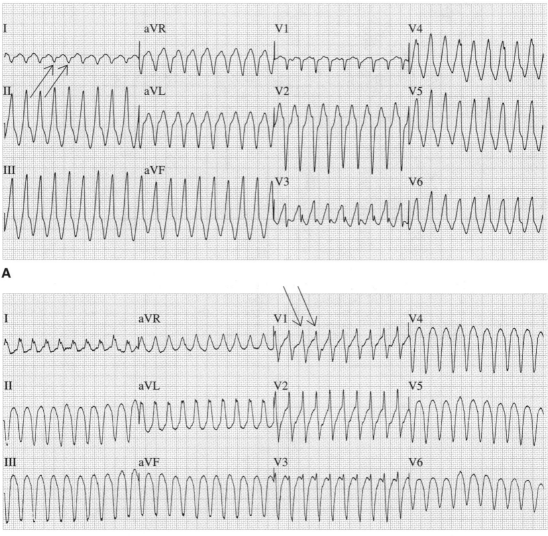

Figure 17.10. **A.** All 12 standard leads of the ECG are presented from the otherwise healthy patient whose ECG is shown in Figure 17.9A. Electrophysiologic mapping and ablation confirmed an origin of VT in the RV outflow area. *Arrows* indicate the negativity of right-axis deviation in lead I. **B.** Twelve-lead ECG from a 61-year-old man who presented after a syncopal episode at home, and then had recurrent syncope after arrival at the emergency department. *Arrows* indicate the broad (≥0.04 sec) initial R waves in lead V1.

In monitoring with a single right-sided lead such as MCL$_1$, the morphology of the initial part of the QRS complex may provide sufficient clues to differentiate VT from an SVT with LBBB. Figure 17.11 provides an example of the development of RVT in the presence of an SVT (atrial fibrillation) with LBB aberration. The typically narrow initial R wave of LBBB is at first apparent, but is replaced by a broad initial R wave when the rate increases and the QRS complex further widens. This characteristic provides the diagnosis of a second tachyarrhythmia (RVT), since the narrow initial R wave would have persisted had the transition from atrial fibrillation to atrial flutter been the reason for the increase in both ventricular rate and QRS duration.

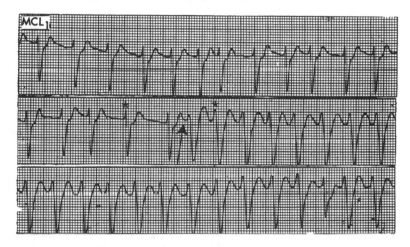

Figure 17.11. A continuous recording of lead MCL$_1$ from a 77-year-old woman with ischemic cardiomyopathy and chronic heart failure. An *arrow* indicates the onset of the VT and *asterisks* indicate contrasting narrow and broad initial R waves in lead MCL$_1$.

Figure 17.12 illustrates schematically the contrast between the initial 0.06 second of the QRS complexes in SVT with LBBB (Fig. 17.12*A* and *B*) and RVT with lead-V1-negative morphology (Fig. 17.12*B* and *C*). LBBB causes a delay in the activation of the left ventricle, and therefore notching or slurring in the terminal part of the QRS complex. The initial part of the QRS complex represents rapid activation of the right ventricle via the unaffected RBB. This is manifested in lead V1 by either a narrow initial R wave (*A*) or a Q wave with a sharp downstroke, which reaches its nadir within 0.06 second (*B*). However, when RVT causes the impulse to originate from a site of microreentry within the ventricles, there is slow movement of the wavefronts of activation throughout the remainder of the ventricular myocardium, and notching or slurring may therefore occur in any part of the QRS complex. Such slow conduction is represented in lead V1 by either a slurred or a notched Q wave, which reaches its nadir later than 0.06 second (*C*), or by a broad (0.04 sec) initial R wave (*D*).[29,30]

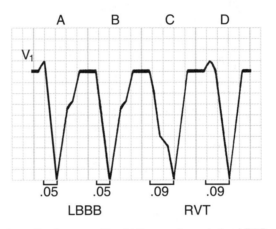

Figure 17.12. A schematic diagram of lead-V1 recordings during LBBB and two varieties of RVT. The *brackets* indicate the durations from the onsets of the QRS complexes to the nadirs of the maximal negative waveforms: 0.05 second in **A** and **B**, and 0.09 second in **C** and **D**.

The slow conduction during VT is also indicated by a slow rise or descent of the initial waveform in lead V6. Drew and Scheinman have observed that if more than 0.07 second is required to reach either the peak of the R wave (Fig. 17.13A) or the nadir of the S wave (Fig. 17.13B), the diagnosis is almost always VT.[31]

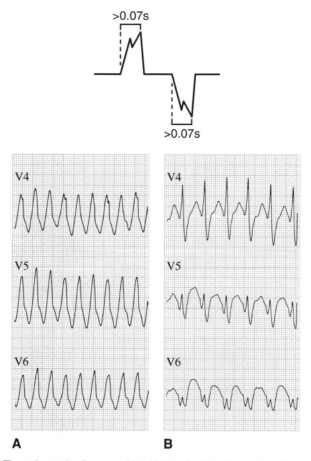

Figure 17.13. The schematic diagram of lead V6, indicating the method for measuring the duration from the onset of the QRS complex to the peak to the R or S wave, and the recordings of the ECG in leads V4 to V6 from two patients illustrate the slow rise of the R wave **(A)** and the slow descent of the S wave **(B)**.

An extreme deviation of the axis of the QRS complex in the frontal plane, into the upper right quadrant between −90 degrees and −180 degrees, very seldom is found with aberrantly conducted beats (exceptions include some complex congenital heart lesions and hearts with multiple infarcts). However, this often appears in VT arising from either ventricle (Fig. 17.6).[19] The presence of extreme axis deviation is therefore strongly suggestive of a diagnosis of VT.

All of the clues described above owed their original recognition to clinical observation and deduction, and were in use for many years before they were confirmed by experimental studies. Their performance in patients with the diagnosis of VT confirmed by invasive electrophysiologic studies is presented in Table 17.4.[19,20]

Table 17.4.   Diagnosis of Ventricular Tachycardia

Lead	QRS Morphology		Incidence
V₁	Single peak	⋀	15/15
	Taller first rabbit ear	⋀	7/7
	QR	⋁⋀	16/17
	RS	⋀⋎	4/4
V₆	rS	⋁	27/31
	QS	⋁	17/17
	QR	⋁⋀	8/8
Axis −30 to −180 degrees[a]			68/75
QRS interval >0.14 sec[a]			59/59

[a] Of little use if previous tracing not available.

LEFT- VERSUS RIGHT-VENTRICULAR TACHYCARDIA

It is generally true that one can distinguish between tachycardia originating in the right versus the left ventricle by observing whether the QRS complexes are lead-V1 positive or lead-V1 negative. However, important exceptions have been identified by observing the morphology of the QRS complex during artificial ventricular pacing[32] and by electrophysiologic identification of the site of origin of clinical episodes of VT. In one study, VT indeed originated from the left ventricle in all of 22 individuals with lead-V1 positivity, but originated from the right ventricle in only three of the 20 subjects with lead-V1 negativity (Table 17.5).[33] The ventricle of origin seemed to vary with the condition of the heart: in the three subjects with normal hearts, lead-V1 negativity was indeed associated with a right ventricular origin of VT, but in all 17 subjects with ischemic heart disease, the VT originated from inside or near the left side of the interventricular septum. It has been hypothesized that areas of infarction sufficiently delay activation of the left ventricle to allow the right ventricle to be activated earlier, producing lead-V1 negativity.[34] In a series of individuals without heart disease, all of the electrophysiologically investigated VTs with lead-V1 negativity originated from the outflow tract of the right ventricle.[35]

Table 17.5. QRS Morphology/Site of Origin

V$_1$	LV	RV
⋀	22/22	0/22
⋁	17/17 (sick)	3/3 (well)

VARIATION OF DURATION OF VENTRICULAR TACHYCARDIA

 VT is usually designated as either *nonsustained VT* or *sustained VT*, depending on whether it persists for longer than 30 seconds.[1] Nonsustained VT has also been defined as VT lasting less than 1 minute[36] and for fewer than 10 beats.[37] Figure 17.14 illustrates two recurrences of VT initiated by ventricular premature beats (VPBs) that satisfy most of these definitions of nonsustained VT. Note that the initial episode continues for many more than 10 beats.

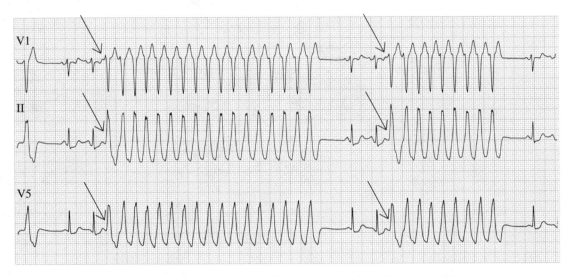

Figure 17.14. Simultaneous recording of leads V1, II, and V5 from a 32-year-old woman who presented with palpitations but no other evidence of heart disease. *Arrows* indicate initiation of the episodes of palpitation by VPBs.

Episodes of nonsustained VT may recur chronically over a period of months to years.[38] However, there are striking differences in incidence and prognosis between RVT and LVT.[39] Patients with LVT tend to be older, to be male, and to have diagnosable heart disease, whereas those with RVT tend to be younger, to be female, and to not have diagnosable heart disease. RVT is more likely to be induced by particular situations, such as moderate exercise, emotional excitement, upright posture, or smoking.[40,41] LVT, associated with either ischemic or idiopathic cardiomyopathy, has also been shown to be exercise induced.[42] RVT is commonly associated with arrhythmogenic right ventricular cardiomyopathy.[1]

VARIATIONS IN THE ELECTROCARDIOGRAPHIC APPEARANCE OF VENTRICULAR TACHYCARDIA—TORSADES DE POINTES

 All of the examples provided in the foregoing sections have been of *monomorphic VT* because of the consistency of their QRS-complex morphologies. However, torsades de pointes represents a commonly occurring VT with variations in morphology (*polymorphic VT*) (Fig. 17.1). This French term translates as "twistings of the points."[25,43,44] Torsades de pointes VT is characterized by undulations of continually varying amplitudes that appear alternately above and below the baseline. The wide ventricular waveforms are not characteristic of either QRS complexes or T waves, and the rate varies from 180 to 250 beats/min (Fig. 17.15).[45] Torsades de pointes VT is usually nonsustained; however, it may persist for longer than 30 seconds, satisfying the definition of a sustained tachyarrhythmia. It may also at times evolve into ventricular fibrillation.

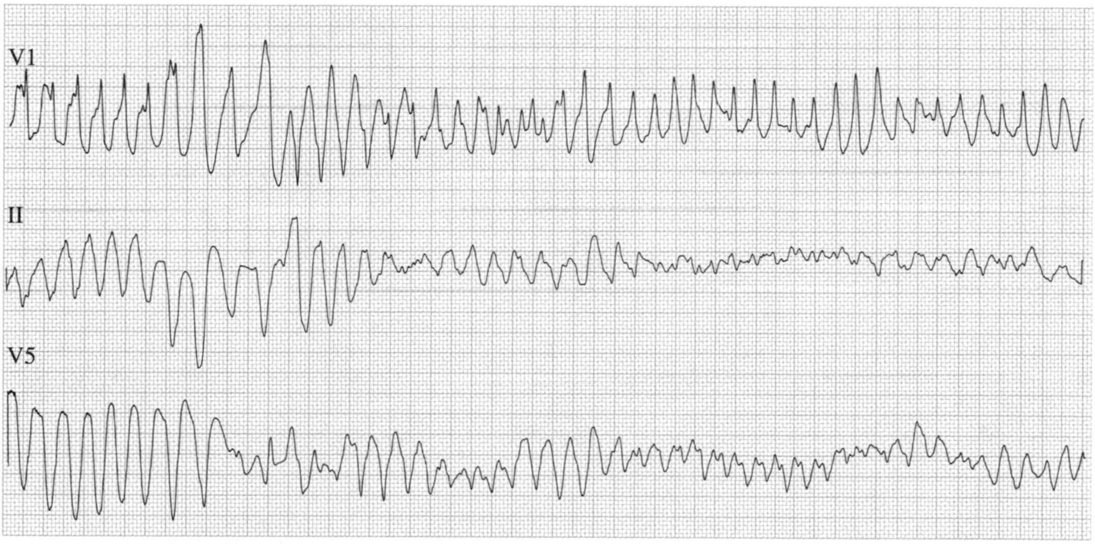

Figure 17.15. Simultaneous recordings of leads V1, II, and V5 from a 62-year-old woman receiving diuretic therapy who presented after experiencing a syncopal episode at home. Syncope recurred in the emergency department during this ECG recording. The patient's serum potassium concentration was 2.3 mEq/L.

Torsades de pointes almost always occurs in the presence of prolongation of the QTc interval.[46,47] This may be caused by the proarrhythmic effect of drugs that prolong ventricular recovery time, including quinidine,[48,49] procainamide,[43,47] disopyramide,[50,51] sotalol,[11] phenothiazines, some antibiotics, some antihistamines, and tricyclic antidepressants.[11] It also occurs with electrolyte abnormalities such as hypokalemia and hypomagnesemia,[11] insecticide poisoning,[52] subarachnoid hemorrhage,[53] congenital prolongation of the QTc interval,[54] ischemic heart disease,[55] and bradyarrhythmias.[3]

VENTRICULAR FLUTTER/FIBRILLATION

Ventricular flutter/fibrillation is a macroreentrant tachyarrhythmia within the ventricular muscle that is analogous to the atrial flutter/fibrillation spectrum discussed in Chapter 15 ("Reentrant Atrial Tachyarrhythmias—The Atrial Flutter/Fibrillation Spectrum") (Fig. 17.16*A*). Neither QRS complexes nor T waves are clearly formed, and the rhythm looks similar when viewed right-side up or upside down. Immediately after the onset of reentry, a regularly undulating baseline is present (Fig. 17.16*B*, top). This *ventricular flutter* looks like a larger version of atrial flutter, but it remains regular and orderly only transiently because the rapid, weak myocardial contractions produce insufficient coronary blood flow (Fig. 17.16*B*, middle). As a result, there is prompt deterioration toward the irregular appearance of *ventricular fibrillation* (Fig. 17.16*B*, bottom). Ventricular flutter has been given various names, including "ventricular tachycardia of the vulnerable period" and "prefibrillation."

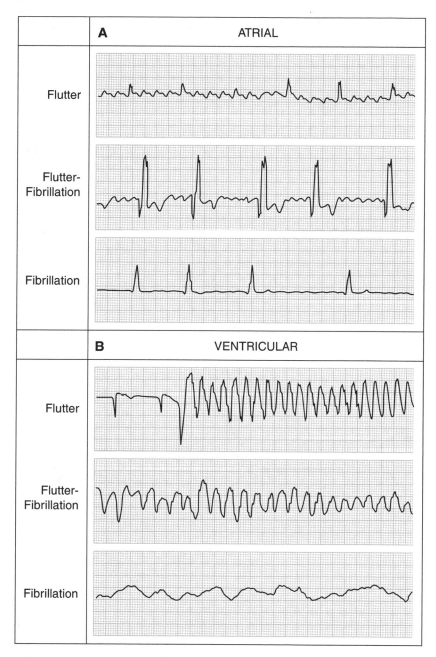

Figure 17.16. The atrial flutter/fibrillation spectrum **(A)** is compared with its ventricular counterpart **(B)**. (From Wagner GS, Waugh RA, Ramo BW. Cardiac arrhythmias. New York: Churchill Livingstone, 1983:22, with permission.)

Clinical Observations

The various factors capable of creating movement along the flutter/fibrillation spectra in the atria and ventricles are presented in Figure 17.17. When the ventricular reentry is electrically induced during cardiac surgery (to decrease the myocardial energy requirement), and coronary blood flow is maintained by an external pump, slow-coarse ventricular flutter persists until it is electrically terminated at the completion of the surgical procedure. When ventricular flutter/fibrillation occurs spontaneously, it soon deteriorates toward the rapid-fine end of the spectrum, and electrical shock is less effective in its termination. This inverse relationship between the coarseness of the rhythm and the strength of the electrical current required for termination of ventricular flutter/fibrillation has clinical applicability. β-Adrenergic agents and calcium are commonly used when, during an episode of ventricular fibrillation-induced cardiac arrest, even the maximal output of the electrical defibrillator fails to terminate the reentry process.

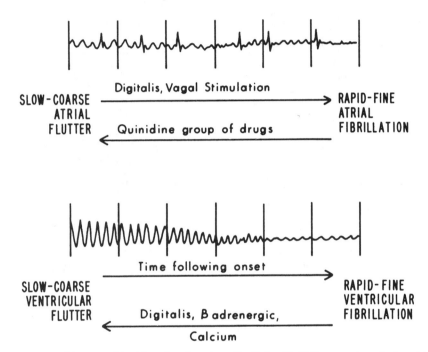

Figure 17.17. Movement in either direction along the flutter/fibrillation spectrum in the atria **(A)** and ventricles **(B)**. The *arrows* indicate the direction in which the various factors tend to affect the rate of the reentry process. (From Wagner GS, Waugh RA, Ramo BW. Cardiac arrhythmias. New York: Churchill Livingstone, 1983:23, with permission.)

A common error in ECG-based diagnosis is mistaking an external electrical artifact (e.g., from skeletal muscle tremor) for ventricular flutter, as illustrated in Figure 17.18. The patient whose ECG is shown in the figure mistakenly received emergency treatment for a ventricular arrhythmia, but close inspection of the rhythm strip reveals the higher frequency, normal QRS complexes superimposed on the artifactual waveforms.

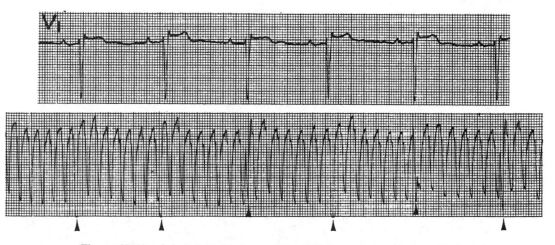

Figure 17.18. Lead V1 from a preoperative ECG is used as a reference for the MCL_1 monitoring lead immediately after cholecystectomy in a 72-year-old woman. The *arrows* indicate the regularly occurring higher-frequency waveforms representing the locations of the patient's normal QRS complexes.

Critical-care nurses have observed that patients with ventricular flutter may remain apparently stable for several seconds after the onset of this arrhythmia, particularly if they do not have a cardiac disease. A firm blow to the chest ("thump-version") may terminate ventricular flutter.[56] It is important to quickly scan the rhythm strip for continuing, regular QRS complexes (as in Figure 17.18) before initiating the emergency therapy.

Holter recordings that fortuitously capture the onset of "sudden death" have confirmed that the cause is usually ventricular fibrillation, as illustrated in Figure 17.19. The onset may be preceded by another reentrant ventricular tachyarrhythmia.[57,58] In patients undergoing continuous bedside monitoring during acute myocardial infarction, the arrhythmias observed just before the onset of ventricular fibrillation have been a single R-on-T VPB, sustained monomorphic VT, nonsustained monomorphic VT with a rate above 180 beats/min, or polymorphic VT.[59] The wide-QRS-complex tachyarrhythmia (in the top and middle strips of Fig. 17.19) could be either LVT or an SVT with RBB aberrancy. In the ECG shown in Figure 17.19, sinus rhythm resumes after termination of the VT; however, the ensuing lengthened cardiac cycle precipitates an R-on-T VPB. This in turn initiates ventricular flutter that rapidly degenerates into fibrillation in the bottom strip.

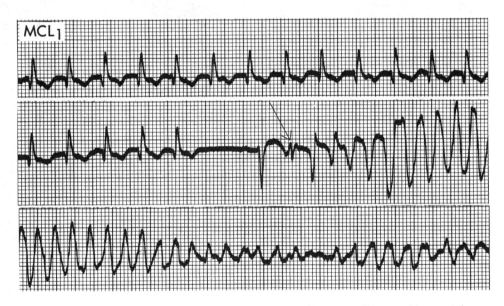

Figure 17.19. Continuous bedside recording of lead MCL$_1$ from a 67-year-old man at the onset of a cardiac arrest. An *arrow* indicates the early-occurring VPB that initiates the ventricular flutter that rapidly deteriorates into ventricular fibrillation.

GLOSSARY

Concordant precordial negative: a term describing abnormally wide QRS complexes that are predominately negative in all six of the precordial leads.

Concordant precordial positive: a term describing abnormally wide QRS complexes that are predominately positive in all six of the precordial leads.

Monomorphic: a single appearance of all QRS complexes.

Monomorphic VT: VT with a regular rate and consistent QRS-complex morphology.

Nonsustained VT: VT of less than 30 second duration.

Polymorphic VT: VT with a regular rate but frequent changes in QRS-complex morphology.

Sustained VT: VT of at least 30 second duration or requiring an intervention for its termination.

Torsades de pointes: a polymorphic ventricular tachyarrhythmia with the appearance of slow polymorphic ventricular flutter without discernible QRS

complexes or T waves. The ventricular activity has constantly changing amplitudes and seems to revolve around the isoelectric line.

Ventricular fibrillation: rapid and totally disorganized ventricular activity without discernible QRS complexes or T waves in the ECG.

Ventricular flutter: rapid organized ventricular activity without discernible QRS complexes or T waves in the ECG.

Ventricular flutter/fibrillation: the spectrum of ventricular tachyarrhythmias that lack discernible QRS complexes or T waves in the ECG; these tachyarrhythmias produce ECG effects that range from gross undulations to no discernible electrical activity.

Ventricular tachycardia: a rhythm originating distal to the branching of the common bundle, with a ventricular contraction rate of at least 100 beats/ min.

REFERENCES

1. Shenasa M, Borggrefe M, Haverkamp W, et al. Ventricular tachycardia. Lancet 1993;341:1512–1519.
2. Akhtar M, Gilbert C, Wolf FG, et al. Reentry within the His Purkinje system: elucidation of re-entrant circuit using right bundle-branch and His bundle recordings. Circulation 1976;58:295.
3. Ben-David J, Zipes DP. Torsades de pointes and proarrhythmia. Lancet 1993;341:1578–1582.
4. Toboul P. Torsade de pointes. In: Wellens HJJ, Kulbertus HE, eds. What's new in electrocardiography. Boston: Martinus Nijhoff, 1981:229.
5. Welch WJ. Sustained macroreentrant ventricular tachycardia. Am Heart J 1982;104:166 160.
6. Lesch M, Lewis E, Humphries JO, et al. Paroxysmal ventricular tachycardia in the absence of organic heart disease: report of a case and review of the literature. Ann Intern Med 1967;66:950–960.
7. Pedersen DH, Zipes DP, Foster PR, et al. Ventricular tachycardia and ventricular fibrillation in a young population. Circulation 1979;60:988–997.
8. Fulton DR, Chung KJ, Tabakin BS, et al. Ventricular tachycardia in children without heart disease. Am J Cardiol 1985;55:1328–1331.
9. Swartz MH, Teichholz LE, Donoso E. Mitral valve prolapse: a review of associated arrhythmias. Am J Med 1977;62:377–389.
10. Wei JY, Bulkley BH, Schaeffer AH, et al. Mitral-valve prolapse syndrome and recurrent ventricular tachyarrhythmias: a malignant variant refractory to conventional drug therapy. Ann Intern Med 1978;89:6–9.
11. Campbell TJ. Proarrhythmic actions of antiarrhythmic drugs: a review. Aust NZ J Med 1990;20:275–282.
12. The Cardiac Arrhythmia Suppression Trial (CAST) Investigators: Preliminary report: effect of encainide and flecainide on mortality in a randomized trial of arrhythmia suppression after myocardial infarction. N Engl J Med 1989;321:406–412.
13. Bolick DR, Hackel DB, Reimer KA, et al. Quantitative analysis of myocardial infarct structure in patients with ventricular tachycardia.Circulation 1986;74:1266–1279.
14. Tchou P, Young P, Mahmud R, et al. Useful clinical criteria for the diagnosis of ventricular tachycardia. Am J Med 1988;284:53–56.
15. Morady F, Baerman JM, DiCarlo LA Jr, et al. A prevalent misconception regarding wide-complex tachycardias. JAMA 1985;254:2790–2792.
16. Marriott HJ. Differential diagnosis of supraventricular and ventricular tachycardia. Geriatrics 1970;25:91–101.
17. Sandler IA, Marriott HJL. The differential morphology of anomalous ventricular complexes of RBBB-type in V1: ventricular ectopy versus aberration. Circulation 1965;31:551.
18. Swanick EJ, LaCamera F Jr, Marriott HJL. Morphologic features of right ventricular ectopic beats. Am J Cardiol 1972;30:888–891.
19. Wellens HJJ, Bar FW, Vanagt EJ, et al. Medical treatment of ventricular tachycardia, considerations in the selection of patients for surgical treatment. Am J Cardiol 1982;49:186–193.
20. Wellens HJJ, Bar FW, Lie KI. The value of the electrocardiogram in the differential diagnosis of a tachycardia with a widened QRS complex. Am J Med 1978; 64:27–33.
21. Switzer DF. Dire consequences of verapamil administration for wide QRS tachycardia. Circulation 1986;74 [Suppl II]:105.
22. Dancy M, Camm AJ, Ward D. Misdiagnosis of chronic recurrent ventricular tachycardia. Lancet 1985; 2:320–323.
23. Stewart RB, Bardy GH, Greene HL. Wide-complex tachycardia: misdiagnosis and outcome after emergent therapy. Ann Intern Med 1986;104:766–771.
24. Vera Z, Cheng TO, Ertem G, et al. His bundle electrography for evaluation of criteria in differentiating ventricular ectopy from aberrancy in atrial fibrillation. Circulation 1972;45[Suppl II]:355.

25. Gulamhusein S, Yee R, Ko PT, Klein GJ. Electrocardiographic criteria for differentiating aberrancy and ventricular extrasystole in chronic atrial fibrillation: validation by intracardiac recordings. J Electrocardiol 1985; 18:41–50.

26. Gozensky C, Thorne D. Rabbit ears: an aid in distinguishing ventricular ectopy from aberration. Heart Lung 1974;3:634–636.

27. Brugada P, Brugada J, Mont L, et al. A new approach to the differential diagnosis of a regular tachycardia with a wide QRS complex. Circulation 1991;83:1649–1659.

28. Rosenbaum MB. Classification of ventricular extrasystoles according to form. J Electrocardiol 1969; 2:289–297.

29. Wellens HJJ. The wide QRS tachycardias. Ann Intern Med 1986;104:879.

30. Kindwall E, Brown JP, Josephson ME. ECG criteria for ventricular and supraventricular tachycardia in wide complex tachycardias with left bundle branch morphology. J Am Coll Cardiol 1987;9:206A.

31. Drew BJ, Scheinman MM. Value of electrocardiographic leads MCL$_1$, MCL$_6$, and other selected leads in the diagnosis of wide QRS complex tachycardia. J Am Coll Cardiol 1991;18:1025–1033.

32. Waxman HL, Josephson ME. Ventricular activation during ventricular endocardial pacing. I. Electrocardiographic patterns related to the site of pacing. Am J Cardiol 1982;50:1–10.

33. Josephson ME, Horowitz LN, Waxman HL, et al. Sustained ventricular tachycardia: role of the 12-lead electrocardiogram in localizing site of origin. Circulation 1981;64:257–272.

34. Josephson ME, et al. Relation between site of origin and QRS configuration in ventricular rhythms. In: Wellens HJJ, Kulbertus HE, eds.What's new in electrocardiography. Boston: Martinus Nijhoff, 1981:200.

35. Buxton AE, Marchlinski FE, Doherty JU, et al. Repetitive, monomorphic ventricular tachycardia: clinical and electrophysiologic characteristics in patients with and patients without organic heart disease. Am J Cardiol 1984;54:997–1002.

36. Vandepol CJ, Farshidi A, Spielman SR, et al. Incidence and clinical significance of induced ventricular tachycardia. Am J Cardiol 1980;45:725–731.

37. Josephson ME, Horowitz LN, Farshidi A, et al. Recurrent sustained ventricular tachycardia. I. Mechanisms. Circulation 1978;57:431–440.

38. Denes P, Wu D, Dhingra RC, Amat-y-leon R, et al. Electrophysiological studies in patients with chronic recurrent ventricular tachycardia. Circulation 1976; 54:229–236.

39. Pietras RJ, Mautner R, Denes P, et al. Chronic recurrent right and left ventricular tachycardia: comparison of clinical, hemodynamic and angiographic findings. Am J Cardiol 1977;40:32–37.

40. Vetter VL, Josephson ME, Horowitz LN. Idiopathic recurrent sustained ventricular tachycardia in children and adolescents. Am J Cardiol 1981;47:315–322.

41. Wu D, Kou HC, Hung JS. Exercise-triggered paroxysmal ventricular tachycardia: a repetitive rhythmic activity possibly related to afterdepolarization. Ann Intern Med 1981;95:410–414.

42. Mokotoff DM. Exercise-induced ventricular tachycardia: clinical features, relation to chronic ventricular ectopy, and prognosis. Chest 1980;77:10–16.

43. Kossmann CE. Torsade de pointes: an addition to the nosography of ventricular tachycardia. Am J Cardiol 1978;42:1054–1056.

44. Smith WM, Gallagher JJ. "Les torsades de pointes": an unusual ventricular arrhythmia. Ann Intern Med 1980; 93:578–584.

45. Strasberg B, Sclarovsky S, Erdberg A, et al. Procainamide-induced polymorphous ventricular tachycardia. Am J Cardiol 1981;47:1309–1314.

46. Kay GN, Plumb VJ, Arcciniegas JG, et al. Torsade de pointes: the long-short initiating sequence and other clinical features: observations in 32 patients. J Am Coll Cardiol 1983;2:806–817.

47. Soffer J, Dreifus LS, Michelson EL. Polymorphous ventricular tachycardia associated with normal and long Q-T intervals. Am J Cardiol 1982;49:2021–2029.

48. Reynolds EW, Vandeer Ark CR. Quinidine syncope and the delayed repolarization syndromes. Mod Concepts Cardiovasc Dis 1976;45:117–122.

49. Roden DM, Thompson KA, Hoffman BF, et al. Clinical features and the basic mechanisms of quinidine-induced arrhythmias. J Am Coll Cardiol 1986;8:73A–78A.

50. Nicholson WJ, Martin CE, Gracey JG, et al. Disopyramide-induced ventricular fibrillation. Am J Cardiol 1979;43:1053–1055.

51. Wald RW, Waxman MB, Colman JM. Torsades de pointes ventricular tachycardia: a complication of disopyramide shared with quinidine. J Electrocardiol 1981;14:301–307.

52. Ludomirsky A, Klein HO, Sarelli P, et al. Q-T prolongation and polymorphous ("torsades de pointes") ventricular arrhythmias associated with organic insecticide poisoning. Am J Cardiol 1982;49:1654–1658.

53. Carruth JE, Silverman ME. Torsades de pointes: atypical ventricular tachycardia complicating subarachnoid hemorrhage. Chest 1980;78:886–888.

54. Jervell A, Lange-Nielsen F. Congenital deaf-mutism, functional heart disease with prolongation of the Q-T interval and sudden death. Am Heart J 1957;54:59.

55. Krikler DM, Curry PVL. Torsades de pointes, an atypical ventricular tachycardia. Br Heart J 1976;38:117–120.

56. Lown B, Taylor J. Thump-version. N Engl J Med 1978;283:1223–1224.

57. Kempf FC, Josephson ME. Cardiac arrest recorded on ambulatory electrocardiograms. Am J Cardiol 1984; 53:1577–1582.

58. Panadis IP, Morganroth J. Sudden death in hospitalized patients: cardiac rhythm disturbances detected by ambulatory electrocardiographic monitoring. J Am Coll Cardiol 1983;2:798–805.

59. Bluzhas J, Lukshiene D, Shlapikiene B, et al. Relation between ventricular arrhythmia and sudden cardiac death in patients with acute myocardial infarction: the predictors of ventricular fibrillation. J Am Coll Cardiol 1986;8[Suppl IA]:69A–72A.

CHAPTER 18

Ventricular Versus Supraventricular With Aberrant Conduction

Having considered all of the commonly occurring tachyarrhythmias, it may help to consider in depth the differential diagnosis of tachyarrhythmias of ventricular origin and tachyarrhythmias of supraventricular origin with aberrant ventricular conduction. The term ventricular *ectopy* is useful for indicating a ventricular origin for a given tachyarrhythmia, since such arrhythmias range from a single wide premature beats (PB) to sustained wide-QRS-complex tachyarrhythmias. The diagnostic differentiation of ventricular ectopy from aberrant conduction must be made whenever the QRS complex is "wide" (duration ≥120 ms), since aberrancy does not always result in a QRS complex sufficiently wide as to "mimic" an arrhythmia of ventricular origin. Indeed, aberrancy often produces only minor distortion of the normal QRS complex, with little or no prolongation (<120 ms).

In its general consideration, "aberrant" ventricular conduction occurs either intermittently or persistently in individuals with abnormalities of intraventricular conduction (Chapter 5, "Intraventricular Conduction Abnormalities"). Ventricular preexcitation (Chapter 6, "Ventricular Preexcitation") is also technically an aberrancy, but is not considered again in this chapter. Aberrancy, as specifically considered with regard to cardiac arrhythmias, occurs in the absence of these abnormal conditions when a supraventricular impulse encounters persistent refractoriness in a part of the ventricular conduction system, usually because of a change in length of the cardiac cycle. The importance of aberrancy rests on two facts:

1. It is common. As Lewis said in 1925, "aberration is known to be frequent in paroxysmal tachycardia."
2. It is often overlooked, with the result that supraventricular arrhythmias are misdiagnosed as ventricular arrhythmias and are treated as such.

Aberration is not a rare curiosity that can be left to the experts in arrhythmias. Almost all physicians are occasionally required to diagnose and treat cardiac arrhythmias, and should therefore have the ability to differentiate between supraventricular and ventricular sites of origin in cases of arrhythmia.

CIRCUMSTANCES PRODUCING ABERRANCY

When any responsive tissue reacts to a stimulus, the reaction is followed by a dormant interval (the refractory period) during which the tissue cannot respond to a similar stimulus. This period of rest is necessary for the tissue to recoup and return to a state in which it can again react normally to the stimulus. Any such period has a finite, measurable duration, and if the tissue is asked to respond during its refractory period, the response will be absent or at least subnormal. Characteristics of the refractory period differ for different portions of the interventricular conduction system. The His-Purkinje system usually exhibits an "all-or-none" response, in contrast to the atrioventricular (AV) node, which exhibits a graded response.

The refractory period of the cardiac conducting pathways is proportional to the length of the preceding cycle (RR interval). Thus, the longer the cycle and slower the rate, the longer the ensuing refractory period, and vice versa. Ventricular aberration can therefore result from a shortened immediate cycle, an extended preceding cycle, or a combination of both (Fig. 18.1). In the case of two regular cycles with normal conduction, as shown in Figure 18.1, the conduction in the third *beat* (beat 3) is also normal. However, the conduction in the third beat may become aberrant (lower two diagrams) if either the second cycle is shortened (Fig. 18.1*B*) or the first cycle is lengthened (Fig. 18.1*C*). Shortening of the cycle (Fig. 18.1*B*) may bring that beat within the refractory period of part of the conducting system. Lengthening of the preceding cycle (Fig. 18.1*C*) will prolong the refractory period so that the next beat, although occurring no earlier than than in the previous cycle, falls within the now longer refractory period.

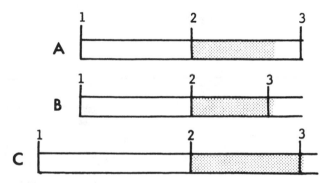

Figure 18.1. In the diagrams, *1*, *2*, and *3* are consecutive beats and the *stippled area* represents the refractory period of some part of the conducting system during the second cycle.

Figure 18.2 illustrates right bundle-branch block (RBBB) aberration of atrial premature beats (APBs). The early impulses have taken the right bundle branch (RBB) "by surprise" (while it is still refractory), and it has been unable to respond and conduct these impulses. The atrial extrasystole arises after three normally conducted beats, and its impulse arrives at the RBB while the latter is still refractory. The extrasystole is therefore conducted with RBBB aberration. In Figure 18.2, the seventh beat is also an extra systole, but it is less premature and is therefore conducted normally.

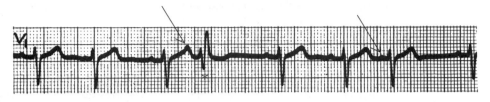

Figure 18.2. A lead-V1 rhythm strip from a 73-year-old woman following gall bladder surgery. *Arrows* indicate the premature P waves initiating the fourth and the seventh cycles, and an *asterisk* indicates the RBB aberrancy during the fourth cycle.

RBBB aberration is much more common (about 80% of all aberration) than is left bundle-branch block (LBBB) aberration.[1,2] In an individual with cardiac disease, however, LBBB aberration constitutes a greater proportion (about 33%) of the aberrant conduction encountered. In a study by Kulbertus and colleagues,[3] in which these investigators were able to produce 116 different aberrant configurations by inducing atrial premature beats in 44 patients, RBBB accounted for only 53% of the experimentally produced aberrancies—a smaller than expected proportion (Table 18.1).

Table 18.1. Patterns of Induced Aberration and Their Incidences

RBBB alone	28	i.e.
RBBB + LAFB	21	RBBB = 53%
RBBB + LPFB	12	LAFB = 32%
LAFB alone	17	LPFB = 19%
LPFB alone	10	LBBB = 15%
LBBB	10	Unclassified = 10%
ILBBB	6	
Unclassified	12	
	———	
	116	

LAFB, left anterior superior fascicular block; LPFB, left posterior inferior fascicular block; ILBBB, incomplete left bundle branch block.

CHARACTERISTICS OF ABERRANCY

Aberrant conduction is a secondary phenomenon, always the result of some primary disturbance, and never requires treatment. At times, the morphology of the aberrant QRS complex is indistinguishable from the pattern in an occurence of ventricular ectopy. At other times, however, the aberrant shapes of the QRS complexes provide broad hints of their having a supraventricular origin.

The first principle in the diagnosis of aberrancy is not to diagnose it unless there is evidence favoring it, since wide QRS complexes are more often produced by beats originating in the ventricular than in the supraventricular regions. An axiom that often proves useful in medical diagnosis is "When you hear hoof beats, think first of a horse rather than a zebra—only consider a zebra if you see its stripes." The six key characteristics of aberration (its "stripes") are presented in Table 18.2.

Table 18.2. The "Stripes" of Aberration

1. Triphasic morphology
   a. rsR' variant in V1
   b. qRs variant in V_6
2. Initial deflection identical to normal beat (if RBBB)
3. Immediately preceding atrial activity
4. Second-in-the-row phenomenon
5. Alternating BBB patterns separated by single normal beat
6. Identical wide QRS pattern previously diagnosed as aberrancy

The first four "stripes" are observable in Figure 18.3, in which the two continuous rhythm strips contain three clusters of rapid beats. Each cluster is initiated by a premature ectopic P wave (Stripe 3). The second beat alone presents a bizarre appearance (Stripe 4). It has a triphasic (rsR') RBBB pattern (Stripe 1), with the initial deflection identical to that of the conducted sinus beats (Stripe 2). These points clinch the recognition of aberration.

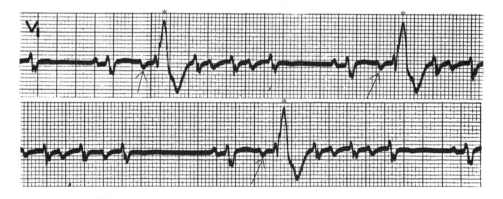

Figure 18.3. A continuous lead-V1 rhythm strip from a 54-year-old man with severe chronic obstructive pulmonary disease. *Arrows* indicate the three premature P waves and *asterisks* indicate the aberrantly conducted premature QRS complexes.

Triphasic Lead-V1/V6 Morphology of the QRS Complex

The shape of the QRS complex is in many cases diagnostic of aberrancy. Triphasic contours (rsR′ in lead V1 and qRs in lead V6) heavily favor the diagnosis of aberration. Figure 18.4 illustrates an atrial tachyarrhythmia with RBBB aberration. The rsR′ pattern in lead V1 and the qRs pattern in lead V6 would each alone be virtually diagnostic of the supraventricular origin of this arrhythmia. Note that the sinus rhythm following termination of the tachyarrhythmia is rapid and irregular, as is typical with severe pulmonary disease (Chapter 14, "Accelerated Automaticity").

Despite the availability of morphologic clues introduced during the past 30 years[2,4,5] and confirmed more recently,[6–9] many authors persist in ignoring them,[10–12] instead continuing to give predominant and undue weight to the presence or absence of independent atrial activity. When independent atrial activity (AV dissociation) is evident, it is a most valuable clue to the diagnosis of ventricular tachycardia (VT). The presence of AV dissociation cannot, however, be relied upon, for three reasons:

1. AV dissociation is present in only a minority of ventricular tachycardias. In one carefully studied series, it was found in only 27 of 100.[13]
2. Even when AV dissociation is present, the independent P waves may be difficult or impossible to recognize in the clinical tracing.
3. Rarely, junctional tachyarrhythmias with bundle-branch block may be dissociated from an independent sinus rhythm (Fig. 17.4).

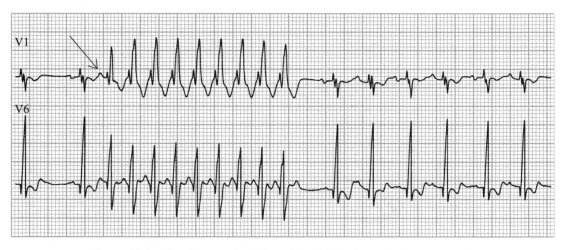

Figure 18.4. Simultaneous lead-V1 and lead-V6 rhythm strips from a 61-year-old woman with severe pulmonary emphysema. An *arrow* indicates the premature P wave.

Initial Deflection of the Abnormal Beat is Identical to Normal Beat

There is no reason for a ventricular impulse to produce an initial deflection identical to that of a normally conducted supraventricular impulse. Conversely, since normal ventricular activation begins on the left side, RBBB does not interfere with initial activation unless there is also block in one fascicle of the left bundle. As a result, if a wide QRS complex has a pattern compatible with RBBB and begins with a deflection identical to that of conducted beats, aberration is probably the diagnosis.

Atrial Activity Immediately Preceding the Abnormal Ventricular Beat

Sometimes, the diagnosis of aberration depends upon the recognition of P waves preceding the abnormal QRS complex. Figure 18.5 illustrates several paroxysms of wide QRS complexes. A careful inspection reveals, however, that each group of three abnormal ventricular beats is preceded by a premature P wave, thereby confirming the diagnosis of aberrant conduction. The wide QRS complexes should be considered triphasic because there is a downward deflection between the r and R′ waves that only sometimes penetrates below the baseline to form an s wave. Note that ventricular conduction becomes aberrant when a short, normal sinus cycle follows a long cycle that is subsequent to an APB, and returns to normal only when a long cycle after an APB follows a short cycle preceding the APB. This example also illustrates the value of recording at least two simultaneous ECG leads, since the P waves in some cycles are visible only in lead V6, where there is minimal evidence of the aberrantly conducted QRS complexes.

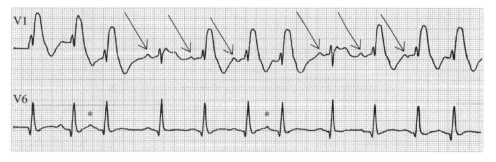

Figure 18.5. Simultaneous lead-V1 and lead-V6 rhythm strips from a 64-year-old woman with chronic angina who presented with severe chest pain. *Arrows* in lead-V1 recording indicate sinus P waves preceding the normally and aberrantly conducted QRS complexes, and *asterisks* in lead V6 indicate premature P waves preceding the final (the third in the group of three) aberrantly conducted beats.

Aberrant Beats Occurring Exclusively as the Second-in-a-Row of Beats

The reason that only the second in a row of beats tends to be aberrant is that it is the only beat that ends a relatively short cycle preceded by a relatively long one (Fig. 18.1). Since the refractory period of the conduction system is proportional to the length of the preceding ventricular cycle, the sequence of a long cycle (lengthening the subsequent refractory period) followed by a short cycle provides conditions for the development of aberration.

Alternating Patterns of Bundle-Branch Block Separated by a Single Normal Beat

When a pattern that could represent either LBBB or RBBB is separated by a single normally conducted beat from a pattern that could represent the other type of bundle-branch block, it should be strongly presumed that there is bilateral aberration rather than ectopy from alternate ventricles. (See text and Figure 18.14 on page 387.)

Identical Wide QRS-Complex Pattern Previously Diagnosed as Aberrancy

If one is lucky enough to have available a previous recording that shows the same wide QRS pattern associated with sufficient "stripes" for the diagnosis of aberrancy, one can then diagnose the arrhythmia in question as a supraventricular tachyarrhythmia (SVT) with aberrancy. Figure 18.6A shows a tachyarrhythmia that, although the

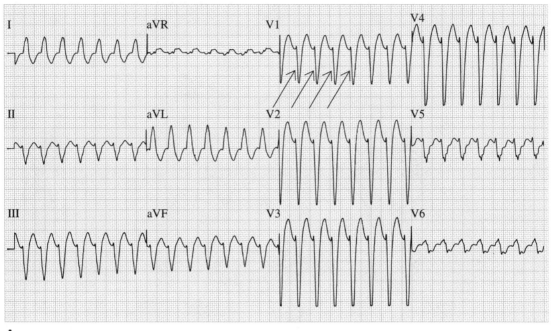

A

Figure 18.6.   Twelve-lead ECGs from a 63-year-old man in the postoperative recovery room after coronary artery bypass surgery. *Arrows* indicate the identical QRS-complex appearances in the short-axis view in lead V1 during tachycardia **(A)** and preoperative normal sinus rhythm **(B)**.

clean downstroke in lead V1 favors left bundle-branch (LBB) aberrancy, could also represent right-ventricular tachycardia (RVT). Figure 18.6*B* is a recording from the same patient taken 1 year earlier. Since this clearly shows sinus rhythm with LBBB, and the QRS complexes of the two recordings are identical, the current tachyarrhythmia can be considered an SVT with LBB aberrancy, most likely atrial flutter with 2:1 AV block.

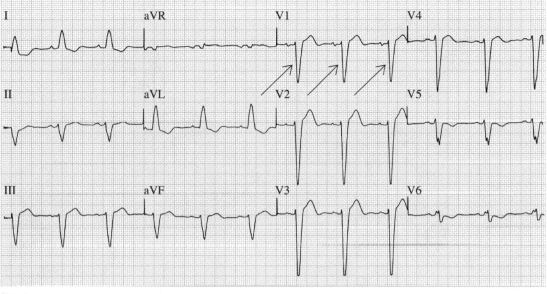

B

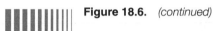

Figure 18.6. *(continued)*

VENTRICULAR ABERRATION COMPLICATING ATRIAL FLUTTER/FIBRILLATION

Ventricular aberration often complicates the atrial macroreentrant tachyarrhythmia of atrial flutter/fibrillation (Chapter 15, "Reentrant Atrial Tachyarrhythmias—The Atrial Flutter/Fibrillation Spectrum"). Interruption of normal intraventricular conduction by wide QRS beats during atrial flutter/fibrillation is more likely to be due to aberration than to a coincidental ventricular premature beat (VPB) or (if there is a series of wide complexes) to VT. Since in the presence of atrial flutter/fibrillation there is no preceding discrete atrial activity to indicate aberrant conduction, one has to rely more heavily on the morphology of the wide QRS complexes to differentiate aberration from ventricular origin. Accordingly, the rsR′ pattern in lead V1 or MCL$_1$ (Fig. 18.7), or the qRs pattern in lead V6, assists in establishing the diagnosis of aberrant conduction. Figure 18.7 provides contrast between an aberrantly conducted beat (the first wide QRS complex) and a VPB (the second wide QRS complex). Note that a long cycle following a short cycle sets the stage for aberrancy.

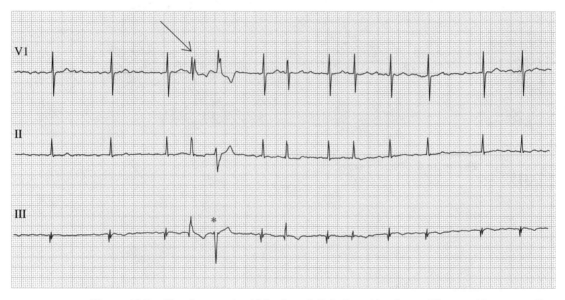

Figure 18.7. Simultaneous lead-V1, -II, and -III rhythm strips from a 75-year-old woman with a recent inferior-wall myocardial infarction. An *arrow* indicates the triphasic RsR′ in lead V1 for the first wide QRS complex, and an *asterisk* indicates the oppositely directed initial deflection in lead III for the second wide QRS complex.

Gouaux and Ashman[1] first drew attention to the fact that aberrant conduction was likely to complicate atrial flutter/fibrillation when a longer cycle was followed by a shorter cycle (Fig. 18.8). Aberration produced by a long–short sequence is sometimes referred to as the Ashman phenomenon. It is important to keep in mind that this cycle sequence cannot be used to differentiate aberration from ectopy because, by the *rule of bigeminy*, a lengthened cycle also tends to precipitate a ventricular extrasystole. Therefore, a long–short cycle sequence ending with a wide QRS complex is as likely to represent a VPB as an aberrant beat. Once again, morphologic clues become important in distinguishing these phenomena. Note that in sinus rhythm, a premature P wave is confirmed only by reference to the normal, biphasic T wave during the first cycle, and that aberrancy occurs only when a long cycle has preceded the short cycle induced by an APB. The fifth premature P wave initiates the atrial flutter/fibrillation.

Several other, minor clues help to differentiate aberration from ventricular ectopy in the presence of atrial flutter/fibrillation.[4] These are discussed in the following sections.

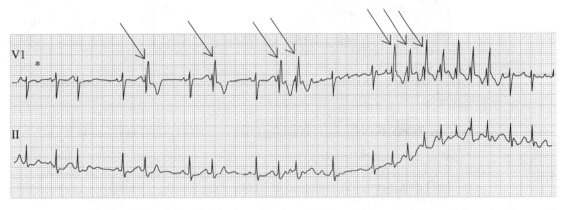

Figure 18.8. A lead-V1 rhythm strip from a 77-year-old woman with a history of paroxysmal atrial fibrillation. An *asterisk* indicates the normal T wave that allows identification of the subsequent premature P waves. *Arrows* indicate similar triphasic QRS-complex morphology (rsR′) for the APBs during sinus rhythm and for the wide beats during atrial flutter/fibrillation.

The Presence of a Longer Returning Cycle

Ventricular ectopy tends to be followed by a longer returning cycle. This is because many ectopic ventricular impulses are conducted backward, into the AV node. If this happens, the AV node is left partly refractory by the retrograde invasion, so that the next several atrial impulses are cannot penetrate it and reach their ventricular destination.

The Absence of a Longer Preceding Cycle

As indicated previously, a long preceding cycle favors both aberration and ectopy, and cannot be used as a point for differentiating the two. On the other hand, the absence of a longer preceding cycle is evidence against aberration, and therefore favors ventricular ectopy (Fig. 18.9).

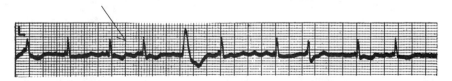

Figure 18.9. A lead-II rhythm strip from an 87-year-old man with chronic atrial flutter/fibrillation who was being evaluated for elective abdominal surgery. An *arrow* indicates the shorter rather than longer preceding cycle.

Comparative Cycle Sequences

If a wide QRS complex ends a longer-shorter cycle sequence, we have seen that differentiation between aberration and ectopy may be difficult. If an even longer cycle followed by an even shorter cycle ends with a normally conducted beat, the evidence against aberration is strong, and the diagnosis of ectopy is favored (Fig. 18.10).

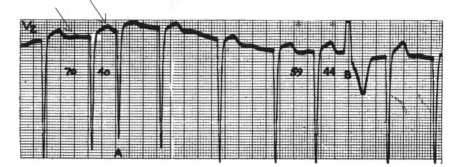

Figure 18.10. A lead-V2 rhythm strip from a 64-year-old man with severe mitral regurgitation. *Arrows* indicate the even longer and even shorter preceding cycles for another normally conducted beat than for the wide beat (*asterisks*).

Undue Prematurity

When so much AV block is present that all conducted cycles are long, the appearance of a wide QRS complex ending a cycle far shorter than any of the normally conducted beats favors the diagnosis of ectopy (Fig. 18.11). It would be very unusual for a poorly conducting AV node to suddenly permit extremely early conduction to the ventricular Purkinje system. Note that the atrial flutter/fibrillation in the example shown in Figure 18.11 is so "fine" that even in lead V1, no atrial activity is visible.

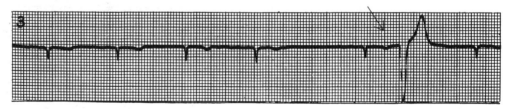

Figure 18.11. A lead-V1 rhythm strip from a 72-year-old woman with a recent anterior infarction. An *arrow* indicates the immediately preceding cycle, which is remarkably short in comparison with all others.

Fixed or Constant Coupling

Fixed or constant coupling as a clue to the distinction of aberration from ventricular ectopy is obviously applicable only if several wide QRS beats are available for comparison. If the interval between the normally conducted beat and the ensuing wide QRS beat is constant to within a few hundredths of a second, ventricular ectopy is favored (Fig. 18.12). In the example, a "coarser" atrial flutter–fibrillation is present, and the absence of conduction with aberrancy is confirmed by variation of the intervals between the onsets of the wide QRS complexes and immediately preceding f waves.

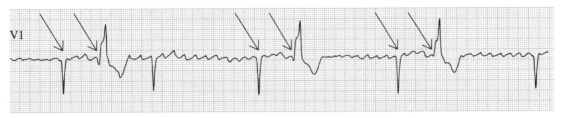

Figure 18.12. A lead-V1 rhythm strip from an 81-year-old man with a recent anterior infarction. *Arrows* indicate the fixed intervals coupling all wide beats with their immediately preceding normally conducted beats.

From a therapeutic viewpoint, an extremely important form of aberration may complicate the flutter end of the atrial flutter/fibrillation spectrum. When uncomplicated and untreated, atrial flutter usually manifests an AV conduction ratio of 2:1. If digitalis, propranolol, or verapamil is then administered, the conduction pattern often changes to alternating 2:1 and 4:1, producing alternately longer and shorter cycles. At this stage, the beats that end the shorter cycles may develop aberrant conduction (Fig. 18.13A), producing the fixed coupling typical of a bigeminal rhythm. If the patient is receiving digitalis, the fixed coupling is likely to evoke a diagnosis of ventricular ectopy and be attributed to digitalis toxicity. The still-needed digitalis is then wrongfully discontinued, when in fact the situation calls for more AV-nodal blockade to further reduce conduction to a constant 4:1 with a normal ventricular rate, which is the appropriate goal of therapy. Figure 18.13B presents an example of fixed coupling occurring when slowing of the flutter rate (180 beats/min) facilitates AV-nodal conduction (3:2). In contrast with Figure 18.12, note the constant interval between the onsets of the wide QRS complexes and immediately preceding flutter waves in both Figure 18.13A and B.

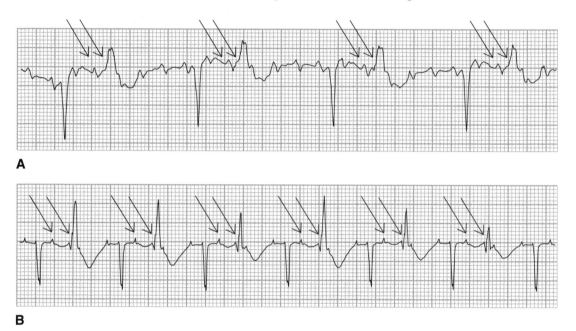

Figure 18.13. Lead-V1 rhythm strips from two patients receiving pharmacologic therapy for atrial flutter complicating chronic heart failure. **A:** Digitalis has been administered to slow the ventricular rate. **B:** Quinidine has been added to the maintenance digitalis to attempt conversion to sinus rhythm. *Arrows* indicate the fixed "F-wave-to-wide-QRS" intervals in both **A** and **B**.

There is a common tendency for an aberrancy of ventricular conduction to be bilateral (Fig. 18.14). There may even be an abrupt switch from one form of aberration to the other (from RBBB to LBBB or vice versa) via a single, intervening, normally conducted beat. Although unexplained, this phenomenon is sufficiently characteristic to assist in differentiating bilateral aberrancy from bifocal ventricular ectopy. In Figure 18.14, the initiating premature P waves before each single wide QRS complex or series of wide QRS complexes assures the supraventricular origin of the ectopy.

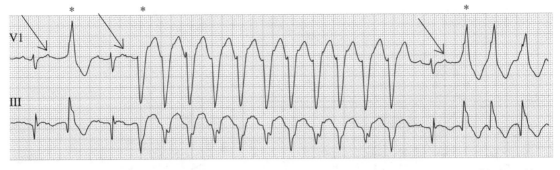

Figure 18.14. Simultaneous lead-V1 and lead-III rhythm strips from a 56-year-old man with an acute inferior-wall myocardial infarction. *Arrows* indicate the premature P waves and *asterisks* indicate first the RBB, then the LBB, and then again the RBB aberrancy.

CRITICAL RATE

Most of the examples of aberration presented in the preceding sections occur because an impulse of supraventricular origin traverses the AV node early, suddenly creating a short ventricular cycle. However, aberration also may appear with the gradual acceleration of sinus rhythm. Figure 18.15 presents two examples of slight sinus acceleration in which the cardiac cycle gradually shortens until it becomes shorter than the refractory period of one of the bundle branches, whereupon aberrant conduction develops. The wide QRS complexes will persist until the cycle lengthens sufficiently for normal conduction to occur. The rate at which the bundle-branch block develops is known as the *critical rate*, and when such block comes and goes with changes in the heart rate, the condition is known as *rate-dependent bundle-branch block* (in this instance, *tachycardia-dependent bundle-branch block*). The tachycardia may be either true (>100 beats/min) or relative (faster than the preexisting rate).

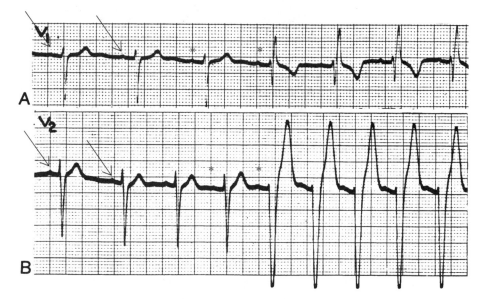

Figure 18.15. Lead-V1 rhythm strips from a 19-year-old woman with palpitations during hospitalization for mononucleosis **(A)** and a 64-year-old man with unstable coronary symptoms **(B)**. *Arrows* indicate the baseline atrial rate during normal condition, and *asterisks* indicate the accelerated rate that produces the RBB **(A)** and LBB **(B)** aberration.

One of the interesting features of tachycardia-dependent bundle-branch block is that the critical rate at which the block develops is faster than the rate at which the block disappears. In Figure 18.16, as the sinus rhythm accelerates, normal conduction prevails at a cycle length of 100 msec (rate of 60 beats/min), and the cycle at which the bundle-branch block develops is 91 msec in duration (rate of 66 beats/min). However, as the rate slows, the bundle-branch block persists at a cycle of 100 msec (rate of 60 beats/min), and for normal conduction to resume, the cycle must lengthen further to 108 in sec (rate of 56 beats/min).

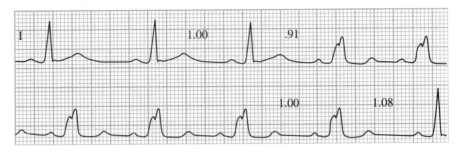

Figure 18.16. A continuous lead-I rhythm strip from an 82-year-old woman with chronic hypertension and cardiac failure. Numbers indicate the intervals between both normally and abnormally conducted beats (1.00 sec), preceding the onset of LBB aberrancy (0.91 sec), and preceding the return to normal conduction (1.08 sec).

There are two reasons for this difference in rate requirement for the development of bundle-branch block during acceleration and deceleration, as follows:

1. Since the refractory period of the ventricular conduction system is proportional to the length of the preceding ventricular cycle, it follows that as the ventricular rate accelerates, the refractory periods become progressively shorter (i.e., the potential for conduction progressively improves, and there is therefore a tendency to preserve normal conduction). The converse is true as the ventricular rate slows: refractory periods get longer, and the potential for conduction diminishes, making aberration more likely.

2. More important, however, is the factor that is diagrammed in Figure 18.17. The shaded area in the RBB indicates the refractory segment that fails to conduct when the impulse first arrives, causing RBBB aberration. An instant later, the refractory segment in the RBB has recovered and is receptive for conduction of the impulse, which has meanwhile negotiated the LBB. For the impulse to travel down the LBB and through the interventricular septum to the distal RBB requires about 0.06 second. Thus, the previously refractory RBB is depolarized about 0.06 second after the beginning of the QRS complex. Thus, as far as the RBB is concerned, its cycle begins about 0.06 second after the beginning of the RBBB QRS complex. The conventional measurement of cycle length from the beginning of the final normal QRS complex to the beginning of ensuing wide QRS complex does not provide an indication of the the time required for RBB recovery, since the cycle of the RBB did not begin until halfway through the wide QRS complex. It follows that for normal conduction to resume, the critical cycle during deceleration must be longer than the critical cycle during acceleration by about 0.06 second. This calculation fits nicely with the observed findings in Figure 18.16.

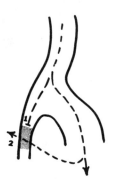

Figure 18.17. Diagram of the two mechanisms responsible for the difference in the critical rate during acceleration and deceleration. *1* indicates the inability of the supraventricular impulse to initially penetrate the RBB, and *2* indicates subsequent penetration of the RBB via the transseptal "detour."

Paradoxical Critical Rate

Abnormal intraventricular conduction sometimes occurs only at the end of a lengthened ventricular cycle. Since one would expect conduction to be better after an extremely long ventricular cycle (because there is ample time for even the prolonged refractory period to be completed), the occurrence of this type of aberration seems paradoxical. It is referred to as *bradycardia-dependent bundle-branch block*, and the bradycardia can be either true (<60 beats/min) or relative (slower than the preexisting rate). The rate at which the bundle-branch block develops is known as the *paradoxical critical rate*. In Figure 18.18, normal conduction is present at a rate of 82 beats/min, and the bundle-branch block develops only if the cycle length increases to a point equaling a rate of 68 beats/min. The sinus rhythm is repeatedly interrupted by atrial extrasystoles. All of the conducted beats ending the lengthened cycles following extrasystolic beats show RBBB, whereas the shorter sinus cycles and the even shorter extrasystolic cycles show more normal intraventricular conduction. As with tachycardia-dependent bundle-branch block, the rate at which bradycardia-dependent bundle-branch block develops is known as the critical rate.

The cause of bradycardia-dependent bundle-branch block is the spontaneous depolarization of pacemaking cells in the bundle branches in an attempt to terminate the prolonged delay in the ventricular cycle. However, a supraventricular impulse arrives before these ventricular Purkinje cells achieve the threshold required for pacemaking or "capturing" the ventricular rhythm. The supraventricular impulse is conducted slowly through these bundle-branch cells because they are no longer in their fully repolarized state. The impulse is therefore conducted more rapidly through the uninvolved bundle branch, creating aberrancy.[17,18]

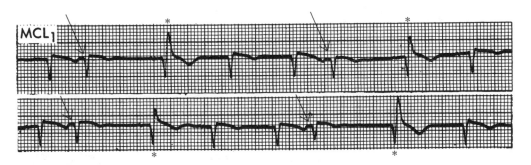

Figure 18.18. Lead-V1 rhythm strip from an 83-year-old woman with acute anterior infarction. *Arrows* indicate the normally conducted APBs and *asterisks* indicate the RBB aberration following the pauses.

MARRIOTT'S GENERAL APPROACH TO THE DIAGNOSIS OF REGULAR WIDE-QRS-COMPLEX TACHYARRHYTHMIAS

In previous editions of this text, Dr. Marriott provided an approach to diagnosis in cases marked by a regular, wide-QRS-complex tachyarrhythmia.

In attempting to distinguish SVT with aberrancy from VT, QRS-complex morphology should receive primary attention. The observation of characteristic features serves the purposes of both accuracy and speed, but if morphologic clues are absent or equivocal, one must look elsewhere.

Although the demonstration of AV dissociation is of considerable diagnostic value, and evidence of it should always be sought, it must not be a point of diagnostic dependence. If P waves are not recognizable even in lead V1, more specialized leads may be informative (Chapter 2, "Recording the Electrocardiogram"). A precordial lead known as S5 may be tried.[19] For this lead, the positive electrode is placed in the fifth right intercostal space, close to the sternal border, and the negative electrode is placed over the manubrium. If this fails, an esophageal[16,20] or intracardiac[21] lead will almost always be successful in displaying P waves. Alternatively, the administration of adenosine intravenously will affect the AV node selectively to reveal the P waves of any atrial tachycardia, or will suddenly terminate a reentrant AV-junctional tachycardia (RJT).[22–23]

With the following principles in mind, we can formulate a systematic approach to identifying the source of a regular tachycardia:

1. First, look at the patient's neck veins and listen to the first heart sound with the patient holding his or her breath. Irregular cannon waves in the neck, and/or variation in the beat-to-beat intensity of the first heart sound, constitutes hemodynamic evidence of dissociation and suggests a ventricular tachycardia. A first heart sound of unvarying intensity and either no cannon waves or regular cannon waves in the neck is evidence against dissociation, and the tachycardia is probably supraventricular (exceptions include VT with retrograde 1:1 conduction and VT with concurrent atrial fibrillation). If an electrocardiograph is available, do not use carotid sinus or other vagal stimulation until after a tracing has been taken, since the vagal maneuver may terminate a tachycardia of supraventricular origin, leaving no graphic record to document the paroxysm.

2. Record a 12-lead ECG and look at the pattern of the QRS complex. If the QRS complex is normal in contour and duration, the tachycardia is supraventricular. If it is widened and bizarre, the tachycardia may be either ventricular or supraventricular with aberrant ventricular conduction. If the QRS complex is widened, study its morphology in leads V1/V6, observe the frontal-plane axis, and look for the other morphologic clues to a supraventricular or ventricular origin of the tachycardia. Try to find a lead in which P waves are identifiable, and look for fusion beats. If previous tracings are available, look for isolated extrasystoles and compare their pattern with that of the tachycardia.

3. If the diagnosis is still in doubt, try carotid sinus massage or other vagal stimulation. If the tachycardia is supraventricular, this may terminate it. In atrial flutter, vagal stimulation may temporarily halve the rate by increasing the AV conduction ratio from 2:1 to 4:1. If the tachycardia is ventricular, it will usually remain unaffected.[24]

4. If there is still doubt, administer adenosine as discussed above.

5. If doubt remains, one may administer procainamide intravenously with appropriate precautions. If the tachycardia is ventricular, this will be a correct treatment.[22]

6. A recording may be made with a precordial S5 esophageal or intraarterial lead.

7. Calcium antagonists should never be administered.

8. If the patient is unstable, administer synchronized direct-current shock.

9. If facilities for performing an electrophysiologic study are available, and the clinical circumstances warrant the procedure, this technique may provide the only certain means of differentiating ventricular aberration from ventricular ectopy and indicating the definitive treatment.[25]

GLOSSARY

Ashman phenomenon: aberration in the intraventricular conduction of an impulse that completes a short cardiac cycle following a long cycle because the long cycle results in delay of repolarization.

Bradycardia-dependent bundle-branch block: an aberration in conduction that develops because of a gradual deceleration of the sinus rhythm.

Critical rate: a cycle length so short that part of the ventricular Purkinje system has not yet recovered from its previous activation, resulting in aberrant conduction of a supraventricular impulse.

Ectopy: any number of beats, ranging from a single PB to a sustained tachyarrhythmia, arising from outside the sinus node.

Paradoxical critical rate: a cycle length so long that part of the ventricular Purkinje system has already begun the process of impulse formation and therefore conducts the supraventricular impulse so slowly that aberrancy occurs.

Rate-dependent bundle-branch block: an aberration that develops as the result of a gradual change in sinus rhythm.

Rule of bigeminy: the likelihood that a VPB will occur after a long cycle because the long cycle results in delay of repolarization, facilitating reentry of the impulse causing the VPB.

Tachycardia-dependent bundle-branch block: an aberration that develops because of a gradual acceleration of sinus rhythm.

REFERENCES

1. Gouaux JL, Ashman R. Auricular fibrillation with aberration simulating ventricular paroxysmal tachycardia. Am Heart J 1947;34:366.
2. Sandler IA, Marriott HJL. The differential morphology of anomalous ventricular complexes of RBBB-type in lead V1; ventricular ectopy versus aberration. Circulation 1965;31:551.
3. Kulbertus HE, de Laval-Rutten F, Casters P. Vectorcardiographic study of aberrant conduction; anterior displacement of QRS, another form of intraventricular block. Br Heart J 1976;38:549–557.
4. Marriott HJL, Sandler IA. Criteria, old and new, for differentiating between ectopic ventricular beats and aberrant ventricular conduction in the presence of atrial fibrillation. Prog Cardiovasc Dis 1966;9:18.
5. Marriott HJL. Differential diagnosis of supraventricular and ventricular tachycardia. Geriatrics 1970;25:91–101.
6. Gulamhusein S, Yee R, Ko PT, Klein GJ. Electrocardiographic criteria for differentiating aberrancy and ventricular extrasystole in chronic atrial fibrillation: validation by intracardiac recordings. J Electrocardiol 1985; 18:41–50.
7. Vera Z, Cheng TO, Ertem G, et al. His bundle electrography for evaluation of criteria in differentiating ventricular ectopy from aberrancy in atrial fibrillation. Circulation 1972;45[Suppl II]:355.
8. Wellens HJJ, Bar FW, Lie KI. The value of the electrocardiogram in the differential diagnosis of a tachycardia with a widened QRS complex. Am J Med 1978;64:27–33.
9. Wellens HJJ, Bar FW, Vanagt EJ, et al. Medical treatment of ventricular tachycardia; considerations in the selection of patients for surgical treatment. Am J Cardiol 1982;49:186–193.
10. Bailey JC. The electrocardiographic differential diagnosis of supraventricular tachycardia with aberrancy versus ventricular tachycardia. Pract Cardiol 1980;6:118.
11. Pietras RJ, Mautner R, Denes P, et al. Chronic recurrent right and left ventricular tachycardia: comparison of clinical, hemodynamic and angiographic findings. Am J Cardiol 1977;40:32–37.
12. Zipes DP. Diagnosis of ventricular tachycardia. Drug Ther 1979;9:83.
13. Niazi I, McKinney J, Caceres J, et al. Reevaluation of surface ECG criteria for the diagnosis of wide QRS tachycardia. Circulation 1987:76(suppl IV):412.
14. Marriott HJL, Bieza CF. Alarming ventricular acceleration after lidocaine administration. Chest 1972;61:682–683.
15. Sherf L, James TN. A new electrocardiographic concept: synchronized sinoventricular conduction. Dis Chest 1969;55:127–140.
16. Kistin AD. Problems in the differentiation of ventricular arrhythmia from supraventricular arrhythmia with abnormal QRS. Prog Cardiovasc Dis 1966;9:1.
17. Gambetta M, Childers RW. Reverse rate related bundle branch block. J Electrocardiol 1973;6:153–157.
18. Massumi RA. Bradycardia-dependent bundle branch block. A critique and proposed criteria. Circulation 1968;38: 1066–1073.
19. Lian, Cassimatis, Hebert. Interet de la derivation precordiale auriculaire S5 dans le diagnostic des troubles du rythme auriculaire. Arch Mal Coeur 1952;45:481.
20. Copeland GD, Tullis IF, Brody DA. Clinical evaluation of a new esophageal electrode, with particular reference to the bipolar esophageal electrocardiogram. II. Observations in cardiac arrhythmias. Am Heart J 1959;57:874.
21. Vogel JHK, Tabari K, Averill KH, et al. A simple technique for identifying P waves in complex arrhythmias. Am Heart J 1964; 67:158.
22. Griffith MJ, Ward DE, Linker NJ, et al. Adenosine in the diagnosis of broad complex tachycardia. Lancet 1998;1:672.
23. Conti JB, Belardinelli L, Curtis AB. Usefulness of adenosine in diagnosis of tachyarrhythmias. Am J Cardiol 1995;75: 952–955.
24. Hess DS, Hanlon T, Scheinman M, et al. Termination of ventricular tachycardia by carotid sinus massage. Circulation 1982; 65:627–933.
25. Damato AN, Lau SH. Clinical value of the electrogram of the conduction system. Prog Cardiovasc Dis 1970;13: 119–140.

CHAPTER 19

Decreased Automaticity

When the automaticity of the sinus node is decreased, the result is a bradyarrhythmia originating either from the sinus node itself or from a "lower" site in the pacemaking and conduction system that spontaneously depolarizes to maintain a cardiac rhythm (Fig. 1.7). When the decelerated rhythm originates from the sinus node, the term *sinus bradycardia* is used to describe it, and when it originates from a lower site the terms *atrial rhythm*, *junctional rhythm*, or *ventricular rhythm* are used. These are not truly arrhythmias, but rather escape rhythms that attempt to compensate for the problem of decreased sinus-node automaticity. Figure 19.1 illustrates the various consequences of the slowing of sinus automaticity to less than 60 beats/min. The automaticity of the distal sites is suppressed if the sinus node is pacemaking normally, but it then returns (escapes) at its own, slower rate when the sinus node fails. Normal escape beats emerge from an atrial (Fig. 19.1A), His bundle (Fig. 19.1B), or ventricular Purkinje (Fig. 19.1C) site after the sinus impulses fail to appear.

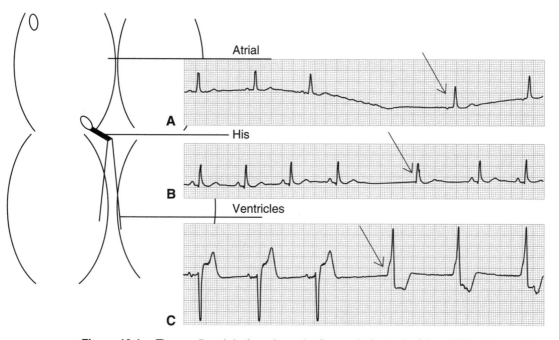

Figure 19.1. The *small ovals* in the schematic diagram indicate the SA and AV nodes, and the common bundle (*His*) and bundle branches are shown to lead toward the ventricles from the AV node. *Arrows* indicate the atrial **(A)**, His-bundle **(B)**, and ventricular escape **(C)** beats that terminate the pauses after the sinus node has failed to maintain its dominant rhythmicity. (From Wagner GS, Waugh RA, Ramo BW. Cardiac arrhythmias. New York: Churchill Livingstone, 1983:4, with permission.)

MECHANISMS OF BRADYARRHYTHMIAS OF DECREASED AUTOMATICITY

 There are three causes of decreased automaticity:

1. Physiologic slowing of the sinus rate.
2. Physiologic or pathologic enhancement of parasympathetic nervous activity.
3. Pathologic pacemaker failure.

Physiologic Slowing of the Sinus Rate

Although a rate of less than 60 beats/min is technically termed a bradyarrhythmia, it is often a normal variation of cardiac rhythm (especially in well-trained athletes, whose heart rates may be as low as in the thirties of beats per minute at rest). The rhythm may be either sinus bradycardia or, as shown in Figure 19.2, a junctional (Fig. 19.2A) or ventricular (Fig. 19.2B) rhythm. Bradycardia is a physiologic reaction to relaxation or sleeping, when the parasympathetic effect on cardiac automaticity dominates over the sympathetic effect. Even during the expiratory phase of the respiratory cycle, there is slowing of the sinus rate, often into the bradycardic range (Fig. 3.13). The lead-V1-positive QRS complexes in Figure 19.2B indicate that the escape site is in the left bundle.

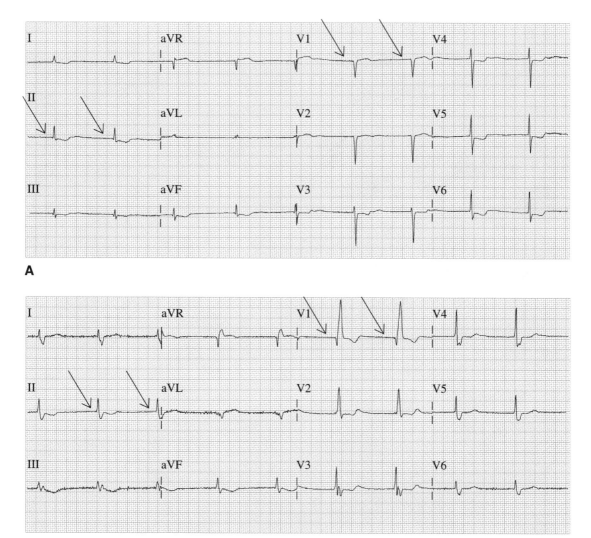

Figure 19.2. Twelve-lead ECGs from **A:** a 72-year-old woman receiving β-adrenergic blocking therapy for ischemic heart disease; and **B:** an otherwise healthy 81-year-old man on the day after prostate surgery. *Arrows* indicate complete absence of P waves preceding the normal **(A)** and abnormally wide QRS complexes **(B)**.

Physiologic or Pathologic Enhancement of Parasympathetic Activity

All cells with pacemaking capability are under some influence of the sympathetic and parasympathetic divisions of the autonomic nervous system. This influence is greatest in the sinus node and diminishes in the lower sites with pacemaking capacity. Usually, the changing autonomic balance causes a gradual increase or decrease in the pacing rate. However, many factors can induce a sudden increase in parasympathetic activity and decrease in sympathetic activity. These factors include:

1. Fright.
2. Carotid sinus massage.
3. Hypersensitivity of the carotid sinus.
4. Straining (i.e., a Valsalva maneuver).
5. Ocular pressure.
6. Increased intracranial pressure.
7. Sudden movement from a recumbent to an upright position.
8. Drugs that cause pooling of blood by dilating the veins.

This increase in parasympathetic activity is termed a *vasovagal reaction* (*vasovagal reflex*) because it has a prominent component of vascular relaxation in addition to cardiac slowing, and because it is mediated by the vagus, the principal parasympathetic nerve. Typical bradyarrhythmias that occur suddenly during a vasovagal reaction are presented in Figure 19.3. An episode of vomiting causes a sudden increase in parasympathetic activity manifested by both slowing of the sinus rate and failure of atrioventricular (AV) conduction (note the nonconducted P wave in the electrocardiogram [ECG] shown in Fig. 19.3). The increase in parasympathetic activity also suppresses escape pacemakers, and the resulting pause is interrupted only by the return of sinus rhythm. The combination of vascular relaxation and cardiac slowing results in a reduction in cardiac output so severe that it may cause dizziness or even loss of consciousness. This is termed *vasovagal syncope* or fainting. It is typically reversed when the individual falls into a recumbent position, thereby increasing venous return to the heart. When fainting occurs with the individual in the recumbent position, it can usually be reversed by elevation of the legs.

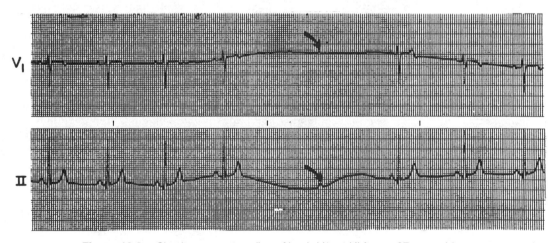

Figure 19.3. Simultaneous recording of leads V1 and II from a 67-year-old woman soon after cholecystectomy. *Arrows* indicate a nonconducted P wave. (From Wagner GS, Waugh RA, Ramo BW. Cardiac arrhythmias. New York: Churchill Livingstone, 1983:208, with permission.)

A single physiologic vasovagal reaction can have severe pathologic consequences if the individual is injured during a consequent fall, or if the change in body position required to restore venous return to the heart is not possible. Indeed, the autonomic reflex itself may become pathologic, resulting in *neurocardiogenic syncope*.[1–3] Repeated, severe, and sudden episodes of bradyarrhythmia with vasodilation require medical intervention to prevent serious injury or death.

Pathologic Pacemaker Failure

When a sudden period of complete absence of P waves appears in the ECG, the term *asystole* is used. The term *sick sinus syndrome* is often applied to this situation, since it is tempting to attribute the problem solely to the sinus node and pathologic pacemaker failure. However, if the problem was in fact limited to the sinus node, it would not produce any serious bradyarrhythmia, because a 1- to 2-second pause in sinus rhythm would be interrupted by escape from a lower site with the capacity for impulse formation, as shown in Figure 19.4. After three sinus beats (Fig. 19.4A), there is no further evidence of atrial activity, but then two junctional escape beats result. The pause following a ventricular premature beat (VPB) (Fig. 19.4B) ends with a junctional escape beat. After three sinus beats (Fig. 19.4C), a nonconducted atrial premature beat (APB) provides a cycle long enough for the ventricular Purkinje system to provide an escape beat.

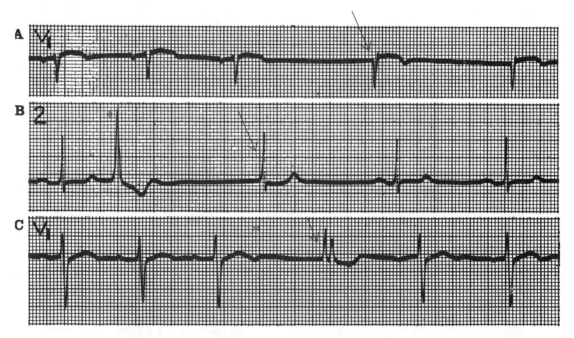

Figure 19.4. Rhythm strips from three individuals during postoperative monitoring: lead V1 **(A and C)** and lead II **(B)**. *Arrows* indicate junctional escape beats in **A** and **B** and the ventricular escape beat in **C**. *Asterisks* indicate the VPB in **B** and nonconducted APB in **C**. (From Marriott HJL. ECG/PDQ. Baltimore: Williams & Wilkins, 1987:171, with permission.)

Therefore, a prolonged atrial pause is caused by either:

1. Enhanced parasympathetic activity.
2. Impairment of all cells with impulse formation capability.

Although "sick pacemaker syndrome" would be a more accurate term, "sick sinus syndrome" is used here because of its general acceptance. Its characteristics are:

1. Bradyarrhythmia at rest.
2. Incapability to appropriately increase the pacemaking rate with increased sympathetic nervous activity.
3. Absence of escape rhythms when the sinus rate slows.
4. Sensitivity to suppression of impulse formation by various drugs.
5. Sensitivity to suppression of impulse formation by a reentrant tachyarrhythmia[4,5] (Fig. 19.5).

Lead II

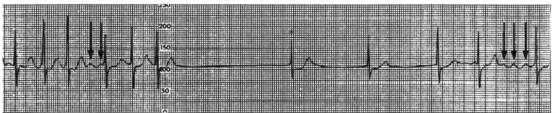

Figure 19.5. A lead-II rhythm strip from a 64-year-old man with paroxysmal atrial fibrillation. *Arrows* indicate the † waves and an *asterisk* indicates the junctional escape after a 2.5-second pause. (From Wagner GS, Waugh RA, Ramo BW. Cardiac arrhythmias. New York: Churchill Livingstone, 1983:210, with permission.)

In the example of atrial flutter/fibrillation shown in Figure 19.5, the arrhythmia terminated abruptly and was followed by a 2.5-second pause. All potential atrial, junctional, and ventricular pacemakers were suppressed during the atrial tachyarrhythmia. An escape junctional pacemaker eventually emerged. After three beats, atrial reentry recurred and atrial flutter/fibrillation reappeared.

Sick sinus syndrome is a part of the *tachycardia–bradycardia syndrome*,[6,7] in which bursts of an atrial tachyarrhythmia, often atrial fibrillation, alternate with prolonged pauses (Fig. 19.6). An irregular atrial tachycardia stops abruptly and is followed by a 4-second pause in sinus rhythm. The junctional rhythm at a rate of 40 beats/min is interrupted by a return of the atrial tachycardia.

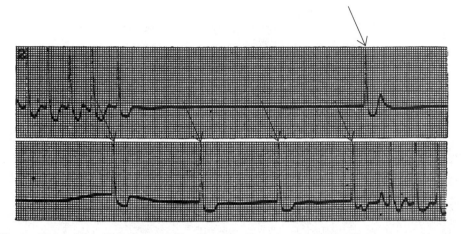

Figure 19.6.   A lead-II rhythm strip from an 82-year-old woman with history of recurrent syncopal episodes. *Arrows* indicate the junctional escape rhythm following the initial failure of emergence of an adequate escape rhythm.

Although sick sinus syndrome predominantly affects the elderly, it has been recognized as early as the first day of life.[8] Temporary and reversible manifestations of the syndrome can be caused by digitalis, quinidine, β-blockers, or aerosol propellants. The chronically progressive sick sinus syndrome was formerly believed to be due to ischemia, but a postmortem angiographic study of the sinus-nodal artery confirmed vascular involvement in less than one-third of 25 subjects with the chronic syndrome.[9] Sick sinus syndrome may result from inflammatory diseases, cardiomyopathy, amyloidosis,[10] collagen disease, metastatic disease, or surgical injury. In many patients, no cause is evident, and the syndrome is therefore classified as idiopathic. In these patients, it may be part of a sclerodegenerative process also affecting the lower parts of the cardiac pacemaking and conduction systems.

Two complications that affect the prognosis of patients with sick sinus syndrome are atrial fibrillation and AV block. During a 3-year follow-up study, atrial fibrillation developed in 16% and AV block developed in 8% of patients.[11]

The diagnosis of sick sinus syndrome can usually be made from the standard ECG or from a 24-hour Holter recording carefully correlated with the patient's clinical history. Pauses of 3 seconds or longer in sinus rhythm, although uncommon, do not necessarily indicate a poor prognosis, cause symptoms, or require artificial pacemaker implantation if the patient is asymptomatic.[12] In some patients, more sophisticated tests may be required. One of the best of these is measurement of the sinus-node recovery time after rapid atrial pacing, which is useful in recognizing sinoatrial (SA) block as the underlying mechanism for sick sinus syndrome.[13–15] Disorders of the sinus-node probably account for half of all implantations of permanent pacemakers.[16]

SINOATRIAL BLOCK

Although SA block is caused by failure of an impulse to emerge from the sinus node, it is often impossible to determine whether this or some other mechanism is responsible for an absent P wave. SA block should be diagnosed only when a mathematical relationship between the longer and shorter sinus cycles can be demonstrated, or when the sinus cycles show the characteristic, classical Wenckebach sequence of Mobitz Type I block. (Chapter 20, "Atrioventricular Block").

SA block is characterized by the intermittent failure of an impulse to emerge from the SA node, resulting in the occasional complete absence of beats (Fig. 19.7). The rhythm strips shown in the figure are continuous. The long cycle at the beginning of each strip is due to an absent sinus beat, in which an entire P-QRS-T sequence is missing. Note that the pauses are approximately equal to twice the observed sinus cycle length. When no such pattern can be established, "sinus pause" is a useful and appropriate term for the abnormally long cycle, accompanied by indication of its duration (e.g., a 4.5-second sinus pause).

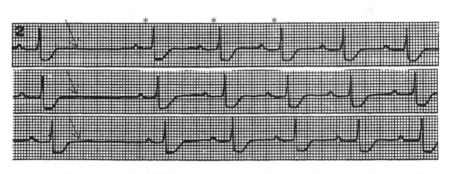

Figure 19.7. A continuous lead-II rhythm strip from a 77-year-old man receiving digitalis therapy for chronic congestive heart failure. *Arrows* indicate the times when P waves should have emerged from the sinus node pacemaker, and *asterisks* indicate the accompanying first-degree AV block (PR interval = 0.28 second).

PERSPECTIVE ON SINUS PAUSES

Although sudden pauses in sinus rhythm are common and important arrhythmias, it is often impossible to determine their etiology with the standard ECG or any other clinical test. When the sinus pauses are brief, the differential diagnosis includes sinus-node failure, SA block, and an APB that fails to conduct to the ventricles (Chapter 13, "Premature Beats"). It is often impossible to reach a conclusion about the etiology of a sudden sinus pause because underlying sinus arrhythmia makes it difficult to determine whether the pause is a precise multiple of the PP interval (Fig. 19.7). Also, when a nonconducted APB is present, the premature P wave is often obscured by a T wave (see Figs. 13.7 and 13.8).

When sudden pauses in sinus rhythm are prolonged, nonconducted APBs are not a consideration, and failure of all pacemaking cells, rather than only of the sinus node, must be considered. The differentiation of abnormal control of these pacemakers by the autonomic nervous system from abnormality within the pacemaking cells themselves is often difficult to make.

When pauses in sinus rhythm are brief, no clinical intervention is required, and the patient may not be at future risk for either the generalized pacemaker failure or autonomic abnormality that produces prolonged pauses. When sinus pauses are prolonged, it may be necessary to proceed with treatment without differentiating between a neurologic and cardiologic etiology.

GLOSSARY

Asystole: A pause in the cardiac electrical activity with neither atrial nor ventricular waveforms present on the ECG.

Atrial rhythm: a rhythm with a rate of less than 100 beats/min, and with abnormally directed P waves (indicating origination from a site in the atria other than the sinus node) preceding each QRS complex.

Escape rhythms: rhythms that originate from sites in the pacemaking and conduction system other than the sinus node, after a pause created by the failure of either normal sinus impulse formation or atrioventricular impulse conduction.

Junctional rhythm: a rhythm with a rate of less than 100 beats/min, with an inverted P wave direction visible in the frontal-plane leads and normally appearing QRS complexes. The P waves may precede or follow the QRS complexes, or may be obscured because they occur during the QRS complexes.

Neurocardiogenic syncope: a condition that occurs when an individual experiences a vasovagal reaction that causes loss of consciousness. It may be diagnosed by using a head-up tilt test.

Sick sinus syndrome: inadequate function of cardiac cells with pacemaking capability, resulting in continuous or intermittent slowing of the heart rate at rest and an inability to appropriately increase the rate with exercise.

Tachycardia–bradycardia syndrome: a condition in which both rapid and slow cardiac rhythms are present. The rapid rhythms tend to appear when the rate slows abnormally, while the slow rhythms are prominent immediately after the sudden cessation of a rapid rhythm.

Vasovagal reaction (reflex): sudden slowing of the heart rate either from decreased impulse formation (sinus pause) or decreased impulse conduction (AV block), resulting from increased activity of the parasympathetic or decreased activity of the sympathetic nervous system. The slowing of the cardiac rhythm is accompanied by peripheral vascular dilation.

Vasovagal syncope: loss of consciousness caused by a vasovagal reaction. Consciousness is almost always regained when the individual falls into a recumbent position, because this results in increased venous return to the heart.

Ventricular rhythm: a rhythm with a rate of less than 100 beats/min, with abnormally wide QRS complexes. There may be either retrograde association or AV dissociation.

REFERENCES

1. Abboud FM. Neurocardiogenic syncope. N Engl J Med 1993;328:1117–1120.
2. Fouad FM, Siitthisook S, Vanerio G, et al. Sensitivity and specificity of the tilt table test in young patients with unexplained syncope. Pace 1993;16:394–400.
3. Thilenius OG, Ryd KJ, Husayni J. Variations in expression and treatment of transient neurocardiogenic instability. Am J Cardiol 1992;69:1193–1195.
4. Lown B. Electrical reversion of atrial fibrillation. Br Heart J 1967;29:469–489.
5. Ferrer MI. The sick sinus syndrome. Mt. Kisco, NY: Futura Publishing, 1974.
6. Kaplan BM, Langendorf R, Lev M, et al. Tachycardia–bradycardia syndrome (so-called "sick sinus syndrome"). Am J Cardiol 1973;31:497–508.
7. Moss AJ, Davis RJ. Brady-Tachy syndrome. Prog Cardiovasc Dis 1974;16:439–454.
8. Ector H, Van der Hauwaert LG. Sick sinus syndrome in childhood. Br Heart J 1980;44:684–691.
9. Shaw DB, Linker NJ, Heaver PA, et al. Chronic sinoatrial disorder (sick sinus syndrome): a possible result of cardiac ischemia. Br Heart J 1987;58:598–607.
10. Evans R, Shaw DB. Pathological studies in sinoatrial disorder (sick sinus syndrome). Br Heart J 1977;39:778–786.
11. Sutton R, Kenny RA. The natural history of sick sinus syndrome. Pacing Clin Electrophysiol 1986; 9:1110–1114.
12. Hilgard J, Ezri MD, Denes P. Significance of ventricular pauses of three seconds or more detected on twenty-four-hour Holter recordings. Am J Cardiol 1984;55:1005.
13. Chung EK. Sick sinus syndrome: current views. Part II. Mod Concepts Cardiovasc Dis 1980;49;61,67–70.
14. Gann D, Tolentino A, Samet P. Electrophysiologic evaluation of elderly patients with sinus bradycardia. Ann Intern Med 1979;90:24–29.
15. Yeh SJ, Lin FC, Wu D. Complete sinoatrial block in two patients with bradycardia–tachycardia syndrome. J Am Coll Cardiol 1987;9:1184–1188.
16. Kaplan BM. Sick sinus syndrome. Arch Intern Med 1978;138:28.

CHAPTER 20

Atrioventricular Block

Atrioventricular (AV) block refers to an abnormality in electrical conduction between the atria and ventricles. The term *heart block* has also been used to describe this abnormality. Normal AV conduction was discussed in Chapter 3 ("Interpretation of the Normal Electrocardiogram"), and the parts of the cardiac pacemaking and conduction system that electrically connect the atrial and ventricular myocardia are illustrated in Figure 20.1. The term *degree* is used to indicate the severity of AV block. This severity can vary from minor (first degree), in which all impulses are conducted with delay, through moderate (second degree), in which some impulses are not conducted, to complete (third degree), in which no impulses are conducted. Any of these three levels of severity of AV block can be caused by conduction abnormality in the AV node (*A*), His bundle (*B*), or both the right bundle branch (RBB) and left bundle branch (LBB) (*C*).

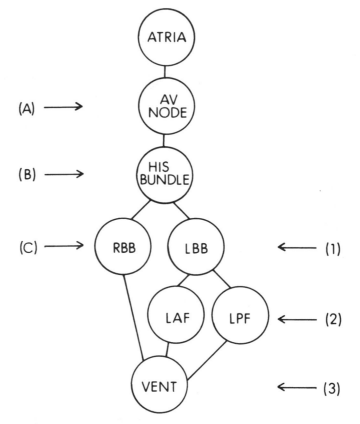

Figure 20.1. Figure 5.1 is reproduced to schematically illustrate the anatomic layers of AV-junctional (AV node *[A]* and His Bundle *[B]*) and ventricular (RBB and LBB *[C]*) structures potentially capable of causing AV block. The numbers *1*, *2*, and *3* are anatomic layers of the ventricles incapable of initiating a narrow (less than 0.12 second) QRS complex.

SEVERITY OF ATRIOVENTRICULAR BLOCK

First-Degree Atrioventricular Block

The "normal" PR interval has a duration of 0.12 to 0.21 second. *First-degree AV block* is generally defined as a prolongation of AV conduction time (PR interval) to longer than 0.21 second. In analyses of records from normal young persons, the incidence of first-degree block by this definition ranged from 0.5%[1] and 2%.[2] In healthy middle-aged men, a prolonged PR interval in the presence of a normal QRS complex was found not to affect prognosis and to be unrelated to ischemic heart disease.[3] Figure 20.2 illustrates two examples of first-degree AV block. The first of these (Fig. 20.2A) is minor, with a PR interval of 0.24 second, while the second (Fig. 20.2B) shows extreme PR lengthening. Note that in Figure 20.2B the P wave is superimposed on the T wave of the preceding cycle.

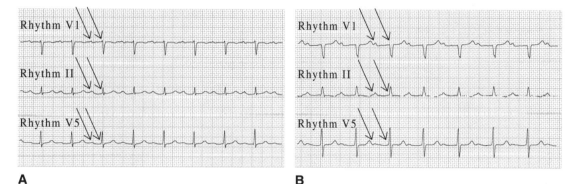

A **B**

Figure 20.2. Simultaneous three-lead (V1, II, and V5) rhythm strips showing examples of first-degree AV block from healthy 69-year-old **(A)** and 72-year-old **(B)** women receiving no medications. *Arrows* indicate PR intervals of 0.25 **(A)** and 0.35 second **(B)**.

Second-Degree Atrioventricular Block

By definition, *second degree AV block* is present when one or more, but not all, atrial impulses fail to reach the ventricles. Examples of atrial premature beats (APBs) that are not conducted simply because they occur early were presented in Chapter 13 ("Premature Beats"; see Figs. 13.7 and 13.8). This situation is not considered AV block because it is not abnormal. Figure 20.3 presents an example of both first- and second-degree AV block in which on-time P waves either have delayed AV conduction (first and second cycles of the series) or no AV conduction (third cycle) .

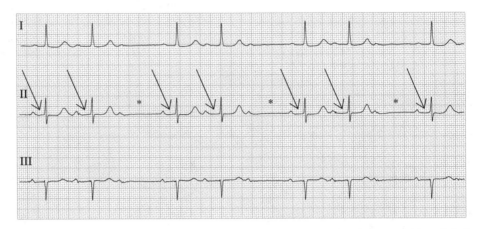

Figure 20.3.   Lead-I, -II, and -III rhythm strips from an 82-year-old woman receiving digitalis therapy for chronic heart failure. *Arrows* indicate first-degree AV block and *asterisks* indicate second-degree AV block.

A second-degree AV block may be intermittent (Fig. 20.4A) or continuous (Fig. 20.4B). Note that in Figure 20.4A, the second-degree block occurs only after a sequence of six conducted beats, of which the first shows no AV block and the latter five show first-degree block (7:6 block). In Figure 20.4B, there is continually alternating first-degree and second-degree AV block (2:1 block).

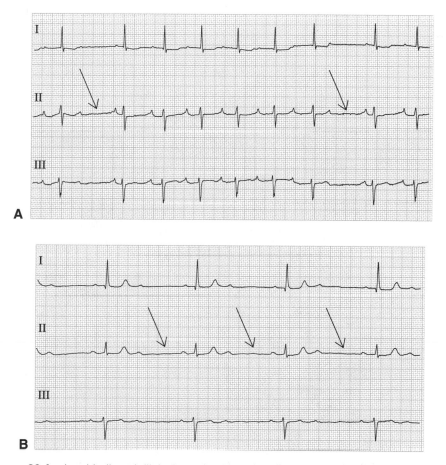

Figure 20.4. Lead-I, -II, and -III rhythm strips from a 51-year-old man with chronic pulmonary disease and receiving digitalis therapy **(A)** and a 77-year-old woman with hypertension and receiving both β-adrenergic and calcium antagonist therapy **(B)**. *Arrows* indicate failure of AV conduction, and therefore the presence of second-degree AV block.

Second-degree AV block may be marked by any ratio of P waves to QRS complexes (Fig.20.5). In Figure 20.5A, there are the commonly appearing 3:2 and 4:3 AV conduction ratios. However, in Figure 20.5B the sinus rate is in the tachycardia range, and the more rapid "bombardment" of the AV node causes the 2:1 ratio to be intermittently increased to 3:1.

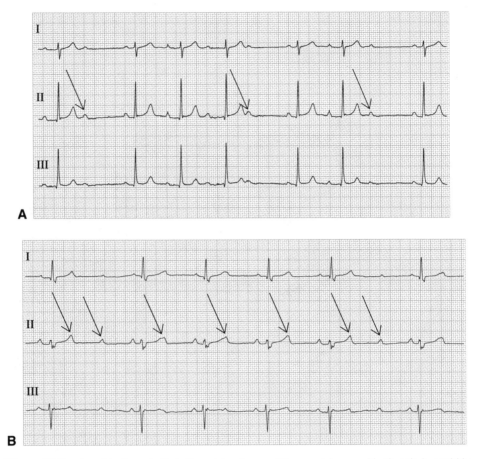

Figure 20.5. Lead-I, -II, and -III rhythm strips from a 57-year-old man with chronic bronchitis and cor pulmonale **(A)** and a 79-year-old woman with acute pulmonary edema **(B)**, both of whom were receiving long-term digitalis therapy for heart failure. *Arrows* indicate P waves that completely fail to conduct to the ventricles.

When determining the clinical significance of second-degree AV block, the atrial rate should be considered. As discussed in Chapter 15 ("Atrial Reentrant Tachyarrhythmias"), conduction of some but not all atrial impulses is essential for clinical stability in the presence of atrial flutter/fibrillation. Chapter 14 ("Accelerated Automaticity"; see Fig. 14.6) indicates that second-degree AV block commonly occurs along with atrial tachycardia, particularly when there is digitalis toxicity. When "AV block" occurs in the presence of an atrial tachyarrhythmia, the block itself is considered a normal occurrence and not an additional arrhythmia (Fig. 20.6A) unless the ventricular rate is reduced into the bradycardic range (Fig. 20.6B).

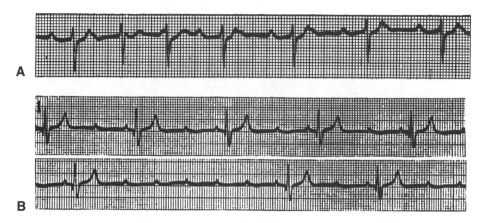

Figure 20.6. Lead-II rhythm strips from elderly patients receiving digitalis therapy. The ventricular rates are in the normal (60 to 100 beats/min) **(A)** and bradycardic (15 to 40 beats/min) **(B)** ranges. Note the prolonged pause in the ventricular rhythm (3.5 second) in **(B)**.

When both second-degree AV block and sinus pauses are present (Chapter 19, "Decreased Automaticity"), the cause is most likely not within the heart itself, but rather in its autonomic nervous control.

Second-degree AV block usually occurs in the AV node,[4,5] and is associated with reversible conditions such as rheumatic fever or the acute phase of an inferior myocardial infarction. It is also associated with treatment with digitalis, a β-adrenergic blocker, or a calcium-channel blocking drug. Since second-degree AV block is generally a transient disturbance in rhythm, it seldom progresses to complete AV block. However, in one study of 16 children manifesting second-degree block, seven developed complete block.[6] Chronic second-degree AV block may occasionally occur in many conditions, including aortic valve disease, atrial septal defect, amyloidosis, Reiter's syndrome, and mesothelioma of the AV node.

Third-Degree Atrioventricular Block

When no atrial impulses are conducted to the ventricles, the cardiac rhythm is termed third-degree AV block, and the clinical condition is determined by the escape capability of the more distal Purkinje cells. The junctional or ventricular escape rhythm in the presence of third-degree AV block is almost always precisely regular, because these sites are not as influenced by the sympathetic/parasympathetic balance as is the sinus node. Figure 20.7A shows quite adequate junctional escape in a case of third-degree AV block, but Figure 20.7B shows less optimal ventricular escape.

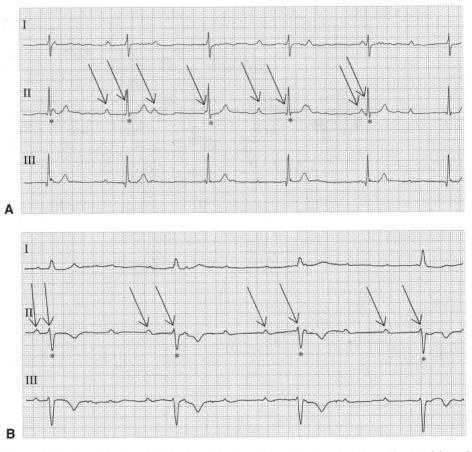

Figure 20.7. Lead-I, -II, and -III rhythm strips from two patients presenting with complaints of dyspnea on exertion. *Arrows* indicate the varying PR-interval relationships and *asterisks* indicate the regular junctional **(A)** and ventricular **(B)** escape rates.

In most clinical instances, complete AV block is at least partly compensated by an escape rhythm originating from an area distal to the site of the block. However, complete AV block of sudden onset may cause syncope with catastrophic results, or even sudden death, when there is no escape rhythm, as in Figure 20.8. As seen in the figure, P waves occur immediately after the T waves, and the first two P waves are conducted without even first-degree block, but the third and all subsequent P waves are not conducted at all. Thus, third-degree AV block may not be preceded by AV block of either of the two lower degrees of severity.

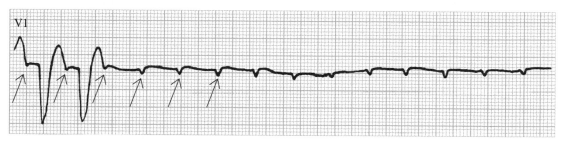

Figure 20.8. A lead-V1 rhythm strip from an 83-year-old woman on telemetry monitoring during hospitalization following an episode of syncope. *Arrows* indicate the continuing sinus tachycardia before and after the onset of complete AV block.

Third-degree AV block always produces AV dissociation, with its independent atrial and ventricular rhythms; however, AV dissociation may result from other sources than third-degree AV block. Decreased sinus automaticity (Chapter 19, "Decreased Automaticity"), increased junctional and ventricular automaticity (Chapter 14, "Accelerated Automaticity"), and reentrant ventricular tachycardia (Chapter 17, "Reentrant Ventricular Tachyarrhythmias") can all produce AV dissociation by creating the condition in which anterograde impulses fail to traverse the AV node because they encounter the refractoriness that follows AV-nodal activation by retrograde impulses. Therefore, AV dissociation caused solely by impaired function of the AV conduction system should actually be termed "AV dissociation due to AV block" (Fig. 20.7A and B), and AV dissociation caused solely by an accelerated distal pacing site should be termed "AV dissociation due to refractoriness" (Fig. 20.9A). Both causes can coexist, producing "AV dissociation due to a combination of AV block and refractoriness," when there are P waves that are obviously not conducted to the ventricles but the ventricular rate is slightly above the upper limit of the bradycardic range of 60 beats/min (Fig. 20.9B). The term "interference" is often used to describe the condition of refractoriness that either causes or contributes to the two types of AV dissociation described here.

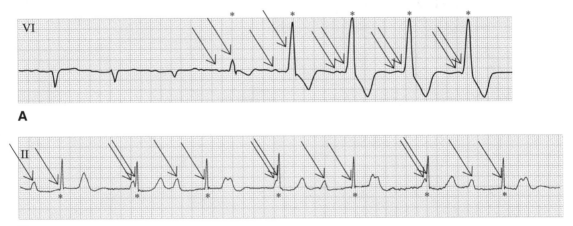

Figure 20.9. Rhythm strips from two patients receiving digitalis therapy for congestive heart failure: **A:** lead V1. **B:** lead II. Note in **A** that the initial independent ventricular beat is a "fusion beat" produced partly by conduction from the atria and partly from the ventricular pacing site. *Arrows* indicate the varying relationships between adjacent P waves and QRS complexes, and *asterisks* indicate the regular ventricular rates. Note that the P waves are unusually small in **A** and unusually large in **B**.

Often, the AV dissociation produced by third-degree AV block is "isoarrhythmic," with similar atrial and ventricular rates and with P waves and QRS complexes occurring almost simultaneously. Insight into the presence or absence of AV block can be attained only when a P wave appears at a sufficiently remote time from a QRS complex that the ventricular refractory period would be expected to have been completed. In Figure 20.10, there is AV dissociation during the first three cycles, when the independent sinus and ventricular rhythms are similar. Then, when variation in rate caused by respiration (sinus arrhythmia) accelerates the sinus rate but does not affect the ventricular escape focus during the fourth cycle, atrial capture occurs. This event proves AV conduction to be possible, and eliminates AV block as a contributor to the AV dissociation.

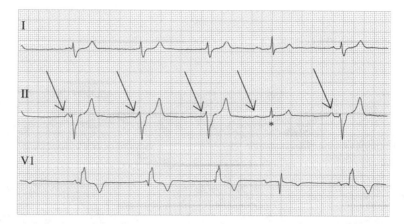

Figure 20.10. Lead-I, -II, and -V1 rhythm strips from an 87-year-old woman receiving digitalis therapy for congestive heart failure. *Arrows* indicate P-wave locations (the irregularity is due to sinus arrhythmia) and an *asterisk* indicates a QRS complex produced by atrial capture.

Block in both the RBB and LBB (level C in Figure 20.1), rather than block at the AV node or in the His bundle, is usually the cause of chronic complete AV block.[7–10] Idiopathic fibrosis, called either Lev's disease or Lenegre's disease, is the most common cause of chronic complete AV block.[7,11] Acute complete AV block within the AV node results from inferior myocardial infarction, digitalis intoxication, and rheumatic fever.[12] Acute complete AV block within the bundle branches results from anterior myocardial infarction.[13,14] Complete AV block may also be congenital, such as when it results from maternal anti-Ro antibodies affecting the AV node.[15]

In the presence of chronic left or right bundle-branch block, the individual is at some risk of suddenly developing complete AV block. After this occurs, the ventricles either remain inactive (ventricular asystole; Fig. 20.8) and the patient experiences syncope or even sudden death, or a more distal pacing site takes over (Fig. 20.7B) and controls the ventricles (ventricular escape). In this event, the atria continue to beat at their own rate and the ventricles beat at a lower tempo or rhythm. This independence (AV dissociation due to AV block) is readily recognized in the ECG recording from the lack of relationship between the slow ventricular complexes and the more frequent P waves. Each maintains its own rhythm without regard for the other.

Differentiation between second- and third-degree AV block is accomplished by considering first the relationship among the ventricular waveforms in a series of cycles (RR intervals), and second the relationship between the atrial and ventricular waveforms in each of these cycles (PR or flutter-R intervals). If the RR interval is irregular, some AV conduction can be assumed, and second-degree block is present. If the RR interval is regular, a constant PR or flutter-R interval indicates second-degree AV block, while a varying PR or flutter-R interval indicates third-degree block with an escape rhythm generated by a lower site. Figure 20.11 presents examples of AV block occurring in the presence of three different atrial tachyarrhythmias: sinus tachycardia (Fig. 20.11A), atrial flutter (Fig. 20.11B), and atrial fibrillation (Fig. 20.11C). Consecutive RR intervals are constant in all of the examples, at 2.84, 1.40, and 1.96 second, respectively. In Figure 20.11A and B, it is obvious that there is third-degree AV block, since the adjacent PR relationships in A and flutter wave-R relationships in B are quite variable. In Figure 20.11C, third-degree AV block can be assumed because the absence of regular atrial activity in atrial fibrillation prohibits any constancy in AV conduction relationships.

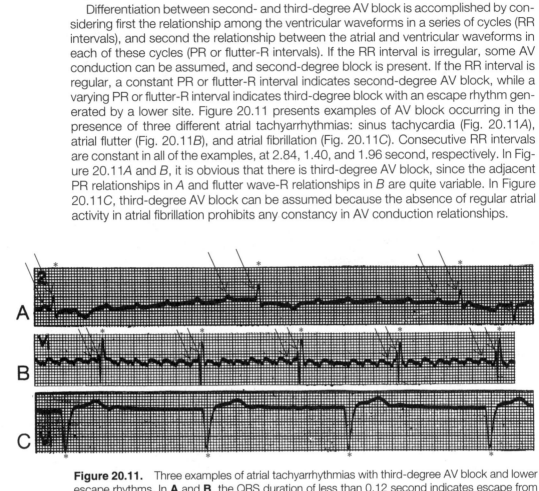

Figure 20.11.   Three examples of atrial tachyarrhythmias with third-degree AV block and lower escape rhythms. In **A** and **B**, the QRS duration of less than 0.12 second indicates escape from the common bundle, but in **C** the QRS duration of 0.16 second indicates either escape from the common bundle accompanied by LBBB or escape from the right bundle branch. *Arrows* indicate the varying P-QRS **(A)** and F-QRS **(B)** intervals, and *asterisks* indicate the constant ventricular rates in all three examples.

LOCATION OF ATRIOVENTRICULAR BLOCK

As discussed in Chapter 5 ("Intraventricular Conduction Abnormalities" and presented schematically in Figure 20.1, AV block can be located in the AV node, the common bundle, or the bundle branches. This distinction is important, because both the etiology and prognosis are quite different with proximal (AV-nodal) versus distal (infranodal) block. Fortunately, block within the common bundle is so rare that the clinical decision about the location of an AV block is essentially limited to the AV node versus the bundle branch.

Two aspects of the electrocardiographic appearance of rhythm may help in differentiating AV block at the AV node versus AV block in a bundle branch: (a) the consistency of the PR intervals of conducted impulses and (b) the width of the QRS complexes of either conducted or escape impulses. Since only the AV node has the ability to vary its conduction time, the Purkinje cells of the common bundle and bundle branches must conduct at a particular speed or not at all. Therefore, when a varying PR interval is present, AV block is most likely to exist within the AV node.

A QRS complex of normal duration (less than 0.12 second) can occur only when the impulse producing the complex has equal access to both the right and left bundle branches. Therefore, when an AV block is located at the bundle-branch level, the conducted or escape QRS complexes must be 0.12 second or longer. The diagnosis is complicated by the possibility of either a fixed bundle-branch block accompanying AV-nodal block or an aberrancy of intraventricular conduction (Chapter 18, "Ventricular versus Supraventricular with Aberrant Conduction"). Consequently, a QRS complex of normal duration confirms that a block has an AV-nodal location, whereas a QRS complex of prolonged duration is not helpful in locating the site of an AV block.

CONSIDERATION OF THE VARIABILITY OF ATRIOVENTRICULAR CONDUCTION TIMES

When the duration of the QRS complex of either conducted or escape beats is within normal limits (less than 0.12 second), the location of an AV block is almost always the AV node. Since the common bundle is so rarely the site of AV block, it should not be a clinical consideration. On the other hand, when the QRS complex is prolonged (0.12 second), it is necessary to observe the pattern of AV conduction times as approximated by PR intervals.

The AV conduction time from beat to beat can be either variable or constant. However, variability in the conduction time can occur only in the AV node: the common bundle and its branches lack the ability to significantly vary their conduction times. The AV node has this ability to vary conduction time because its cells have uniquely prolonged periods of partial refractoriness as they return from their depolarized to their repolarized states. Therefore, in cases of less than complete AV block, a nodal versus an infranodal (bilateral bundle) location can be determined by observing whether the PR interval is variable, as in the first case, or constant, as in the second.

AV conduction patterns can be considered only when some conduction is present (first- or second-degree AV block). No differentiation between an AV-nodal and an infranodal location is possible in the case of a complete (third-degree) block with wide escape QRS complexes (Fig. 20.7*B*).

ATRIOVENTRICULAR-NODAL BLOCK

Electrocardiographically, the classic form of AV-nodal block is reflected by the *Wenckebach sequence*, in which the PR interval may begin within normal limits but is usually somewhat prolonged. With each successive beat, the PR interval then gradually lengthens until there is failure to conduct an impulse and a ventricular beat is dropped (Figs. 20.3, 20.4A, and 20.5A). Following the nonconducted P wave, the PR interval reverts to normal (or near normal) and the sequence is repeated. At times, the PR interval may stretch to surprising lengths (0.80, 0.90, or even to more than 1.0 second).

Progressive lengthening of the PR interval occurs in the Wenckebach sequence because each successive atrial impulse arrives progressively earlier in the relative refractory period of the AV node, and therefore takes progressively longer to penetrate the node and reach the ventricles. This is a physiologic mechanism during atrial flutter/fibrillation, but its occurrence at normal heart rates implies impairment of AV conduction.[16] The progressive lengthening of the PR interval usually follows a predictable pattern: the maximal increase in the PR interval occurs between the first and second cardiac cycles, and the increase between subsequent cycles then becomes progressively smaller. The reason for this pattern is illustrated in Figure 20.12, an idealized diagram of an AV-nodal Wenckebach sequence. The largest increase in duration of the PR interval (+0.12 second) is in the second (0.34 second) over the first (0.22 second) cycle. Thus, although the PR interval becomes progressively longer (0.22, 0.34, 0.39, and 0.42 second), the increase in its duration becomes progressively smaller (+0.12, +0.05, and +0.03 second).

This phenomenon leaves its mark on the rhythm of the ventricles. After the pause produced by complete failure of AV conduction, the RR intervals in the ECG tend to decrease progressively, and the long cycle (the one containing the nonconducted beat) is of shorter duration than two of the shorter cycles because it contains the shortest PR interval (Fig. 20.12). The RR interval is composed of the RP interval plus the incremental increase in the PR interval, and it therefore decreases progressively from 0.92 to 0.85 to 0. 83 second. The RR interval surrounding the nonconducted P wave (1.40 second) is less than twice the length of the shortest cycle (0.83 second) because instead of containing a PR increment, it contains a PR decrement (−0.2 second). The long cycle is therefore 0.80 + 0.80–0.20 = 1.40 second.

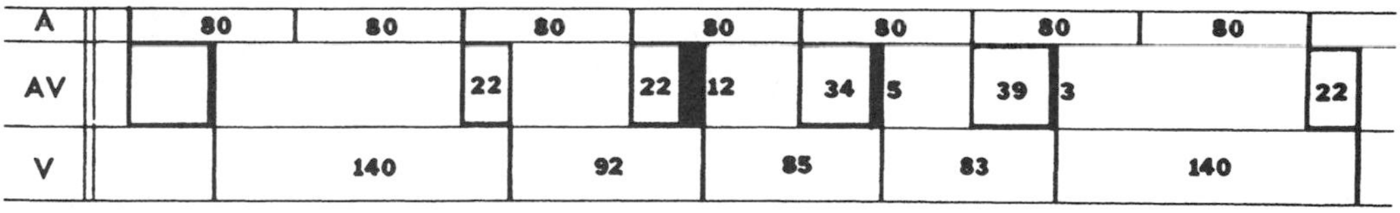

A		80		80		80		80		80		80		80		
AV					22		22	12	34	5		39	3			22
V			140			92			85		83			140		

Figure 20.12. Measurements are indicated in hundredths of a second on this ladder diagram. The regular PP intervals are indicated in Level A, the abnormal nodal conduction in Level AV, and the resulting irregular RR intervals in Level V.

This pattern of progressively decreasing RR intervals preceding a pause in AV conduction that lasts for less than twice the duration of the shortest RR interval is of only-academic interest in the case of AV-nodal block, but a similar pattern of PP intervals may provide the only clue to the presence of sinus-nodal exit block (Chapter 19, "Decreased Automaticity").

In summary, three characteristic features of the cardiac cycle. which can be figuratively referred to as the *footprints of the Wenckebach sequence*, occur with AV-nodal block: (a) the beats tend to cluster in small groups, particularly in pairs, because 3:2 P-to-QRS ratios are more common than 4:3 ratios, which are more common than 5:4 ratios, and so forth; (b) in each group of ventricular beats, the first cycle is longer than the second cycle, and there is a tendency for progressive shortening to occur in successive cycles; and (c) the longest cycle (the one containing the dropped ventricular beat) is less than twice the length of the shortest cycle (Fig. 20.13).

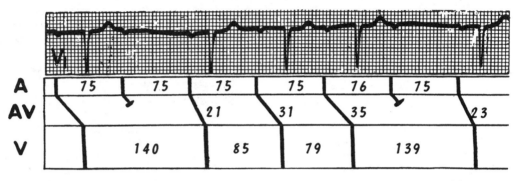

Figure 20.13. A lead-V1 rhythm strip accompanied by a ladder diagram with atrial (A) AV-nodal (*AV*), and ventricular (*V*) levels. The various intervals are indicated in hundredths of a second.

The footprints of the Wenckebach sequence are apparent in Figure 20.14, although only the P waves that occur during the long cycles are visible. The beats are grouped in pairs and trios. In three of the four trios, the first cycle is longer than the second cycle, and the longest cycles separating the groups are less than twice the length of the shortest cycles.

When second-degree AV block appears during an acute inferior myocardial infarction, the elevation of the ST segment in the ECG may obscure many of the P waves, as seen in Figure 20.14. The visible P waves with prolonged PR intervals during the pauses allow diagnosis of first-degree block, but only the typical RR-interval pattern allows a diagnosis of second-degree AV-nodal block.

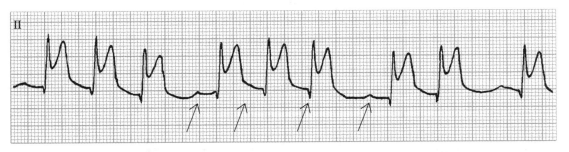

Figure 20.14. A continuous recording of lead II from a 63-year-old man with acute inferior myocardial infarction. *Arrows* indicate both the obvious and the assumed locations of sinus-originated P waves.

The features described above are typical of a classic Wenckebach period, but AV-nodal block rarely fits this pattern because both the sinus rate and AV conduction are under the constant influence of the autonomic nervous system.[17,18] Among common divergences from the classic pattern are that: (a) the first increment may not be the greatest; (b) the PR intervals may not lengthen progressively; (c) the last PR increment may be the longest of all; and (d) a nonconducted atrial beat may not occur.[17] The only criterion needed to identify the form of AV block that typically occurs in the AV node is a variation in the PR intervals. The term *Mobitz type I* or simply *type I* AV block is used when variation of the PR intervals is virtually diagnostic of block in the AV node.

The earlier an impulse arrives during the prolonged partial refractory period of the AV node, the longer the time required for conduction of the impulse through to the ventricles. Therefore, once the AV node is in its refractory period, the shorter the interval between a conducted QRS complex and the next conducted P wave (*RP interval*), the longer is the following conduction time (PR interval). This inverse or reciprocal relationship between RP and PR intervals is illustrated schematically in Figure 20.15.

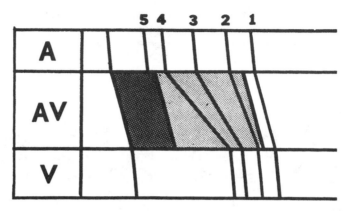

Figure 20.15. A ladder diagram illustrating the effect of progressively earlier entry of atrial impulses (*1–5*) into the AV node (*AV*). The *light stippled area* indicates the AV node's relative refractory period, during which Impulses *2, 3,* and *4* encounter progressively slower conduction. The *dark stippled area* indicates the node's absolute refractory period, during which Impulse *5* cannot be conducted to the ventricles.

Figure 20.16 presents an example of this *RP/PR* reciprocity. There is no AV block at all during the first three beats of sinus rhythm. The APB is analogous to Impulse 4 in Figure 20.15, and the next three successive sinus beats are analogous to Impulses 3 and 2. Only when the sinus beat has a sufficiently long RP interval to avoid the relative refractory period of the AV node can this beat be conducted with a normal PR interval, analogous to Impulse 1 in Figure 20.15. This rhythm should not be considered as AV block, but rather as a physiologic AV-nodal delay resulting from the effect of a single APB.

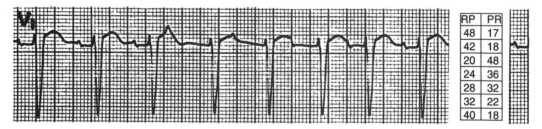

RP	PR
48	17
42	18
20	48
24	36
28	32
32	22
40	18

Figure 20.16. The table of associated RP and PR intervals in hundredths of a second at left indicates reciprocal relationships during Cycles 2 through 8 on the rhythm strip. The initial cardiac cycle is not included because the RP interval preceding its PR interval has not been recorded on the rhythm strip.

The need to consider the variability in AV conduction times in order to determine the location of an AV block is illustrated in Figure 20.17. There is normal sinus rhythm with second-degree AV block and RBBB. For the initial complete cardiac cycles, the RP intervals are constant (1.36 second) and the PR intervals are also constant (0.24 second). It is tempting to locate the AV block below the AV node because the PR intervals do not vary and there is an obvious intraventricular conduction problem. However, the possibility of AV-nodal block has not been eliminated because, with a constant RP interval, the AV node would be expected to conduct with a constant PR interval. Only when the conduction ratio changes from 2:1 (P waves 1–4) to 3:2 (P waves 5–7) is a change produced in the RP interval (from 1.36 to 0.56 second). This shorter RP interval is accompanied by a reciprocally greater PR interval (from 0.24 to 0.36 second), identifying the AV node rather than the ventricular Purkinje system as the location of the AV block.

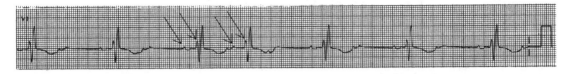

Figure 20.17. A lead-V1 rhythm strip from a 77-year-old woman receiving digitalis therapy for congestive heart failure. *Arrows* indicate the varying PR intervals during the third and fourth cycles that prove the capacity for variable conduction times.

INFRANODAL (PURKINJE) BLOCK

 Although infranodal (i.e., occurring in the Purkinje system) block is much less common than AV-nodal block, it is much more serious than the latter. It is almost always preceded by a bundle-branch block pattern for the conducted beats, with the nonconducted beats resulting from intermittent block in the other bundle branch.[4,5] Continuous block in the other bundle branch results in syncope or heart failure if ventricular escape occurs, and sudden death if there is no ventricular escape. *Infranodal block is almost always due to bilateral bundle-branch block* (Level C in Figure 20.1) rather than His-bundle block (Level B). First-degree AV block may or may not accompany the bundle-branch block, but there is usually no stable period of second-degree AV block. Infranodal block is typically characterized by a sudden progression from no AV block to third-degree (complete) AV block. Since it occurs in the distal part of the pacemaking and conduction system, the escape rhythm may be too slow or too unreliable to support adequate circulation of blood, thereby causing serious and even fatal clinical events.

Unlike the cells in the AV node, those in the Purkinje system have an extremely short relative refractory period. Therefore, they either conduct at a particular speed or not at all. Infranodal block is characterized by a lack of lengthening of the PR interval preceding the nonconducted P wave, and a lack of shortening of the PR interval in the following cycle. This is termed *Mobitz type II* or simply *type II* AV block. It should be diagnosed whenever there is second-degree AV block with a constant PR interval despite a change in the RP interval. Indeed, the distinction between types I and II block does not require the presence of a nonconducted P wave, and can therefore be made in the presence of first-degree AV block alone.

The cardiac rhythm shown in Figure 20.18A should be compared to that in Figure 20.18B. The consistent 3:2 AV ratio provides varying RP intervals. However, in Figure 20.18A, the PR intervals remain constant at 0.20 second, in contrast with Figure 20.18B, in which the varying PP intervals result in varying PR intervals. Therefore, the AV block producing the rhythm shown in Figure 20.18A is in a location that is incapable of varying its conduction time even when it receives impulses at varying intervals. The PR intervals are independent of, rather than reciprocal to, their associated RP intervals. This type II block in Figure 20.18A is indicative of an infranodal (Purkinje) site of failure of AV conduction, in contrast to type I block in Figure 20.18B that is indicative of an AV-nodal site.

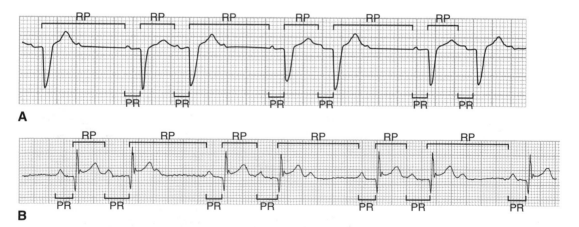

Figure 20.18. Lead-II rhythm strips from a 79-year-old woman with recurrent presyncopal episodes **(A)** and a 59-year-old man with an acute inferior myocardial infarction **(B)**. *Brackets* indicate the variable RP/constant PR pattern typical of type II AV block in **A** and the variable RP/variable PR pattern typical of type I AV block in **B**.

Figure 20.19 presents another example of type II block. Note that the PR intervals remain unchanged despite longer and shorter RP intervals (i.e., there is no RP/PR reciprocity). The recording shown in Figure 20.19 illustrates the two sources of variation in RP intervals: a change in the atrial:ventricular conduction ratio (from 1:1 to 2:1), and the presence of a ventricular premature beat (VPB). Note that no bracket appears in the vicinity of the VPB because it cannot be determined when the AV node is activated retrogradely by the VPB.

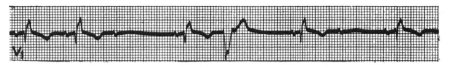

Figure 20.19. A lead-V1 rhythm strip from an 82-year-old man with chronic congestive heart failure. There is a lack of increase in the PR interval when a decrease occurs in the RP interval.

A stepwise method for determining the location of AV block is illustrated in Figure 20.20. This algorithm does not consider the localization of AV block within the common bundle because of the rarity of AV block in this location. (Such a location should be considered only when a QRS complex of normal duration [Step 1] is accompanied by a pattern characteristic of type II block [Step 4].) Note that both Steps 2 and 4 may lead to situations in which it is impossible to determine the location of a block from a particular ECG recording. In this case, additional recordings should be obtained. If these are also nondiagnostic, the patient should be managed as though the block were

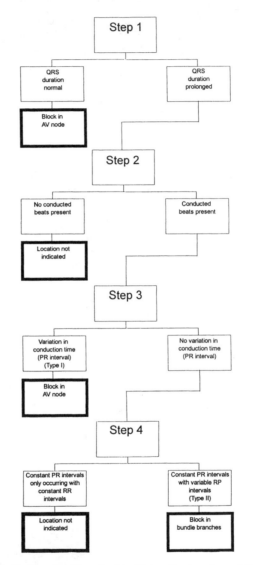

Figure 20.20. The four-step algorithm for identifying the location of AV block from an ECG recording: Step 1: Consider the duration of the QRS complex. Step 2: Consider whether conducted beats are present. Step 3: Consider whether there is variation in the conduction times. Step 4: Consider whether there are constant PR intervals with changing RP intervals. Situations that indicate an endpoint in the algorithm are indicated by *boxes with accentuated borders*.

located in the bundle branches, because such a location has the most serious clinical consequences. This usually requires insertion of a temporary pacemaker, which provides time for further studies to determine the location of the AV block. His-bundle electrograms can be obtained via intracardiac recordings. A prolonged atrial-to-His interval (from the onset of the atrial signal to the time of the His bundle signal), or the absence of a signal from the His bundle, indicates block in an AV-nodal location, while a prolonged His-to-ventricle interval (from the His-bundle signal to the onset of the ventricular signal), or absence of a signal from the ventricles after a His signal, indicates block in a bilateral bundle branches location (Fig. 12.11).

GLOSSARY

Atrioventricular (AV) block: a conduction abnormality located between the atria and the ventricles. Both the severity and the location of the abnormality should be considered.

Degree: a measure of the severity of AV block.

First-degree AV block: conduction of atrial impulses to the ventricles with PR intervals of longer than 0.21 second.

Footprints of the Wenckebach sequence: the pattern of clusters of beats in small groups, with gradually decreasing intervals between beats, preceding a pause that is less than twice the duration of the shortest interval.

Heart block: another term used for AV block.

His-bundle electrograms: intracardiac recordings obtained via a catheter positioned across the tricuspid valve adjacent to the common or His bundle. These recordings are used clinically to determine the location of AV block when this is not apparent from the surface ECG recordings.

Infranodal block: AV block that occurs distal to or below the AV node, and therefore within either the common bundle or in both the right and left bundle branches.

Mobitz type I (type I): a pattern of AV block in which there are varying PR intervals. This pattern is typical of block within the AV node, which has the capacity for wide variations in conduction time. Wenckebach sequences are the classic form of type I block.

Mobitz type II (type II): a pattern of AV block in which there are constant PR intervals despite varying RP intervals. This pattern is typical of block in the ventricular Purkinje system, which is incapable of significant variations in conduction time.

RP interval: the time between the beginning of the previously conducted QRS complex and the beginning of the next conducted P wave.

RP/PR reciprocity: the inverse relationship between the interval of the last previously conducted beat (RP interval) and the time required for AV conduction (PR interval). This occurs in type I AV block.

Second-degree AV block: The conduction of some atrial impulses to the ventricles, with the failure to conduct other atrial impulses.

Stokes-Adams attacks: syncopal episodes caused by periods of cardiac arrest.

Third-degree AV block: failure of conduction of any atrial impulses to the ventricles. This is often referred to as complete AV block.

Wenckebach sequence: the classic form of type I AV block, which would be expected to occur in the absence of autonomic influences on either the SA or AV nodes.

REFERENCES

1. Johnson RL, Averill KH, Lamb LE. Electrocardiographic findings in 67,375 asymptomatic individuals. VII. A-V block. Am J Cardiol 1960;6:153.
2. Van Hemelen NM, Robles de Medina EO. Electrocardiographic findings in 791 young men between the ages of 15 and 23 years; I. Arrhythmias and conduction disorders. (Dutch). Ned Tijdschr Geneeskd 1975; 119:45–52.
3. Erikssen J, Otterstad JE. Natural course of a prolonged PR interval and the relation between PR and incidence of coronary heart disease. A 7-year follow-up study of 1832 apparently healthy men aged 40–59 years. Clin Cardiol 1984;7:6–13.
4. Damato AN, Lau SH. Clinical value of the electrogram of the conduction system. Prog Cardiovasc Dis 1970;13:119–140.
5. Narula OS. Wenckebach type I and type II atrioventricular block (revisited). Cardiovasc Clin 1974;6:137–167.
6. Young D, Eisenberg R, Fish B, et al. Wenckebach atrioventricular block (Mobitz type I) in children and adolescents. Am J Cardiol 1977;40:393–393.
7. Lenegre J. Etiology and pathology of bilateral bundle branch block in relation to complete heart block. Prog Cardiovasc Dis 1964;6:409.
8. Lepeschkin E. The electrocardiographic diagnosis of bilateral bundle branch block in relation to heart block. Prog Cardiovasc Dis 1964;6:445.
9. Rosenbaum MB, Elizari MV, Kretz A, et al. Anatomical basis of AV conduction disturbances. Geriatrics 1970;25:132–144.
10. Steiner C, Lau SH, Stein E, et al. Electrophysiological documentation of trifascicular block as the common cause of complete heart block. Am J Cardiol 1971;28: 436–441.
11. Louie EK, Maron BJ. Familial spontaneous complete heart block in hypertrophic cardiomyopathy. Br Heart J 1986;55:469–474.
12. Rotman M, Wagner GS, Waugh RA. Significance of high degree atrioventricular block in acute posterior myocardial infarction. The importance of clinical setting and mechanism of block. Circulation 1973;47:257–262.
13. Hindman MC, Wagner GS, JaRo M, et al. The clinical significance of bundle branch block complicating acute myocardial infarction. I. Clinical characteristics, hospital mortality, and one year follow-up. Circulation 1978; 58:679–688.
14. Hindman MC, Wagner GS, JaRo M, et al. The clinical significance of bundle branch block complicating acute myocardial infarction. II. Indications for temporary and permanent pacemaker insertion. Circulation 1978;58: 689–699.
15. Ho SY, Esscher E, Anderson RH, et al. Anatomy of con-

genital complete heart block and relation to maternal anti-Ro antibodies. Am J Cardiol 1986;58:291–294.

16. Brodsky M, Wu D, Denes P, et al. Arrhythmias documented by 24 hour continuous electrocardiographic monitoring in fifty male medical students without apparent heart disease. Am J Cardiol 1977;39:390–395.

17. Denes P, Levy L, Pick A, et al. The incidence of typical and atypical atrioventricular Wenckebach periodicity. Am Heart J 1975;89:26–31.

18. Narula OS. His bundle electrocardiography and clinical electrophysiology. Philadelphia: FA Davis, 1975:146–160.

CHAPTER 21

Artificial Cardiac Pacemakers

Wesley K. Haisty, Jr.
Scott A. Robertson
Galen S. Wagner

Artificial cardiac pacemakers are most commonly used in the management of symptomatic bradyarrhythmias caused by abnormal cardiac impulse formation or conduction.[1,2] Pacemakers may also be used in patients with tachyarrhythmias when: (a) necessary pharmacologic therapy carries a risk of causing bradyarrhythmias; or (b) electrical stimuli are required to stop the tachyarrhythmia. In the latter situation, a device with the added capability of *defibrillation* may be required.[3,4]

Figure 21.1 illustrates the components of an implantable artificial pacemaking system. Electronic impulses originate from a *pulse generator* surgically placed subcutaneously in the pectoral area, and which is connected to transvenous leads with small electrodes mounted at their distal ends. These electrodes are positioned adjacent to the endocardial surfaces of the right atrium and right ventricle. Temporary pacing can be achieved with an external pulse generator connected either to transvenous leads positioned like those for permanent pacing or to large precordial electrodes (Zoll device). After open heart surgery, temporary epicardial electrodes may be placed on the atria or ventricles.

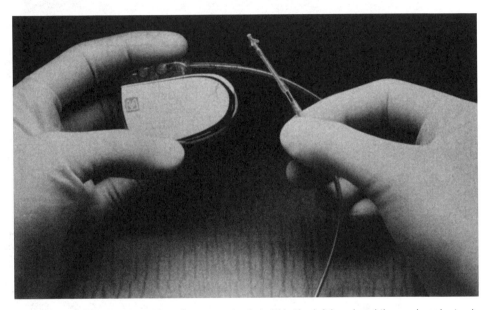

Figure 21.1. The implantable pulse generator is held in the left hand and the pacing electrode in the right.

BASIC CONCEPTS OF THE ARTIFICIAL PACEMAKER

When the cardiac rhythm is initiated by the impulses from an artificial pacemaker, *pacemaker artifacts* can usually be detected on an electrocardiogram (ECG) recording as positively or negatively directed vertical lines, as indicated by arrows in Figure 21.2. Fixed-rate pacing of the ventricles (Fig. 21.2*A*) and the atria (Fig. 21.2*B*) is illustrated. Note that this pacing system has no capability of "sensing" the patient's intrinsic rhythms, and continues to generate impulses despite the resumption of sinus rhythm. Thus, the patient's sinus rhythm (Fig. 21.2*A*) is competing with a fixed-rate ventricular pacemaker. The regular rhythm of the pacemaker spikes is not disturbed by the intrinsic beats of the heart. The atrial pacemaker (Fig. 21.2*B*) competes with sinus rhythm and initiates atrial premature beats (APBs) that fail to conduct until the fourth APB impulse conducts with a long PR interval. Modern pacemakers contain sophisticated sensing capabilities, and "fixed-rate" systems such as that just described are no longer used.

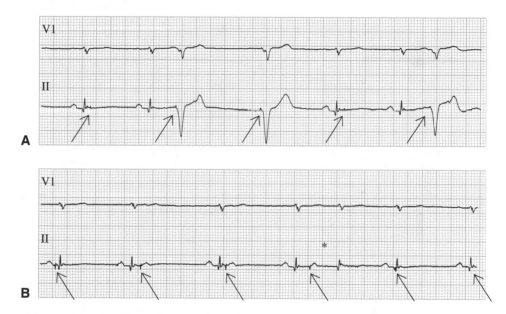

Figure 21.2. Lead-V1 and -II rhythm strips from a 73-year-old man undergoing electrophysiologic study for ventricular arrhythmias to demonstrate the function of fixed rate ventricular (**A**) and atrial (**B**) pacing systems. *Arrows* indicate the very small pacing artifacts at a rate of 50 beats/min occurring continuously in competition with sinus rhythm. In **A**, the second, third, and fifth pacemaker impulses capture the ventricles, while in **B** the second, third, and fourth impulses capture the atria, and the final artificially paced P wave is conducted to the ventricles with a prolonged PR interval (*asterisk*).

As illustrated in Figure 21.3, the amplitude of pacemaker artifacts in the ECG varies among leads, and the artifacts may not be apparent at all in a single-lead recording. The pacing artifacts are prominent in many leads (V2 to V6) but minimal in others, and entirely absent in lead II. If only lead II were observed, there would be no evidence that the cardiac rhythm was artificially generated. The amplitude of the pacing spike also depends on the programmed output and configuration of the pacing system. The amplitude of the spike is increased when unipolar pacing is used, and may vary from beat to beat when digital ECG recording systems are used (as illustrated in Figure 21.3).

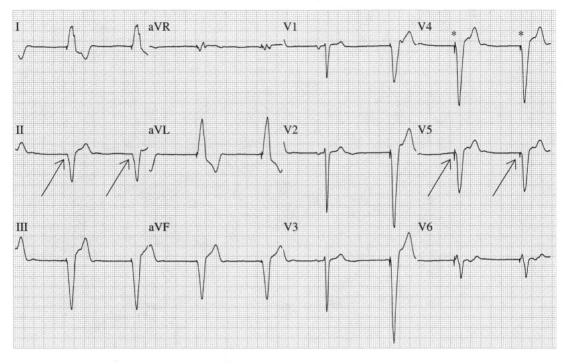

Figure 21.3. A 12-lead ECG from a 67-year-old woman with a permanent transvenous pacemaker for treatment of sick sinus syndrome. *Arrows* indicate the contrasting prominent (lead V5) and absent (lead II) pacing artifacts in different leads, and *asterisks* indicate the varying artifact amplitudes in a single lead (V4) characteristic of digital ECG recordings.

All current artificial pacemakers have a built-in standby or *demand mode* because the rhythm disturbances that require their use may occur intermittently.[5] Figure 21.4 illustrates an example of a normally functioning demand pacemaker. In this mode, the device senses the heart's intrinsic impulses and does not generate artificial impulses while the intrinsic rate exceeds the rate set for the pulse generator. If the intrinsic pacing rate falls below the set artificial pacing rate, all cardiac cycles are initiated by the artificial pacemaker, and no evaluation of its sensing function is possible. In this example, the pacemaker cycle length is 840 msec (0.84 second). Intrinsic beats occur in leads aVR, aVL, and aVF, and in the lead-V1 rhythm strip, and are appropriately sensed by the demand pacemaker.

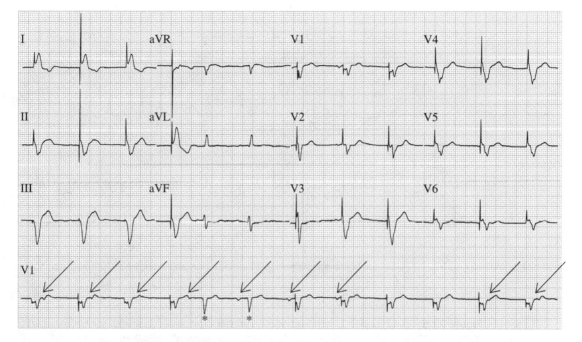

Figure 21.4. A 12-lead ECG and lead-V1 rhythm strip from a 76-year-old man with an implanted demand ventricular pacemaker admitted to the hospital with acute chest pain. *Arrows* in the lead-V1 rhythm strip indicate the P waves of the patient's intrinsic sinus rhythm, and *asterisks* indicate the QRS complexes of intrinsic ventricular activation that inhibit impulse generation from the demand pacemaker. Note the prolonged PR interval (0.32 second) required for the first intrinsic ventricular activation.

If the intrinsic rate is greater than that of the artificial pacemaker, the pacing capability of the demand device may not be detectable on an ECG recording. The activity of the device can only be observed when a bradyarrhythmia occurs (Fig. 21.5) or when a magnet is applied. The magnet converts the pacemaker to fixed-rate pacing. Most current pacemakers will also increase their pacing rate during magnet application, to minimize competition with the patient's intrinsic rhythm. In the example shown in Figure 21.5, the patient's sinus bradycardia is interrupted by magnet application, causing an increase in the pacemaker rate to 100 beats/min.

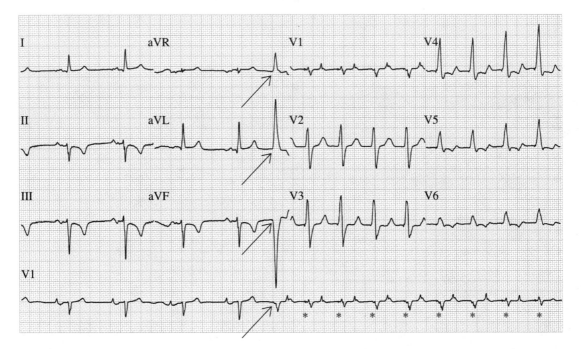

Figure 21.5. A 12-lead ECG and lead-V1 rhythm strip from an 87-year-old woman who had a demand ventricular pacemaker inserted for recurrent presyncopal episodes resulting from high-degree AV-nodal block. Because the symptoms were intermittent, a low pacemaker rate of 50 beats/min was programmed to preserve the patient's intrinsic sinus rhythm. Magnet application (*arrows*) causes fixed-rate pacing (extremely small pacing artifacts are visible in lead V3) at 100 beats/min. The rapid magnet-induced pacing rate (*asterisks* on the lead-V1 rhythm strip) prevents competition with the intrinsic rhythm. Note the P waves following the pacemaker-induced QRS complexes, indicating 1:1 ventricular-to-atrial conduction.

PACEMAKER MODES AND DUAL-CHAMBER PACING

 The North American Society of Pacing and Electrophysiology Mode Code Committee and the British Pacing and Electrophysiology Group jointly developed the NASPE/BGEP Generic (NBG) Code for artificial pacemakers.[6] This code, presented in Table 21.1 and described below, includes three letters to designate the bradycardia functions of a pacemaker, a fourth letter to indicate the pacemaker's programmability and rate modulation, and a fifth letter to indicate the presence of one or more anti-tachyarrhythmia functions.

The first three letters of the NBG code can be easily remembered by ranking pacemaker functions from most to least important. Pacing is the most important function of such an instrument, followed by sensing and then by the response of the pacemaker to a sensed event. The first letter designates the cardiac chamber(s) that the instrument paces. The second letter designates the chamber(s) that the pacemaker senses. Entries for pacing and sensing include "A" for atrium, "V" for ventricle, "D" for dual (atrium and ventricle) and "O" for none. The third letter in the NBG code designates the response to sensed events. Entries for this third letter include "I" for inhibited, "D" for both triggered and inhibited, and "O" for none. The fourth letter describes two different functions: (a) the degree of programmability of the pacemaker ("M" for multiprogrammability, "P" for simple programmability, and "O" for no programmability) and (b) the presence of rate responsiveness ("R" for the presence, and omission of a fourth letter for the absence of rate responsiveness). The fifth letter of the NBG code is seldom used.

Commonly used pacemakers include those with the VVI, AAI, and DDD modes, with VVIR, AAIR, and DDDR designating the rate-modulated modes.[7] VVI pacemakers (Figs. 21.3, 21.4, and 21.5) pace the ventricle, sense the ventricle, and are inhibited by sensed intrinsic events. These instruments represent the classic ventricular demand pacemaker that paces at the programmed rate unless the instrument senses intrinsic ventricular activity at a faster rate. The VVI pacemaker has only a single rate (usually called the minimum rate) to be programmed. By analogy with VVI pacemakers, AAI pacemakers pace the atrium, sense the atrium, and are inhibited by sensed atrial beats. AAI pacemakers also have only a single programmable rate.

Table 21.1. The NASPE/BPEG Generic (NBG) Pacemaker Code

Position	I	II	III	IV	V
Category	Chamber(s) paced	Chamber(s) sensed	Response to sensing	Programmability, rate modulation	Antitachyarrhythmia function(s)
	0 = None	0 = None	0 = None	0 = None	0 = None
	A = Atrium	A = Atrium	T = Triggered	P = Simple Programmable	P = Pacing (antitachyarrhythmia)
	V = Ventricle	V = Ventricle	I = Inhibited	M = Multiprogrammable	S = Shock
	D = Dual	D = Dual	D = Dual	C = Communicating	D = Dual
	(A + V)	(A + V)	(T + I)	R = Rate Modulation	(P + S)

Note: Positions I through III are used exclusively for antibradyarrhythmia function.

DDD pacemakers pace both the atria and ventricles and sense atrial and ventricular impulses. They are *triggered* by P waves to pace the ventricle at the programmed atrioventricular (AV) interval, and are *inhibited* by ventricular sensing to not compete with the patient's underlying rhythm. DDD pacing varies according to the patient's underlying atrial rate. If the patient's atrial rate is below the minimum tracking rate in the DDD mode, the pacemaker will show "minimum rate behavior," pacing both the atrium and the ventricle (Fig. 21.6*A*). If the sinus rate is above the minimum rate in the DDD mode, the pacemaker will track atrial activity and pace the ventricle at the programmed AV interval (Fig.21.6*B*). To prevent tracking of rapid atrial rhythms, the DDD pacemaker requires a programmed maximum tracking rate. More rapid atrial rates will be sensed, but ventricular pacing will be limited to the programmed upper tracking rate ("maximum-rate behavior") (Fig.21.6*C*). If the pacemaker is programmed appropriately, AV intervals following the sensed atrial activity will vary, and will resemble those in AV-nodal block.

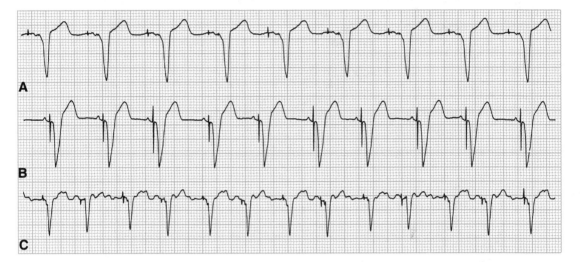

Figure 21.6. Three lead-V1 rhythm strips from a 78-year-old woman with a history of both sick sinus syndrome and atrial flutter. These examples indicate **A:** atrial and ventricular minimum-rate-behavior pacing; **B:** ventricular pacing at the atrially tracked rate with the programmed AV interval; and **C:** ventricular pacing at varying intervals following sensed atrial flutter waves exhibiting maximum-rate behavior.

Figure 21.7 shows the normal function of three DDD pacemakers when the atrial rate is above the programmed minimum rate and below the programmed maximal tracking rate of the pacemaker. The DDD pacemaker is best understood by knowing that it approximates normal AV function and conduction, and that its function closely approximates normal cardiac physiology. The AV intervals provided by DDD pacemakers may shorten with an increased pacing rate. The DDD pacemaker will track both sinus arrhythmia and APBs (Fig. 21.7A), and will sense and be reset by ventricular premature beats (VPBs) (Fig. 21.7B). The pacemaker may lengthen the AV interval for closely coupled APBs, but may not sense very closely coupled APBs when they occur in its atrial refractory period (Fig. 21.7C).

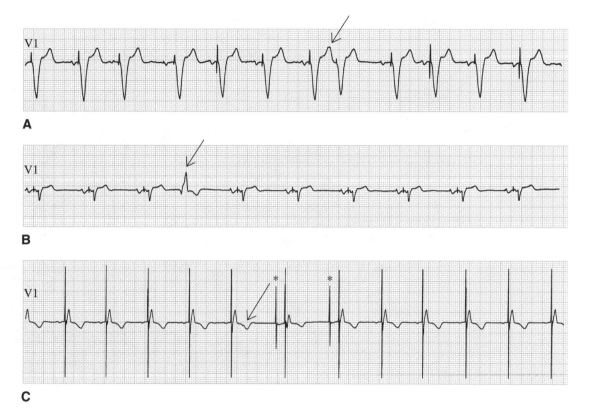

Figure 21.7. Lead-V1 rhythm strips from three patients with syncope due to intermittent AV block followed in a pacemaker clinic. *Arrows* indicate in **A:** a sensed APB occurring at the peak of a T wave, triggering ventricular pacing; **B:** a sensed VPB resetting the pacemaker; and **C:** an unsensed APB occurring before the T wave and thus within the pacemaker's atrial refractory period. *Asterisks* in **C** indicate minimum-rate AV pacing following the APB-induced pause and continuing until intrinsic sinus rhythm exceeds this minimum pacing rate.

VVIR and DDDR pacemakers have the capacity for rate modulation by having their minimum rate automatically increased through an activity sensor. Common sensors include a piezoelectric crystal (activity), accelerometer (body movement), or impedance sensing device (sensing of respiratory rate or minute ventilation). Pacemakers with rate modulation have programmed maximal sensor rates and may have programmable parameters for sensitivity and rate of response.

DDDR pacing and modulation of the minimum rate through sensor activity is shown in Figure 21.8A. Consecutive beats with both atrial and ventricular pacing confirm minimum-rate pacing. The minimum rate has been "modulated" and increased to 84 beats/min as a result of sensor activity. Figure 21.8B shows the same pacemaker tracking the same patient's sinus rhythm at a rate faster than that with the sensor-driven pacing shown in Figure 21.8A. Thus, the DDDR pacemaker can increase the rate of ventricular pacing either through an increased rate of atrial pacing driven by the sensor, or through sensing of an increased intrinsic sinus rate. Maximal sensor rate and maximal tracking rate may be independently programmed in dual-chamber pacemakers.

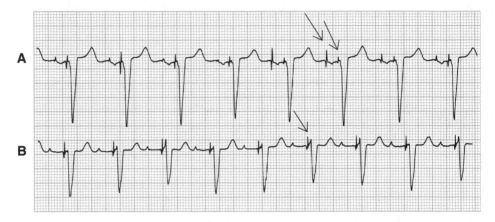

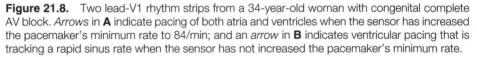

Figure 21.8. Two lead-V1 rhythm strips from a 34-year-old woman with congenital complete AV block. *Arrows* in **A** indicate pacing of both atria and ventricles when the sensor has increased the pacemaker's minimum rate to 84/min; and an *arrow* in **B** indicates ventricular pacing that is tracking a rapid sinus rate when the sensor has not increased the pacemaker's minimum rate.

Pacemaker systems may include antitachycardia pacing (ATP), but current practice usually limits ATP to supraventricular tachyarrhythmias. However, Figure 21.9 presents an example of the use of ATP to terminate a monomorphic ventricular tachycardia.

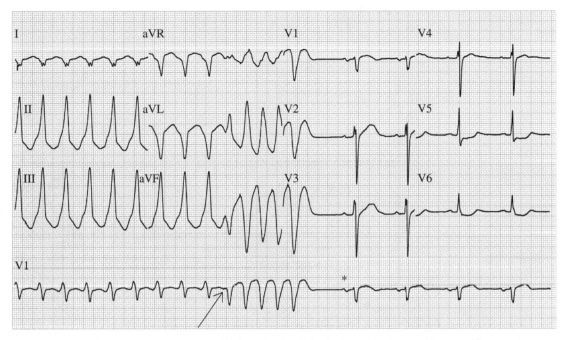

Figure 21.9. A 12-lead ECG and a lead-V1 rhythm strip from a 61-year-old man who presented to the emergency room with brief episodes of palpitations and dizziness that were less severe than those before pacemaker implantation. This recording was begun immediately after recurrence of symptoms. A monomorphic ventricular tachycardia at a rate of 130 beats/min was documented. An *arrow* indicates the beginning of a five-beat pacing train that terminates the tachycardia (the very small pacing artifacts are visible in lead aVF). An *asterisk* indicates the return of sinus rhythm.

ATP for ventricular tachycardia is usually included in an implantable cardioverter defibrillator (ICD). This complex device protects the patient from acceleration of a tachyarrhythmia or even induction of ventricular fibrillation as a complication of ATP. As seen in Figure 21.10, ICD systems incorporating ATP also include AV sequential pacing to protect against bradyarrhythmias.

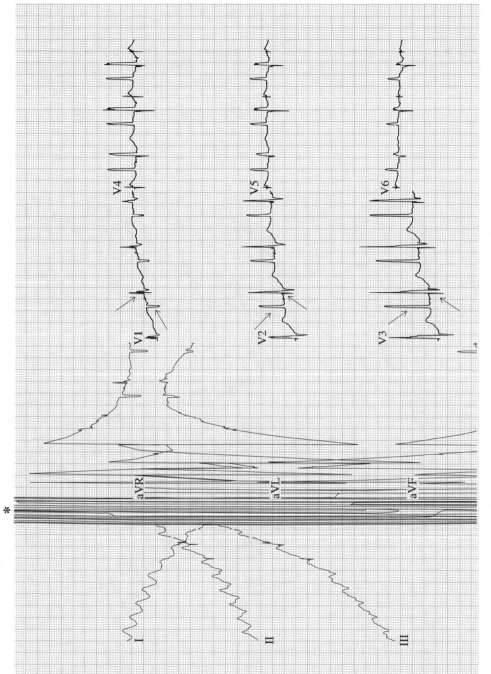

Figure 21.10. A 12-lead ECG from a 69-year-old man during testing of ICD function under anesthesia. A polymorphic ventricular tachycardia at a rate of 250 beats/min had been induced. The high-energy ICD artifact (*asterisk*) terminates the tachycardia. *Arrows* indicate the return of dual-chamber pacing. The atrial pacing artifacts have been distorted by the ICD discharge.

PACEMAKER EVALUATION

The initial aspect of evaluation of any pacemaker system is the assessment of its pacing and sensing functions. Pacing failure is indicated by the absence of atrial or ventricular capture after a pacing artifact, and a pacemaker system may also exhibit either under- or oversensing.

Figure 21.11 shows the typical appearance of failure of both the pacing and sensing functions of a pacemaker. Only a single incidence of ventricular capture occurs. Failure of the sensing function is apparent from the absence of pacemaker inhibition by the patient's intrinsic ventricular beats.

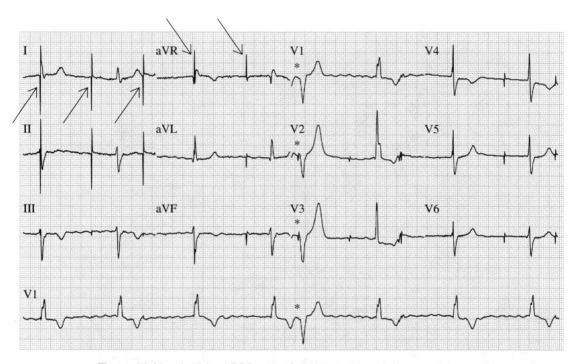

Figure 21.11. A 12-lead ECG with a lead-V1 rhythm strip from an 84-year-old man who returned to a pacemaker clinic with dizziness 11 years after implantation of a VVI pacemaker. *Arrows* show pacing artifacts continuing regularly (68/min) not sensing for the patient's intrinsic beats and not producing paced beats. The *asterisks* indicate the single incidence of ventricular capture by the pacemaker.

The evaluation of dual-chamber pacing systems must assess both atrial and ventricular capture and sensing.[8] Figure 21.12 demonstrates failure only of atrial capture; the ventricular pacing function is intact. Effective atrial sensing is indicated by the tracking of the first two sinus beats, with ventricular pacing at the sinus rate. Effective ventricular sensing is indicated by inhibition of ventricular pacing after the VPB.

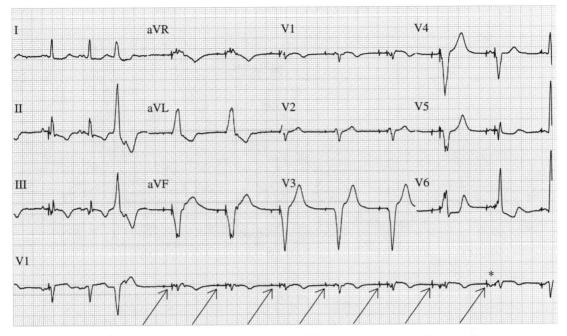

Figure 21.12. A 12-lead ECG with a lead-V1 rhythm strip from a 73-year-old man seen in a pacemaker clinic 6 months after implantation of a DDD pacemaker. During the pause after the VPB, minimum-rate pacing occurs (*the first six arrows*), but with failure of atrial capture. An *asterisk* and the *last arrow* indicate the single incidence of atrial capture by the pacemaker.

Figure 21.13 shows three examples of sensing dysfunction: atrial undersensing (Fig. 21.13A) and ventricular oversensing (Fig. 21.13B and C). In normal pacemaker function, ventricular sensing inhibits the pacemaker activity and atrial sensing triggers the pacemaker activity. The failure of atrial sensing in Figure 21.13A causes failure of the P wave (arrow) to trigger ventricular activity. The abnormal sensing of either skeletal muscle activity (Fig. 21.13B) or noise from a broken lead (Fig. 21.13C) pathologically inhibits the pacemaker activity.

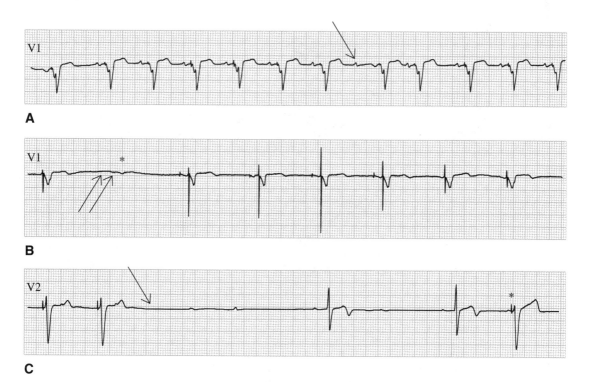

Figure 21.13. Lead-V1 rhythm strips from three patients complaining of palpitations several years after pacemaker implantation; a DDD device was present in **A** and **B** and a VVI device in **C**. The arrow in **A** indicates the single undersensed P wave. The *arrows* in **B** show the expected locations of the atrial and ventricular pacing artifacts. The absence of both artifacts is caused by abnormal sensing of pectoralis muscle activity via the ventricular lead. An *asterisk* indicates a P wave that fails to conduct because of the patient's underlying AV block. The *arrow* in **C** shows the expected location of the next ventricular pacing artifact. The prolonged pause (continuing for more than 6 seconds) is typical of abnormal sensing occurring with broken pacemaker leads. The reappearance (*asterisk*) of the pacing artifact indicates that the lead break is only intermittent.

"Failure to sense" may be incorrectly suspected when the pacing system has not had sufficient time to sense an intrinsic beat.[9,10] This occurs when the patient's intrinsic rate is similar to the instrument's minimum pacing rate, as in Figure 21.14. A period of more than 0.04 second is required for intrinsic activation to reach the pacemaker lead in the right-ventricular apex and to be sensed by the pacemaker. The apparent abnormality in fact represents normal pacemaker function.

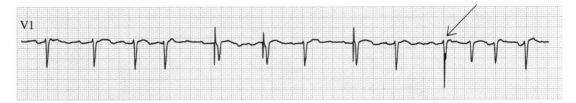

Figure 21.14. An arrhythmia service was consulted for suspected pacemaker malfunction in a 79-year-old woman, indicated by this lead-V1 rhythm recording. The rhythm is atrial fibrillation with intermittent slowing and ventricular pacing. Pacemaker artifacts occur intermittently. An *arrow* shows the pacemaker artifact 0.04 second into an intrinsic QRS complex.

At times, both the pacing and sensing functions of a pacemaker may occur normally in patients with symptoms that are typically associated with pacemaker dysfunction. Figure 21.15 documents normal pacing by a VVI pacemaker. Absence of competing intrinsic activity prevents evaluation of the instrument's sensing function. However the occurrence of 1:1 ventricular-to-atrial conduction leads to the clinical probability that *pacemaker syndrome*[11]—vasovagal syncope caused by atrial dilation produced by the occurrence of atrial contraction during ventricular contraction—is causing the patient's symptoms.

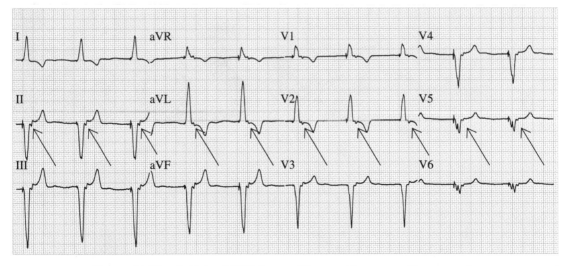

Figure 21.15. A 12-lead ECG from a 63-year-old woman with recurrent syncope several months after implantation of a VVI pacemaker. The *arrows* show the retrograde P waves of 1:1 ventricular-to-atrial conduction that may be associated with a pacemaker syndrome.

In Figure 21.16, both the pacemaker's pacing and sensing functions are evident. However, reversal of the atrial and ventricular leads during their connection to the temporary pacemaker becomes obvious from observing ventricular capture by the initial rather than the second of each pair of pacing artifacts.

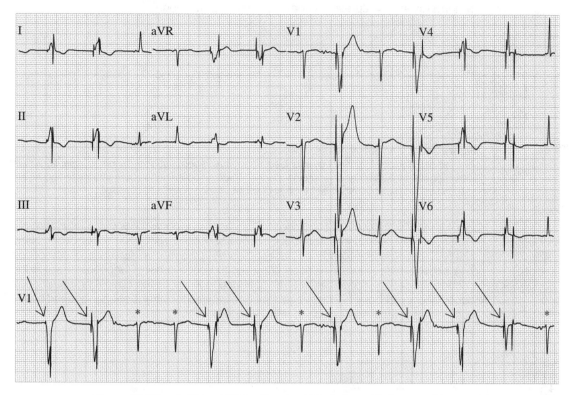

Figure 21.16. A 12-lead ECG with a lead-V1 rhythm strip from an 84-year-old woman at 20 minutes after admission to the recovery room after mitral valve replacement. The pacemaker service was consulted because of the patient's unusual ECG appearance and mild hypotension. *Arrows* show effective ventricular capture by the first of two closely coupled pacing artifacts. The second of each of the pairs occurs either in the QRS complex or in the ST segment of the paced beats. *Asterisks* indicate five intrinsic beats that inhibit the pacemaker, proving normal ventricular sensing function.

MYOCARDIAL LOCATION OF THE PACING ELECTRODE

The spread within the heart of the wavefronts of depolarization from a pacemaker depends on the location of the stimulating electrode. Currently, most endocardial electrodes are positioned near the right ventricular apex. This produces sequential right- and then left-ventricular activation, and therefore a left bundle-branch block pattern on the ECG. As activation proceeds from the right ventricular apex toward the base, the frontal axis is superior producing extreme LAD (Fig. 21.17A). Endocardial electrodes placed in the right-ventricular outflow tract produce activation beginning at the base and directed inferiorly. The frontal axis is then vertical (Fig. 21.17B).

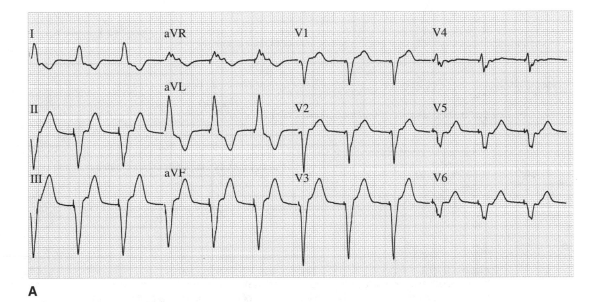

A

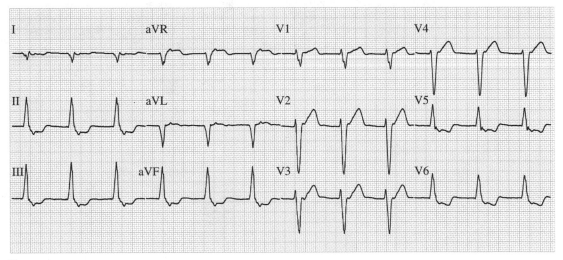

B

Figure 21.17. Twelve-lead ECGs obtained at the time of pacemaker implantation in a 61-year-old man with a history of syncope. The ECG shown in **A** was recorded during pacing of the right-ventricular apex, and the ECG in **B** was recorded during pacing of the right-ventricular outflow tract.

Left-ventricular epicardial electrodes or electrodes placed in the distal coronary sinus pace the left ventricle. This produces sequential left- and then right-ventricular activation, and therefore a right bundle-branch block pattern on the ECG. Usually, pacing a single ventricle produces a wide QRS complex, but pacing of both ventricles simultaneously may narrow the QRS complex, as seen in Figure 21.18.

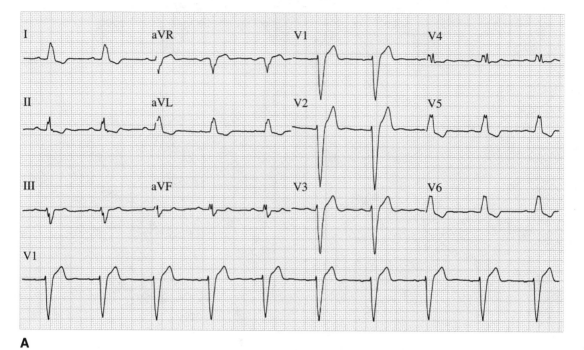

A

Figure 21.18. Three 12-lead ECGs with lead-V1 rhythm strips from a 54-year-old man with heart failure caused by cardiomyopathy and LBBB, with a QRS duration of 190 msec **(A)**. Recordings **(B** and **C)** were obtained at the time of implantation of a DDD pacemaker with pacing electrodes in both the right-ventricular apex and distal coronary sinus. Biventricular pacing **(B)** narrowed the QRS duration from 190 msec to 155 msec. An *arrow* indicates the ventricular pacing artifact tracking sinus rhythm. Intermittent right-ventricular pacing alone **(C)** extended the QRS duration to 210 msec *(asterisks)*, in contrast to the biventricular pacing effect.

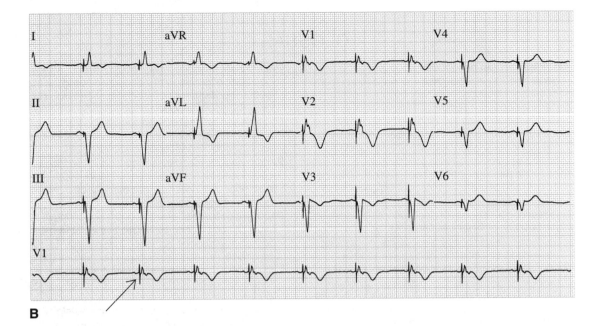

B

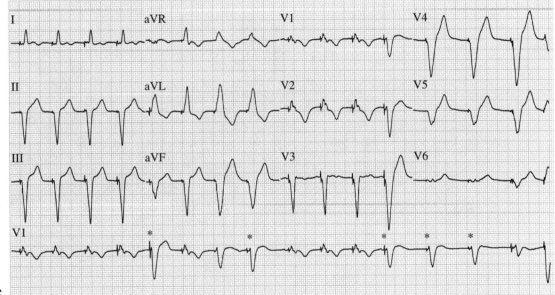

C

Figure 21.18. *(continued).*

GLOSSARY

Artificial cardiac pacemakers: devices capable of generating electrical impulses and delivering them to the myocardium.

Defibrillation: termination of either atrial or ventricular fibrillation by an extrinsic electrical current.

Demand mode: a term describing an artificial pacemaking system with the ability to sense and be inhibited by intrinsic cardiac activity.

Fixed-rate pacing: artificial pacing with the capability only to generate an electrical impulse, without sensing of the heart's intrinsic rhythm.

Oversensing: abnormal function of an artificial pacemaker in which electrical signals other than those representing activation of the myocardium are sensed and inhibit impulse generation.

Pacemaker-induced tachyarrhythmia: a rapid heart rate produced by an artificial pacemaker. A paced impulse occurring when the myocardium is vulnerable to induction of a reentrant circuit because it is just emerging from total refractoriness.

Pacemaker-mediated tachyarrhythmia: a rapid heart rate occurring with a dual-chambered pacing system, using intrinsic VA conduction and artificially paced AV conduction.

Pacemaker artifacts: high-frequency signals appearing on an ECG and representing impulses generated by an artificial pacemaker.

Pacemaker syndrome: a reduction in cardiac output caused by activation by an artificial pacemaker that does not produce an optimally efficient sequence of myocardial activation.

Pacing electrodes: electrodes that, in contrast to the electrodes used to record the ECG, are designed to transmit an electrical impulse to the myocardium. In pacing systems with sensing capability, these electrodes also transmit the intrinsic impulses of the heart to the pacemaking device.

Pulse generator: a device that produces electrical impulses as the key component of an artificial pacing system.

REFERENCES

1. Furman S, et al. A practice of cardiac pacing. New York: Futura, 1986.
2. Gillette PC, Griffin JC. Practical cardiac pacing. Baltimore: Williams & Wilkins, 1986.
3. Dreifus LS, Fisch C, Griffin JC, et al. Guidelines for implantation of cardiac pacemakers and antiarrhythmia devices. A report of the American College of Cardiology/American Heart Association Task Force on Assessment of Diagnostic and Therapeutic Cardiovascular Procedures (Committee on Pacemaker Implantation). Circulation 1991; 84:455–467.
4. Wood M, Ellenbogen KA. Bradyarrhythmias, emergency pacing, and implantable defibrillation devices. Crit Care Clin 1989;5:551–568.
5. Barold SS. Modern cardiac pacing. New York: Futura, 1985.
6. Bernstein AD, Camm AJ, Fletcher RD, et al. NASPE/BPEG Generic pacemaker code for antibradyarrhythmia and adaptive-rate pacing and antitachyarrhythmia devices. Pace 1987;10:794–799.
7. Bernstein AD, Parsonnet V. Survey of cardiac pacing in the United States in 1989. Am J Cardiol 1992;69:331–338.
8. Barold SS, Falkoff MD, Ong LS, et al. The third decade of cardiac pacing: multiprogrammable pulse generators. Br Heart J 1981;45:357–364.
9. Castellanos A Jr, Agha AS, Befeler B, et al. A study of arrival of excitation at selected ventricular sites during human bundle branch block using close bipolar catheter electrodes. Chest 1973;63:208–213.
10. Vera Z, Mason DT, Awan NA, et al. Lack of sensing by demand pacemakers due to intraventricular conduction defects. Circulation 1975;51:815–822.
11. Furman S. The present status of cardiac pacing. Herz 1991;16:171–181.

CHAPTER 22

Dr. Marriott's Systematic Approach to the Diagnosis of Arrhythmias

DR. MARRIOTT'S SYSTEMATIC APPROACH TO THE DIAGNOSIS OF ARRHYTHMIAS

Dr. Marriott evolved the following approach to the analysis of arrhythmias during his first eight editions of *Practical Electrocardiography*: Regarding this approach, he observed that "After analyzing the reasons for the mistakes I have made and those that I have repeatedly watched others make, this system is designed to avoid the common errors of omission and commission. Undoubtedly, we make most mistakes because of failure to apply reason and logic, not because of ignorance."

Many disturbances of rhythm and conduction are recognizable at first glance. Supraventricular arrhythmias are characterized by normal QRS complexes (unless complicated by aberrant ventricular conduction), while ventricular arrhythmias produce bizarre QRS complexes with prolonged QRS intervals. One can usually also immediately spot atrial flutter with 4:1 conduction or atrial fibrillation with a rapid ventricular response (Chapter 15, "Reentrant Atrial Tachyarrhythmias—The Atrial Flutter/Fibrillation Spectrum"). However, if the diagnosis fails to fall into your lap, then the systematic approach is in order.

The steps in the systematic approach are as follows:

Know the Causes of the Arrhythmia

The first step in any medical diagnosis is to know the causes of the presenting symptom. For example, if you want to be a superb headache specialist, the first step is to learn the 50 causes of a headache—which are the common ones, which are the uncommon ones, and how to differentiate between them. This is because "you see only what you look for, you recognize only what you know."[1] Knowing the causes of the various cardiac arrhythmias is part of the equipment that you carry with you and are prepared to use when faced with an unidentified arrhythmia.

Milk the QRS Complex

When a specific arrhythmia confronts you, you should first "milk" the QRS complex. There are two reasons for this. The first is an extension of the Willie Sutton law: "I robbed banks because that's where the money is." Second, milking the QRS complex keeps us in the healthy frame of mind of giving priority to ventricular behavior. It matters comparatively little what the atria are doing, as long as the ventricles are behaving normally. If the QRS complex is of normal duration in at least two leads of the electrocardiogram (ECG) (Fig. 22.1), then the rhythm is supraventricular. If the QRS complex is wide and bizarre, you are faced with the decision of whether this is of supraventricular origin with ventricular aberration, or whether it is of ventricular origin. If you know your QRS waveform morphology, you know what to look for and you will recognize it if you see it.

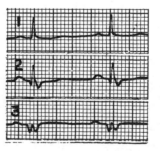

Figure 22.1. In lead I (*1*), the QRS complex appears to be of normal duration, but leads II (*2*) and III (*3*) reveal the true duration of the complex to be 0.12 second.

During the past four decades, the diagnostic morphology of the ventricular complex has come into its own. This began with clinical observation and deduction in which acute coronary-care nurses played an important role.[2-6] These observations have been confirmed by electrophysiologic studies by Wellens and his colleagues, who found that inspection of the pattern of the QRS complex in the clinical ECG tracing afforded the correct diagnosis in 52 of 56 consecutive cases of wide-QRS tachycardia.[7] Despite the availability, simplicity, and accuracy of this method, some authorities persist in ignoring its potential.[8,9]

Cherchez le P

If the answer to the source of an arrhythmia is not provided by the shape of the QRS complex, the next step is "cherchez (look for) le P." In the past, the P wave has certainly been overemphasized as the key to arrhythmias. A lifelong love affair with the P wave has afflicted many an electrocardiographer with the so-called "P preoccupation syndrome." However, there are times when the P wave holds an important diagnostic clue and must therefore be accorded the starring role.

In one's search for P waves, there are several clues and caveats to bear in mind. One technique that may be useful is to employ an alternate lead placement (Chapter 2, "Recording the Electrocardiogram") with the positive electrode at the fifth right intercostal space close to the sternum, and the negative electrode on the manubrium. This will sometimes greatly magnify the P wave, rendering it readily visible when it is virtually indiscernible in other leads. Figure 22.2 illustrates this amplifying effect and makes the diagnosis of atrial tachycardia with 2:1 block immediately apparent. If it succeeds, this technique is a great deal kinder to the patient than introducing an atrial wire or an esophageal electrode to corral elusive P waves.

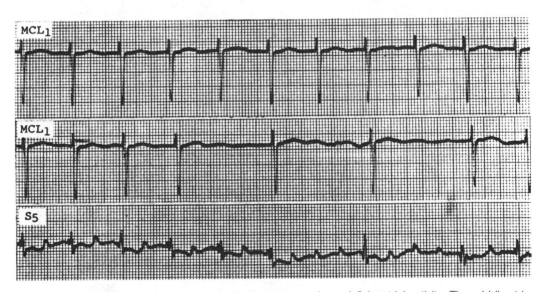

Figure 22.2. The top rhythm strip does not reveal any definite atrial activity. The middle strip shows the effect of carotid sinus stimulation with decreased AV conduction following the fourth QRS complex revealing the slightly irregular baseline typical of fine atrial fibrillation. In contrast, there is obvious atrial activity following the sixth QRS complex in the bottom strip, identifying an atrial tachyarrhythmia (probably PAT) with delayed AV conduction. However, the P waves are halfway between the QRS complexes and, indeed, carotid sinus massage reveals additional P waves concealed within each QRS complex.

Another clue to the incidence of P waves is contained in the "Bix rule," named after the Baltimore cardiologist Harold Bix, who observed: "Whenever the P waves of a supraventricular tachycardia are halfway between the ventricular complexes, you should always suspect that additional P waves are hiding within the QRS complex."

In the top strip of Figure 22.3, the P wave is halfway between the QRS complexes and is therefore a good candidate for the Bix rule. It may be necessary to apply carotid sinus stimulation or another vagal maneuver to bring the alternate atrial waves out of the QRS complex. In the case in Figure 22.3, however, the patient obligingly altered his conduction pattern (middle strip) and spontaneously exposed the flutter waves. It is clearly important to know whether there are twice as many atrial impulses as are apparent, because there is the ever-present danger that the ventricular rate may double or almost double, especially if the atrial rate were to slow somewhat. It is better to be forewarned and take steps to prevent such potentially disastrous acceleration.

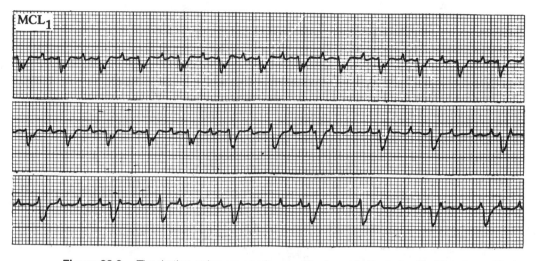

Figure 22.3. The rhythm strips are continuous. The top strip illustrates the Bix rule, and in the middle strip the AV conduction spontaneously decreases, revealing that the atrial rate is twice the ventricular rate.

The "haystack principle" can be of great diagnostic importance when you are searching for difficult-to-find P waves. When you have to find a needle in a haystack, you would obviously prefer a small haystack. Therefore, whenever you are faced with the problem of finding elusive items, always give the lead that shows the least disturbance of the ECG baseline (the smallest ventricular complex) a chance to help you. Some leads would intuitively seem not to be helpful when trying to identify the source of an arrhythmia (e.g., lead aVR). However, the patient whose ECG is illustrated in Figure 22.4 died because his attendants did not know or did not apply the haystack principle and make use of lead aVR. This patient had a runaway pacemaker at a discharge rate of 440 beats/min, with a halved ventricular response at 220 beats/min. Lead aVR was the lead with the smallest ventricular complex, and was the only lead in which the pacemaker blips were plainly visible (arrows). The patient went into shock and died because none of the attempted therapeutic measures affected the tachycardia when all that was necessary was to disconnect the wayward pulse generator.

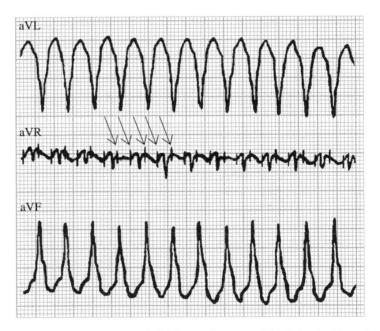

Figure 22.4. Only the prominent, wide QRS complexes are visible in leads aVL and aVF. However, in lead aVR, where the QRS complexes are much smaller, the extremely rapid rate (420 beats/min) of a "runaway" artificial pacemaker (*arrows*) with 2:1 conduction to the ventricles is revealed.

Mind Your P's

The next caveat in identifying the source of an arrhythmia is to "mind your P's." This means to be wary of things that look like P waves (Fig. 22.5), and P waves that look like other things (Fig. 22.6). This particularly applies to P-like waves that are adjacent to QRS complexes, which may turn out to be part of the QRS complexes. This is a trap for someone who suffers from the "P preoccupation syndrome," to whom anything that looks like a P wave is a P wave. Many competent ECG interpreters, given the strip of lead V1 or V2 in Figure 22.5, would promptly and confidently diagnose a supraventricular tachycardia for the wrong reasons. In lead V1, the QRS complex seems not very wide and appears to be preceded by a small P wave. In lead V2, an apparently narrow QRS complex is followed by an unmistakable retrograde P wave. However, the P-like waves in both of these leads are part of the QRS complex. If the duration of the QRS complex is measured in lead V3, it is found to be 0.14 second. In order to attain a QRS complex of that width in leads V1 and V2, the P-like waves need to be included in the measurement.

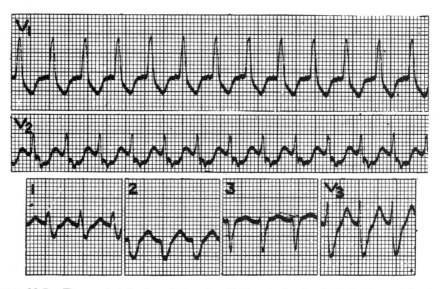

Figure 22.5. The small deflections before (lead V1) and after (lead V2) the large deflections, which are obviously from the ventricles, have the appearances of P waves. However, when the true width of the QRS complexes is revealed in leads I, II, and V3, it is apparent that the small deflections seen in leads V1 and V2 are really almost isoelectric parts of the QRS complexes.

Whenever a regular rhythm is difficult to identify, it is always worthwhile to seek and focus on any interruption in the regularity—a process that can be condensed into the three words "dig the break." It is at a break in the rhythm that you are most likely to find the solution to the source of an arrhythmia. For example, in the beginning strip of Figure 22.6, where the rhythm is regular at a rate of 200 beats/min, it is impossible to know whether the tachyarrhythmia is atrial or junctional. A third possibility is that the small positive waveform is part of the QRS complex and not a P wave at all. Further along the strip, there is a break in the rhythm, in the form of a pause. The most common cause of a pause is a nonconducted atrial premature beat (APB), and this culprit is indicated by the arrow. As a result of the pause, the mechanism of the arrhythmia is immediately obvious. When the rhythm resumes, the returning P wave is in front of the first QRS complex, indicating that the tachyarrhythmia is evidently an atrial tachycardia.

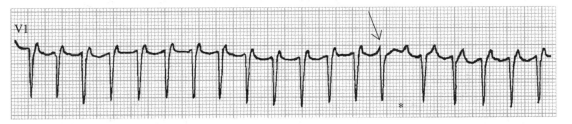

Figure 22.6. At the beginning of the rhythm strip, the small positive waveform following the large negative QRS waveform could be: (a) a part of a wide QRS complex, (b) a retrograde P wave closely following a narrow QRS complex, or (c) an anterograde P wave with prolonged conduction to a narrow QRS complex. This sequence is broken during the fourteenth cycle (*arrow*), where the beginning of a small positive waveform is seen preceding the large negative QRS waveform, and in the fifteenth cycle there is no QRS complex (*asterisk*). The pause (*asterisk*) produced by the blocked PAC is terminated by a normally conducted (PR interval = 0.20 second) beat.

Who's Married to Whom?

The next step is to establish relationships, or ask yourself "Who's married to whom?" This is often the crucial step in arriving at a firm diagnosis in a case of arrhythmia. Figure 22.7 illustrates this principle in its simplest form. A junctional rhythm is dissociated from sinus bradycardia. On three occasions, there are bizarre early beats with a qR configuration that is nondiagnostic. The early beats could be ventricular premature beats (VPBs), but the fact that they are seen only when a P wave is emerging beyond the preceding QRS complex tells us that they are "married to" the preceding P waves. This therefore establishes the beats as conducted or capture beats with atypical right bundle-branch block (RBBB) aberration.

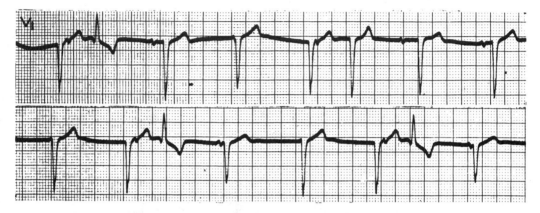

Figure 22.7. The rhythm strips are continuous. All of the early QRS complexes, but only some of the later QRS complexes, are preceded by P waves. The use of calipers reveals dissociation between the atria (which have a regular rate of about 50 beats/min) and the ventricles (the later QRS complexes have a regular rate of about 60 beats/min). The presence of P waves before each early QRS complex suggests intermittent capture of the ventricular rhythm by the atrial rhythm.

Pinpoint the Primary Diagnosis

Figure 22.8 illustrates both the previous principle and the final one: "pinpoint the primary diagnosis." One must never be content to let the diagnosis rest on a secondary phenomenon such as atrioventricular (AV) dissociation, escape, or aberration. Each of these is always secondary to some primary disturbance in rhythm that must be sought out and identified. The ECG shown in Figure 22.8 was obtained from a patient shortly after admission to a coronary care unit (CCU). The basic rhythm (Fig. 22.8A) is sinus rhythm with first- and second-degree AV block. The ECG showed wide QRS complexes that gave the CCU staff concern. One faction contended that the QRS complexes represented ventricular escape beats, while another thought they were conducted from the atria with a paradoxical aberration in the critical rate (bradycardia-dependent bundle-branch block). If you ask yourself, "Who's married to whom?" it becomes obvious that the wide QRS complexes in question are not related to the P waves. The PR intervals preceding the last two wide QRS complexes are strikingly different, measuring 0.32 and 0.20 second respectively, indicating that they are ventricular escape beats. When the patient's AV conduction improves to only occasional second-degree block (Fig. 22.8B), there is never a sufficiently long pause for an escape beat to occur. These observations pinpoint the primary diagnosis as second-degree AV block. The normal ventricular escape beats are only secondary.

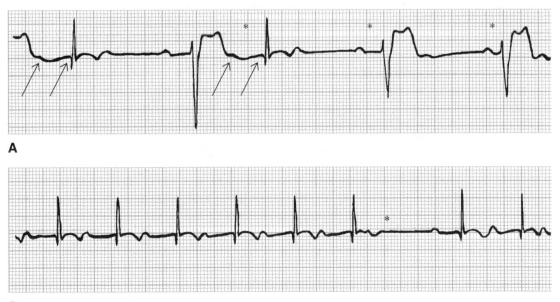

A

B

Figure 22.8. Lead-II rhythm strips from a 74-year-old woman with a recent inferior infarction. In **A,** *arrows* indicate the constant PR interval preceding each narrow QRS complex, and *asterisks* indicate the varying PR intervals preceding the wide QRS complexes. In **B,** an *asterisk* indicates the failure of conduction of P wave that identifies the single episode of second-degree AV block.

REFERENCES

1. Grodman PS. Arrhythmia surveillance by transtelephonic monitoring; comparison with Holter monitoring in symptomatic ambulatory patients. Am Heart J 1979;98: 459.
2. Judson P, Holmes DR, Baker WP. Evaluation of outpatient arrhythmias utilizing transtelephonic monitoring. Am Heart J 1979; 97:759–761.
3. Goldreyer BN. Intracardiac electrocardiography in the analysis and understanding of cardiac arrhythmias. Ann Intern Med 1972;77:117–136.
4. Brodsky M, Wu D, Denes P, et al. Arrhythmias documented by 24-hour continuous electrocardiographic monitoring in 50 male medical students without apparent heart disease. Am J Cardiol 1977;39:390–395.
5. Kantelip JP, Sage E, Duchene-Marullaz P. Findings on ambulatory monitoring in subjects older than 80 years. Am J Cardiol 1986;57:398–401.
6. Harrison DC. Contribution of ambulatory electrocardiographic monitoring to antiarrhythmic management. Am J Cardiol 1978;41:996–1004.
7. Michelson EL, Morganroth J. Spontaneous variability of complex ventricular arrhythmias detected by long-term electrocardiographic recording. Circulation 1980; 61:690–695.
8. Fleg JL, Kennedy HL. Cardiac arrhythmias in a healthy elderly population: detection by 24-hour ambulatory electrocardiography. Chest 1982;81:302–307.
9. Orth-Gomer K, Hogstedt C, Bodin L, et al. Frequency of extrasystoles in healthy male employees. Br Heart J 1986;55: 259–264.

Subject Index

Page numbers in italics denote figures; those followed by "t" denote tables.

Atrioventricular block—*continued*
proximal, 419
second-degree, 315, 408, 410–413, 418, 423, 430, 463, *463*
severity, 408
with sinus pause, 413
third-degree, 315, 408, 414–418, 430
variability of conduction times, 420, 425
Atrioventricular dissociation, 255, 293–294, 319
assessment, 392
in atrioventricular block, 416–417
causes, 416
clinical significance, 392
isoarrhythmic, 417
ventricular tachycardia and, 347, 351, 378
Atrioventricular node, 12, *140*
accelerated junctional rhythm, 293–294
atrioventricular block in, 408, *408, 413, 419, 420, 421–425, 421–425*
in atrioventricular conduction, 126, *126*
conduction in atrial fibrillation, 306
conduction in atrial flutter, 305, *312, 312–313, 313*
defined, 22
P wave, 15
PR interval and, 49
premature beats in, 259, 260
atrial, 263, 265
ventricular, 269–272
reentrant junctional tachyarrhythmias, 328, 330, 331t, 332
retrograde atrial activation, 344
tachycardia, 336, 344
forms of, 341
vs. AV-bypass tachycardia, 337–340
Automaticity, 237, 255
accelerated
accelerated atrial rhythm, 291, 297
accelerated junctional rhythm, 286t, 287, 293–294, 297, 320
accelerated ventricular rhythm, 286t, 287, 295–296, 297, 320, 346
arrhythmias, 286
atrial tachycardia, 201–202, 286t, 287
ECG characteristics, 286
rate ranges, 286, 286t
sinus tachycardia, 286t, 288–290
tachyarrhythmias, 286, 346
decreased
causes of, 397
enhancement of parasympathetic activity in, 399–400
pathologic pacemaker failure, 400–402, *400–402*
problems of, 396
sinus rate slowing in, 398
digitalis effects, 291, 320

normal, 286
problems of, 238–239
premature beats, 261, 261t
Autonomic nervous system, 68
in rate of impulse formation, 288
sinoatrial node in regulation of, 12
aV lead(s), 40
defined, 28
function, 28–29
placement, *28, 29*
voltage calculations, 29
aVF lead, 28, *28, 29, 29*
distortions due to incorrect placement, 33, *34*
T wave amplitude, 174t
aVL lead, 28, *28, 29, 29*
distortions due to incorrect placement, 33, *34*
T wave amplitude, 174t
aVR lead, 27–29, *28, 29*
Axillary line, anterior, 31, *31,* 40
Axis
in atrial enlargement, 75
defined, 68
extreme deviation, 68
left deviation, 68
P wave, 48, 65
QRS complex, 53–56
right deviation, 68
in right-ventricular hypertrophy, 79
T wave, 59–60, *60*
tilt, *4–5*

Base–apex view. *See* Long-axis recording
Base of heart, 22
Baseline negative electrical potential, 7
Baseline noise, *35*
Baseline shift, 35, *35*
Baseline wander
cause, 35
defined, 40
Bedside ECG, 36–37
Bigeminy, 259
atrial, 263, *263*
defined, 282
rule of, 383, 393
ventricular, 274, *274,* 279, *279*
Bix rule, 458
Block
complete, 240
defined, 240, 255
partial, 240
sinoatrial, 403
See also Bundle-branch blocks
Blood volume abnormalities, 72, 76, *76*
Bradyarrhythmia
of decreased automaticity, 396–397
defined, 236, 255, 398
vasovagal reaction, 399–400
Bradycardia
defined, 68
intermittent bundle-branch block and, 120, *120,* 121
sinus. *See* Sinus bradycardia
Bradycardia-dependent bundle-branch block, 391, 393

Bundle-branch blocks
aberration, 379
bilateral, 107, 121, 379
bradycardia-dependent, 120, *120, 121, 391, 393*
catheterization-induced, 117, *117*
causes, 117–118
complete, 82, 90, 97–98
ECG indications, 101, *102*
coronary atherosclerosis and, 118, *118*
critical rate in formation of, 388–390
fibrosis of Purkinje fibers and, 117
incomplete, 82, 90, 98
defined, 93
ECG indications, 101, *101*
vs. ventricular enlargement, 78, 82, 98
intermittent, 119–120
left, 90, 351
causes, 107–108
complete, 97–98
criteria, 108t
incidence of aberration, 376t
incomplete, 98
indications of, 97, *97,* 380–381
left-ventricular hypertrophy and, 113, *113,* 114
postdivisional, 107–108, 121
predivisional, 107–108, 121
with supraventricular tachycardia, 381–382
vs. ventricular enlargement, 82, 98
vs. ventricular tachycardia, 353, 354, 356, 358, *358,* 359, 360, *360*
waveform patterns, 107, *107–109,* 108, 112
paradoxical critical rate in formation of, 391
rate-dependent, 388, 393
right, 90, *244*
complete, 97–98
criteria, 101t
ECG indications, 100–101, *100–102,* 112, 378
incidence of aberration, 376t
incomplete, 98
indications of, 97, *97*
with left anterior fascicular block, 110
with left posterior fascicular block, 111
vs. ventricular tachycardia, 353, 354, 355, 356
systematic analysis, 112–115
tachycardia-dependent, 119, *119,* 388–389, 393
vs. ventricular preexcitation, 125, 133
Bundle branches, 12, *140*
accelerated automaticity, 286t
atrioventricular block in, 408, *408,* 417, 419
defined, 22
fascicular blocks in, 98–99
intraventricular conduction delay, 21, *21*

Thrombosis
   defined, 145
   epicardial injury and recovery,
      171–172, *171–172*
   ischemia in, 141
Thyroid disorders, 220–221
Thyrotoxicosis, 220, 233
Time intervals of electrical events, *17,*
   18
   determining cardiac rate and
      regularity, *46,* 46–47
   grid markings of ECG paper, 44, *44*
   P wave morphology, 48, *48*
   PR interval, 49
   QRS complex duration, 51–53, *52,*
      53
   QT interval, 62
   ST segment, 57
   T wave, 59
Torsades de pointes, 346, *346*
   defined, 233, 371
   ECG characteristics, 365
   hypokalemia and, 223
Total electrical alternans, 212, 233
TP junction, 63
   defined, 68
   in emphysema, 216
TP segment, 162
Transesophageal recording, 249
Transitional lead, *54*
   defined, 68
Transmural, defined, 145
Transtelephonic monitoring, 247, 255
Transverse plane view, *6*
   distortions due to electrode
      placement errors, 34, *34*
   lead placement, 30–32, *30–32*
   normal ECG, 33, *33*
   QRS axis, 56
   T wave axis, *60*
Triaxial reference system, 27
Tricuspid valve disease, *73*
Trigeminy, 259, 263, *263*
   defined, 282
   ventricular, 279, *279*
Triphasic, defined, 23
TU junction, 61, 63
   defined, 68

U wave, 17
   cardiac rhythm assessment, 67, *67*
   defined, 23
   in hypokalemia, 222, 223
   morphology, 61
   source, 61
   T wave fusion, 61, 63, 68
Unifascicular block, 121
   defined, 99, 100
   left fascicular, 103–106, *103–106*
   right bundle-branch block, 100–101,
      100–102

V1 lead
   distortions due to incorrect
      placement, 33, *34*
   localizing premature ventricular
      beats, 275–276, *275–277*
   modified, 40
   placement, 30–31, *30–32*

purpose, 30
QRS complex segment
   in epicardial injury, 176, *176*
   in ventricular premature beats,
      275, *275,* 282
ST segment in epicardial injury, 165,
   168, 169t, 170, *170*
T wave amplitude, 174t
V2 lead
   distortions due to incorrect
      placement, 33, *34*
   placement, 31, *31, 32*
   QRS complex segment in epicardial
      injury, *175,* 176, *176*
   ST segment in epicardial injury, 165,
      168, 169t, 170, *170*
   T wave amplitude, 174t
V3 lead
   placement, 31, *31, 32*
   QRS complex segment in epicardial
      injury, 176, *176*
   ST segment in epicardial injury, 165,
      168, 169t, 170, *170*
   T wave amplitude, 174t
V4 lead
   placement, 31, *31, 32*
   QRS complex segment in epicardial
      injury, *176*
   ST segment in epicardial injury, 168,
      170, *170*
   T wave amplitude, 174t
V5 lead
   in exercise stress testing, 37
   placement, 31, *31, 32*
   QRS complex segment in epicardial
      injury, *176*
   ST segment in epicardial injury, 168
   T wave amplitude, 174t
V6 lead
   placement, 31, *31, 32*
   QRS complex segment in epicardial
      injury, *176*
   ST segment in epicardial injury, *168*
   T wave amplitude, 174t
V lead(s)
   augmented. *See* aV lead(s)
   for continuous monitoring, 36
   defined, 27, 40
   placement, 30–32, *30–32*
   placement alternatives, 36
Vagal maneuver, 290, 297
   tachyarrhythmia assessment, 336
Vasovagal reaction, 399–400, 405
Vasovagal syncope, 405
   in pacemaker syndrome, 449, *449*
Ventricles of heart
   accelerated impulse formation,
      295–296
   cardiac impulse formation and
      conduction, 12
   defined, 23
   delayed activation, 21, *21*
   diagnostic approach, 456
   electrical events in cardiac cycle,
      17
   position of, 4, *5, 6*
   QRS complex waveforms, 16, 18,
      20, *20*
   T wave, 17

Ventricular aberrancy
   atrial activity preceding, 379, *379*
   with atrial flutter/fibrillation, 382–387,
      382–387
   bilateral, 387
   causes, 375
   clinical significance, 374
   critical rate, 388–390
   defined, 374
   ECG characteristics, 374, 377–381,
      377–381
   incidence, 376, 376t
   paradoxical critical rate, 391
   patterns, 376, 376t
   second beat-aberrancy, 379
   treatment, 377
   vs. ventricular ectopy, 374,
      383–387
Ventricular aneurysm, 197, 201
Ventricular contraction, premature,
   441
Ventricular dilation
   in cor pulmonale, 214
   left, 82, *83–84*
   right, 78, 214
Ventricular enlargement
   atrial enlargement and, 76
   axis deviation and, 54
   causes, 76
   congenital disorders, 92
   left, 76–77, *77,* 82, 90, 98
   localizing, 21
   R wave patterns, 51
   right, 76–77, *77,* 78, 90, 98
   systematic ECG evaluation, 90,
      91t
   vs. incomplete bundle block, 78, 82,
      98
   waveform characteristics, 76–77,
      77, 90
   See also Ventricular dilation;
      Ventricular hypertrophy
Ventricular flutter/fibrillation, 346, *346,*
   371
   clinical characteristics, 368
   ECG characteristics, 366, *367,* 369,
      369
   induced by premature beat, 276,
      280
   onset, 370, *370*
   termination, 368
Ventricular hypertrophy
   combined left- and right-, 86–87,
      86–89
   left, 84, *84–85*
   right, 36, 79–81, *79–81*
   systematic ECG evaluation, 90, 91t
Ventricular preexcitation, 66
   activation pathways, 126
   age at onset, 125
   atrial flutter/fibrillation with, 321–323,
      322
   atrial reactivation in, 129
   clinical perspective, 125–130
   defined, 68, 125
   diagnostic approach, 132–133
   ECG abnormalities in, 126–132,
      126–133
   historical conceptualizations, 124

indications, 97–98, *98*
in infants, 333
pathway ablation, 136, *136*
pathway localization, 134–135, *134–135*
with reentrant junctional tachyarrhythmia, 328
vs. bundle-branch block, *125, 125–126*, 133
Ventricular rhythm, 396, 398, *398,* 405
Ventricular septal defect, 92
Ventricular strain, 79, 82, 90, 155, 162
defined, 93
in left-ventricular hypertrophy, 84
Ventricular tachyarrhythmia
accelerated ventricular rhythm, 286t, 287, 295–296, 297, 320, 346
reentrant
heart rate in, 346
mechanisms, 346
See also Torsades de pointes; Ventricular flutter/fibrillation;

Ventricular tachycardia
types of, 346, *346*
Ventricular tachycardia, *245*
atrioventricular dissociation and, 347, 351, 378
cardiac rhythm in, 352–362
defined, 346, 347, 371
diagnosis, 351–362
challenges, 349
QRS morphology, 350, *350*
drug-related, 348
duration, 364
etiology, 348
hemodynamic changes in, 349
left, 353, 354, 363, 364
localizing, 363
monomorphic, 352, 371
polymorphic, 365, 371
QRS morphology, *98*
reentry circuit, 347
right, 354, 358, 360, 363, 364
slow, 297
sustained/nonsustained, 347, 364, 371

vs. atrial flutter/fibrillation, 323
vs. supraventricular tachyarrhythmias, 349, 350–351, 352
vulnerable period, 280, 287
Verapamil, 349, 352, 386
Viewpoints, 26
Voltage measurement, 3, 39
Volume overload, 72, 93
Vulnerable period
atrial, 307
ventricular, 280, 282

Waveform, defined, 23
Wenckebach sequence, 421, 422–423, 430
Wolff–Parkinson–White syndrome, 124, 328
activation pathways, 126
age at onset, 125
defined, 137
ECG abnormalities in, 130

Xiphoid process, 40